The Little B

Third Edition

The Little Black Book of Neurology

THIRD EDITION

Editor
ALAN J. LERNER, M.D.

Assistant Professor of Neurology
Case Western Reserve University School of Medicine
Director, Division of Neurology
Saint Luke's Medical Center
Cleveland, Ohio

Contributors

Mohamed M. Al-Jaberi, M.D.
Cynthia C. Bamford, M.D.
Isabelita R. Bella, M.D.
Jordan A. Brooks, M.D.
Mohan S. Chandran, M.D.
Yoni Dokko, M.D.
Lawrence S. Goldstein, M.D.
Jacob L. Gordon, M.D., M.S.
Steven J. Grosser, M.D.
Peter Hedera, M.D.
R. Edward Hogan, M.D.
Andrew T. Kuntz, M.D.

Wassim Nasreddine, M.D.
Erica M. New, M.D.
Allen D. Pettee, M.D.
Naji J. Riachi, M.D.
Susan L. Scarberry, M.D.
Howard M. Schecht, M.D.
Jason Soriano, M.D.
Joshua J. Sunshine, M.D.
Marle Tani, M.D.
Tina M. Thomas-McCauley, M.D.
Joel Vandersluis, M.D.
Leonard M. Weinberger, M.D.

From the Neurology House Staff of Case Western Reserve University,
University Hospitals of Cleveland, MetroHealth Medical Center,
Cleveland V.A. Medical Center, Cleveland, Ohio

Illustrations by Sundee L. Morris, M.D.

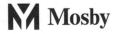 Mosby

St. Louis Baltimore Berlin Boston Carlsbad Chicago London Madrid
Naples New York Philadelphia Sydney Tokyo Toronto

Managing Editor: Laura DeYoung
Project Manager: Peggy Fagen
Production: Graphic World Publishing Services
Manufacturing Supervisor: Betty Richmond
Cover Design: Jeanne Wolfgeher

Copyright © 1995 by Mosby–Year Book, Inc.

Printed in the United States of America.
Composition by Graphic World, Inc.
Printing/binding by Malloy

Mosby–Year Book, Inc.
11830 Westline Industrial Drive
St. Louis, Missouri 63146

Library of Congress Cataloging-in-Publication Data

The little black book of neurology
  —3rd ed. / [edited by] Alan J. Lerner.
      p.   cm.
   Includes bibliographical references.
   ISBN 0-8151-5440-2
   1. Nervous system—Diseases—Handbooks, manuals, etc.
2. Neurology—Handbooks, manuals, etc.   I. Lerner, Alan J.
   [DNLM: 1. Nervous System Diseases—handbooks.
WL   39   L778   1994]
RC355.L58   1994
616.8—dc20
DNLM/DLC
for Library of Congress   94-22738
                                                                    CIP

95 96 97 98 99 / 9 8 7 6 5 4 3 2 1

FOREWORD

Early in 1984, Year Book Medical Publishers, now Mosby, having achieved decades of success with *The Harriet Lane Handbook* in pediatrics, asked me whether the neurology house staff at Case Western Reserve University School of Medicine (University Hospitals of Cleveland/VA Medical Center/MetroHealth Medical Center) would write a similar book in neurology. Like the *Harriet Lane*, it would be a book "by residents for residents" and had to fit in the pocket of a white coat. After meetings with my house staff and representatives from Year Book, we signed the contract in the summer of 1984.

Having carried a black, loose-leaf book in my white coat pocket since my student days, I decided that our handbook should be organized to replace or supplement such loose-leaf books that house officers and students compile for themselves. What followed was the A to Z organization that, with sufficient cross-referencing, eliminated the need for a table of contents and index. Since eponyms abound in neurology and tend to intimidate trainees, we introduced an eponym index. I assigned topics to the PG-3 and PG-4 resident staff and, as might have been predicted, despite my insistence that the writing be crisp and tight, they generated material that could fill large volumes. I didn't have the time for the editing and formatting, and Steven E. Thurston, M.D., then a PG-5 Fellow in Neuro-Ophthalmology, carried the process to fruition. The first edition was published in 1987. The second edition, edited by Drs. James and Jo Bonner, was published in 1991.

We anticipate that this substantially updated third edition, edited by Alan J. Lerner, M.D., will continue to serve house staff and students caring for neurological patients. We welcome comments and criticisms from our readers to assist us in future improvements.

Robert B. Daroff, M.D.
Chief of Staff and former Director of Neurology
University Hospitals of Cleveland
Professor, and former Chairman of Neurology,
Case Western Reserve University School of Medicine
Cleveland, Ohio

PREFACE

The third edition of *The Little Black Book of Neurology* continues to evolve with the rapid changes in neurology, but retains the basic format established in earlier editions. During the process of updating the second edition, the aim has been to streamline the text and cross-references, and provide additional useful tables. Nearly all topics have been updated, and many have been completely rewritten. New topics have been added, ranging from Alzheimer's disease and Creutzfeldt-Jakob disease to gait disorders, sepsis, and Moya-Moya.

I would like to thank the faculty and the staff of the department of neurology at Case Western Reserve University for their support, input, and review of material, especially Robert Friedland, Robert Ruff, Steve Collins, and David Geldmacher. Manuscript preparation was aided by the efforts of Nancy Catalani, Peggy Evans, and Spring Galloway, with editorial support at Mosby by Laura DeYoung

Finally, I would like to thank Dr. Robert Daroff for his support and tireless editing input. And without the support of my wife, Erica New, and my family, this project would never have gone through.

Alan J. Lerner, M.D.

The Little Black Book of Neurology

Third Edition

ABDUCENS NERVE   (see Cranial Nerves, Eye Muscles, Ophthalmoplegia)

ABSCESS, BRAIN

The neurologic manifestations of brain abscesses usually resemble other space-occupying intracranial lesions. Fever occurs in only 50% of cases. A progressive increase in intracranial pressure may lead to bradycardia, confusion, drowsiness, and stupor. The clinical features of cerebellar dysfunction frequently appear late in the natural history of the disease.

Brain abscess develops in three clinical situations: direct extension from contiguous infections; blood-borne spread from distant sites of infection; or after head trauma with skull fracture.

Middle ear infections extend into the temporal lobe or cerebellum, and frontal sinusitis usually extends into the anterior frontal lobe; these are the most common contiguous infections causing brain abscess. Common sources of metastatic brain abscesses have a route of vascular access to the brain that bypasses the pulmonary microcirculation. The single most common cause of metastatic brain abscess is chronic infection of the pleura or lungs (including bronchiectasis, empyema, and lung abscess). Congenital heart malformations with right to-left shunt strongly predispose to brain abscess. Endocarditis can cause multiple small brain abscesses (<1 cm) but rarely causes large isolated abscesses. Penetrating trauma to the skull, including compound depressed skull fractures, basal skull fractures with cerebrospinal fluid (CSF) fistulae, and previous craniotomy, can cause brain abscess formation, sometimes years after the acute event.

Usual bacteriologic isolates from abscesses are related to the site of origin, as follows (organisms listed in order of significance):

1. Middle ear infection: Aerobic and anaerobic streptococci, *Bacteroides fragilis*, and Enterobacteriaceae.
2. Sinusitis: As in middle ear infections, but also including *Staphylococcus aureus* and *Hemophilus* species.
3. Penetrating head trauma: *S. aureus*, streptococci, Enterobacteriaceae, and *Clostridium* species.

Acquired immunodeficiency syndrome (AIDS) is associated with *Toxoplasma* species infection.

The histopathologic stages of abscess formation are characterized as follows. (1) Early cerebritis (days 1 to 3) with a local inflammatory response around a necrotic center. (2) Late cerebritis (days 4 to 9), characterized by increased necrosis and inflammation, with initial fibroblastic formation of the collagen capsule. (3) The early encapsulation stage (days 10 to 13) shows further development of the collagen capsule, which is typically thinner on the less vascular ventricular side. (4) The late capsular stage (days 14 and onward) shows five distinct histologic layers: the necrotic center; inflammatory cells and fibroblasts; the collagen capsule; a neovascular layer; and surrounding edema and reactive gliosis.

Radiologic findings on computed tomography (CT) correlate well with the histopathologic stages. In the cerebritis stage, CT without contrast shows the necrotic center as a hypodensity. Ring enhancement begins in the later stages of cerebritis. In the capsular stages the capsule becomes visible on CT without contrast as a faint ring of hyperintensity as compared to the hypointense necrotic center. Contrast produces a well-defined capsular ring, which is thinner on the ventricular side. Magnetic resonance imaging (MRI) findings are less documented than the CT findings but also reflect histologic changes. Arteriography demonstrates an avascular mass, "ring blush," or "luxury" collateral perfusion around an avascular mass and is especially helpful if mycotic aneurysm is suspected. Electroencephalography (EEG) abnormalities include focal slowing, seizure activity, and evidence of diffuse encephalopathy. If brain abscess is suspected, LP should not be performed because organisms rarely grow in the CSF and the risks of herniation seem greater with abscesses than with other mass lesions.

Treatment requires a combination of antimicrobials, neurosurgical drainage or excision, and eradication of the primary infective focus. Antibiotics should be given based on the route of infection. When the cause is otogenic or unknown, the patient should receive penicillin (PCN) 20 million units per day intravenously (IV), metronidazole 500 mg IV q 6 hr, and a third-generation cephalosporin. For paranasal sinus sources administer PCN and metronidazole. Treatment for posttraumatic cases is vancomycin 1 g IV q 12 hr and a third-generation cephalosporin. Treatment should persist for 6 weeks.

Mortality rates range from 5% to 20%. Poor prognosis is associated with very young or old age, severely altered sensorium, increased size of abscess, acute clinical presentation, metastatic abscess, abscesses of the cerebellum or deep structures, recovery of anaerobic organisms from the abscesses, rupture into the ventricle or subarachnoid space, and concomitant pulmonary infections.

REF: Osenbach RK, Loftus CM: *Neurosurg Clin N Am* 3:403, 1992.

ABSCESS, EPIDURAL

Epidural abscesses usually become evident when spinal and radicular pain progresses to weakness over hours to days. Occasionally a more protracted course occurs. *Staphylococcus* and gram-negative organisms are the most common causes. If the diagnosis is suspected, emergency imaging is indicated. Treatment consists of surgical drainage and appropriate antibiotic coverage.

ACALCULIA

The acquired impairment of arithmetic skills typically occurs in three forms: (1) number alexia, an inability to read numbers; (2) spatial acalculia, a misalignment of numbers in appropriate columns that usually occurs with right hemisphere lesions; and (3) anarithmetria, or loss of calculation skill, often associated with left parietal lobe lesions. Acalculia rarely occurs in isolation; it commonly accompanies aphasia and is a component of Gerstmann's syndrome.

REF: Mesulam MM: *Principles of behavioral neurology*, Philadelphia, 1985, FA Davis.

ACIDOSIS   *(see Electrolyte Disorders)*

ACOUSTIC NERVE   *(see Calorics, Cranial Nerves, Hearing, Vertigo)*

ACROMEGALY   *(see Carpal Tunnel Syndrome, Pituitary)*

ACUTE INTERMITTENT PORPHYRIA   *(see Porphyria)*

ADRENOLEUKODYSTROPHY   *(see Degenerative Diseases of Childhood)*

AGNOSIA

Impaired recognition of sensory stimuli that cannot be attributed to sensory loss, language disturbance, or global cognitive deficit.

Some divide visual agnosia into apperceptive and associative. The first is a deficit of visual processing in which abnormal percepts are formed and may occur after bilateral injury to the primary visual cortex.

Such patients are unable to copy or match visually presented items. In associative visual agnosia, the deficit lies after percept formation but before meaning has been associated. Object agnosia (inability to recognize objects), prosopagnosia (loss of recognition of specific members of a generic group; distinguishing and recognizing faces, cars, houses, etc.) and achromatopsia (inability to perceive color) are all visual agnosias occurring with occipital-temporal lesions, usually bilateral.

Auditory agnosia is an inability to recognize sounds that cannot be attributed to a hearing deficit. It may be restricted to nonspeech sounds (selective auditory agnosia) or to speech sounds (pure word deafness) or involve both (generalized auditory agnosia).

Tactile agnosia, such as astereognosis (inability to recognize objects placed in the hand), is not well characterized in the absence of a primary sensory loss and may not be a true agnosia. Less well-understood problems are anosognosia (lack of awareness of a deficit), anosodiaphoria (failure of mood recognition), and simultanagnosia (inability to perceive more than one object at a time).

REF: Mendez MF, Geehan GR: Cortical auditory disorders: clinical and psychoacoustic features, *J Neurol Neurosurg Psychiatry* 51:1–9, 1988.

Mesulam MM: *Principles of behavioral neurology*, Philadelphia, 1985, FA Davis.

AGRAPHIA

The acquired inability to write occurs in five clinical forms. (1) Pure agraphia (no other language abnormality present) has been described with lesions of the second frontal convolution (Exner's area), superior parietal lobule, and the posterior sylvian region. (2) Aphasic agraphia is the writing disturbance of aphasics that usually resembles their spoken speech. Dominant angular gyrus lesions produce (3) agraphia with alexia. Superior parietal lobule lesions in the dominant hemisphere lead to (4) apractic agraphia, in which the production of letters and words is abnormal, whereas nondominant parietal lesions lead to (5) spatial agraphia with abnormalities of spacing letters and maintaining a horizontal line.

Neuropsychologists have defined two systems of writing. The phonological system decodes speech sounds (phonemes) into letters. In phonological agraphia, produced by lesions of supramarginal gyrus or the insula medial to it, the patient is unable to spell non-words but is capable of spelling familiar words. The lexical system retrieves visual word images when spelling. Lexical agraphia is marked by errors in spelling irregular words, but these errors are phonologically correct (rough—ruf). Lexical agraphia occurs with lesions at the junction of the posterior angular gyrus and parieto-occipital lobule.

REF: Heilman KM, Valenstein E: *Clinical neuropsychology*, ed 3, New York, 1993, Oxford University Press.

AIDS

The acquired immunodeficiency syndrome (AIDS) is caused by the human immunodeficiency virus (HIV), a retrovirus. Neurologic manifestations of AIDS can be due to the HIV virus itself, associated infections, neoplasms, or complications of treatment and can affect any level of the central or peripheral nervous system. Twenty percent to 40% of HIV-infected patients have clinically apparent neurologic disease; in 80%, autopsy findings show neurologic disease.

I. Primary HIV infection.
   A. *Aseptic meningitis* occurs in 5% to 10% of HIV-infected patients; it occurs commonly at the time of seroconversion but may recur later in the illness. Clinical features include fever, headache, meningeal signs, and occasional encephalopathy. Cranial nerves V, VII, and VIII may be involved. Cerebrospinal fluid (CSF) mononuclear pleocytosis occurs (20 to 300 cells); glucose level is normal, and protein levels may reach 100 mg/dl.
   B. *AIDS dementia complex* (ADC) (AIDS encephalopathy) is the most common central nervous system (CNS) complication of AIDs, affecting from 25% to 75% of HIV-infected patients. It occurs at any time during the course of the syndrome and may be its presenting and sole manifestation. The course of ADC is slowly progressive over several months to a year but may progress rapidly over days. Psychomotor retardation, forgetfulness, and inattention are initial findings and may be difficult to distinguish from depression. Later, motor dysfunction, frontal release signs, tremor, myoclonus, pyramidal tract signs, ataxia, and seizures are common. Differential diagnosis includes other causes of infectious, neoplastic, or medication-related encephalopathies. Neuroimaging studies show atrophy in nearly all patients. MRI may show patchy white-matter signal changes. Cerebral calcifications are common in children. CSF shows increased levels of protein, and 25% of patients have a mononuclear pleocytosis. HIV-p24 antigen

titers correlate with disease presence and progression of encephalopathy. Histopathologic features of ADC include diffuse gliosis, foci of tissue necrosis, focal demyelination, and multinucleated giant cells. Zidovudine may help reverse early neuropsychologic deficits.

C. *Vacuolar myelopathy* occurs in 11% to 22% of AIDS patients. The lateral and posterior columns are primarily affected. Progressive spastic paraparesis and incontinence develop over weeks to months, and most patients have coincident dementia.

D. *Peripheral neuropathy.*
   1. Distal symmetric polyneuropathy is the most common neuropathy. Painful dysethesia is the most common complaint. Nerve conduction studies show axonal or mixed axonal and demyelinating features.
   2. Acute and chronic inflammatory demyelinating polyradiculoneuropathy may occur at the time of seroconversion or later during the course of HIV infection. CSF pleocytosis is more common than in the idiopathic forms of Guillain-Barré syndrome or chronic inflammatory demyelinating polyradiculopathy.
   3. Mononeuropathy multiplex.
   4. Brachial plexitis associated with seroconversion and an exanthematous rash has been described.
   5. Cranial neuropathies associated with aseptic meningitis.

E. *Muscle disease.*
   1. Polymyositis can precede seroconversion. Steroids may be beneficial.
   2. Proximal myopathy may develop in patients with AIDS or AIDS-related complex (ARC). Muscle biopsy specimens show atrophy of type 2 fibers. The myopathy may result from poor nutrition or prolonged bed rest, or it may be a remote effect of coexistent malignancy.

II. Secondary infections.
   A. *Toxoplasmosis* is the most common CNS infection in patients with AIDS, affecting 5% to 15% of patients. It becomes evident as single or multiple mass lesions but can also cause a subacute meningoencephalitis. Contrast-enhancing lesions with edema are seen on CT in nearly all patients. The major differential diagnosis of enhancing *Toxoplasma* species lesions is cerebral lymphoma. An indirect diagnostic method is a therapeutic trial of pyrimethamine 25 mg qd with sulfadiazine 2 to 6 g daily divided qid, supplemented by folinic acid 10 mg qd.

Clinical improvement in toxoplasmosis is usually rapid, sometimes within 24 to 48 hours, and improvement can be seen
on CT scans within 1 to 2 weeks. If a response occurs, therapy
must be continued indefinitely.

B. *Fungal* infections include cryptococcosis (most common),
coccidioidomycosis, histoplasmosis, candidiasis, and aspergillosis. CSF study, India ink exam, and titers are helpful in
diagnosis. Treatment is with amphotericin B or fluconazole;
5-flucytosine is often poorly tolerated in AIDS patients.
Chronic fluconazole therapy may help prevent relapse.

C. *Mycobacterium* species include *M. tuberculosis*, *M. kansasii*,
and *M. avium-intracellulare*. CNS involvement is relatively
rare.

D. *Viral* infections.
   1. Progressive multifocal leukoencephalopathy. Diagnosis is
      often suggested by multiple nonenhancing white-matter
      lesions and progressive neurologic deficits. Definitive di-
      agnosis requires brain biopsy (see Encephalitis). Therapy
      with cytosine arabinoside has been attempted.
   2. CMV (encephalitis, meningitis, retinitis, myelopathy, po-
      lyradiculitis). Medications for CMV infections include
      gancyclovir and foscarnet.
   3. Herpes simplex (encephalitis, myelitis).
   4. Varicella zoster (encephalomyelitis, Ramsay Hunt syn-
      drome).

E. *Neurosyphilis* is becoming more common. The course of neurosyphilis is more aggressive with coexistent HIV infection (see
Syphilis).

F. *Bacterial* infections are less common but occur.

III. Neoplasms.
A. *Lymphoma* occurs in 2% of AIDS patients. Almost all cases
are of B-cell origin. Therapy is with whole-brain radiation.
Death usually occurs within 3 months.

B. *Kaposi's sarcoma* rarely involves the CNS.

C. *Non–Hodgkin's lymphoma* may metastasize to the leptomeninges.

IV. Pediatric AIDS. Neurologic complications occur in up to 90% of
pediatric AIDS patients. The spectrum of complications, however,
is somewhat different. Neuropsychologic abnormalities, especially
resulting from AIDS dementia complex, are more common in
children, while CNS opportunistic infections and neoplasms are
less common. In children of affected mothers, microcephaly may

occur if the infection is acquired early in gestation. Postnatally development may be slowed, and corticospinal tract dysfunction may be evident, with spasticity, paraparesis, or quadriparesis.

V. Medication effects. Zidovudine is associated with a myopathy that may be mitochondrial in origin. The myopathy improves with medication withdrawal. Didanosine and zalcitabine can cause a painful neuropathy.

REF: Brew B, Rosenblum M, Price RW: Central and peripheral nervous system complications of HIV infection and AIDS. In De Vita VT Jr et al, eds: *AIDS: Etiology, diagnosis, treatment and prevention, ed 2*, Philadelphia, 1988, Lippincott.

Tucker T: Central nervous system AIDS, *J Neurol Sci* 89:119–133, 1989.

AKATHISIA *(see Neuroleptics)*

AKINETIC MUTISM *(see Coma)*

AKINETIC-RIGID SYNDROME *(see Parkinson's Disease, Parkinsonism)*

ALCOHOL *(see also Nutritional Deficiency Syndrome)*

Neurologic effects of alcohol are due to a combination of its neurotoxic effects or metabolites, nutritional factors, and genetic predisposition. Complications include intoxication, withdrawal syndromes, Wernicke-Korsakoff syndrome, nutritional deficiency states, and other conditions.

Intoxication with alcohol correlates roughly with blood alcohol concentrations. Cognitive dysfunction tends to occur early, whereas cerebellar, autonomic, and vestibular symptoms tend to occur at higher blood alcohol levels. Positional vertigo may result from alcohol diffusing into the cupula when the recumbent position is assumed. As the alcohol concentration rises to a certain level, the intoxication is greater than when it falls to the same level. Blackouts are periods of amnesia, usually during binge drinking, and occur in persons with and without alcoholism.

Withdrawal syndromes occur because of the physical dependence on alcohol and result from either decreased intake or cessation of drinking. The syndromes may be early or late appearing. Most common are the early symptoms, which begin 12 to 24 hours after decreased intake. Tremulousness is common and may be accompanied by nausea, vomiting, insomnia, and hallucinations (visual, tactile, or auditory). Treatment consists of sedation with benzodiazepines. Auditory hallucinations may persist, necessitating the use of neuroleptics. Withdrawal seizures are typically generalized tonic-clonic and begin within the first 24 hours but may occur after several days. Focal seizures imply a structural lesion and should not be attributed to alcohol withdrawal. Treatment of withdrawal seizures is controversial, since they are usually self-limited. Initial loading with phenytoin and slowly tapering off after several days is one approach. Thiamine is routinely given, and hypomagnesemia, if present, is treated. Late withdrawal symptoms, referred to as delirium tremens, are a serious complication and have a peak incidence 72 to 96 hours after decreased alcohol intake. Severe confusion, agitation, vivid hallucinations, tremors, and increased autonomic activity (tachycardia, fever, sweating, and orthostatic hypotension) are characteristic. Symptoms can last for 1 to 3 days and can have a high mortality rate. Treatment consists of sedation with benzodiazepines, hydration with IV fluids, and administration of thiamine, multivitamins, and magnesium (if indicated).

Wernicke-Korsakoff syndrome is the most common deficiency syndrome resulting from chronic alcoholism. Wernicke's syndrome represents the acute phase and classically has the triad of encephalopathy, ataxia, and ocular motor disturbance (nystagmus, ophthalmoplegia, and gaze palsy). Often, however, a complete triad of signs is not present. Atrophy of the mammillary bodies is common. Korsakoff's syndrome is a more chronic condition and includes anterograde amnesia (the inability to incorporate ongoing experience into memory). Both syndromes are attributed to thiamine deficiency and therefore can also be seen in nonalcoholic malnutrition states, although much less commonly. Treatment consists of thiamine, 100 mg per day for 3 days parenterally, followed by oral thiamine indefinitely. IV glucose should never be given without thiamine to a chronic alcoholic because of the risk of precipitating Wernicke's encephalopathy. As with most alcohol related syndromes, supplemental vitamins and magnesium may be beneficial.

Other alcohol-related syndromes include cerebellar degeneration, peripheral neuropathy, optic neuropathy, and myopathy. *Cerebellar degeneration* invariably involves the anterior vermis and paravermian regions with resultant truncal and gait ataxia. A "dying back" sensorimotor neuropathy usually is heralded by complaints of numb, burning feet. Minor motor signs may evolve. *Nutritional amblyopia* (previously called tobacco-alcohol amblyopia) consists of gradual visual loss. It is due to poor nutrition and is not a direct toxic effect of alcohol. In contrast, *alcoholic myopathy* is believed to be caused by the toxic effects of alcohol and improves with abstinence. It may occur as an acute necrotizing disorder with muscle pain and rhabdomyolysis or as a more slowly progressive disease with proximal weakness. The combination of thiamine, multivitamins, and abstinence is the treatment of choice for these syndromes.

Conditions of somewhat uncertain origin occurring in chronic alcoholics include central pontine myelinolysis, Machiafava-Bignami syndrome, and cortical atrophy. *Central pontine myelinolysis* is a rare cerebral white-matter disorder associated with a basis pontis lesion with resultant progressive quadriparesis, horizontal gaze palsy, and obtundation leading to coma. It occurs with excessively rapid correction of hyponatremia. *Machiafava-Bignami syndrome* is a rare demyelinating disease of the corpus callosum and adjacent subcortical white matter associated with excessive consumption of crude red wine. Patients can have cognitive impairment, spasticity, dysarthria, and impaired gait. *Cortical atrophy*, which causes dementia not explained by Korsakoff's syndrome in chronic alcoholics, is not accepted by most authorities. The appearance of "atrophy" or "parenchymal volume loss" on the CT scan is probably related to fluid shifts in the brain and may reverse with abstinence.

Alcoholics have an increased incidence of stroke related to a variety of factors, including rebound thrombocytosis, altered cerebral blood flow, and hyperlipidemia.

REF: Adams RD, Victor M: *Principles of neurology*, ed 5, New York, 1993, McGraw-Hill.

Victor M. In Joynt RJ, ed: *Clinical neurology*, Philadelphia, 1992, Lippincott.

ALEXIA

The loss of a previously acquired reading ability occurs in three forms: (1) anterior alexia, usually seen in association with Broca's aphasia, characterized by impaired comprehension of syntactic structure, (2) central alexia (alexia with agraphia), usually seen in association with visual field deficits but may exist in isolation, and (3) posterior alexia (alexia without agraphia), seen with infarction of the dominant occipital lobe and splenium of the corpus collosum, which results in loss of visual input to the language areas.

ALKALOSIS   *(see Electrolyte Disorders)*

ALZHEIMER'S DISEASE   *(see also Dementia)*

Alzheimer's disease (AD) is the most common dementia. Incidence is 1% per year for individuals over 65 years of age, and prevalence in persons 85 years of age and older is estimated to be 50%. Age is the most important risk factor for AD; less important risk factors are female gender, family history of AD or Down's syndrome, and low educational level. A genetic risk factor, apolipoprotein E4, has been observed for late-onset familial AD. All individuals with Down's syndrome develop pathologic evidence of AD if they live past 35 years of age. Some families are known with clearly autosomal dominant inheritance. Pathologic hallmarks of AD are neurofibrillary tangles, neuritic plaques with amyloid deposition, amyloid angiopathy, and neuronal loss; the secondary association cortex is most heavily involved. The most widespread neurochemical change is a cholinergic deficit.

Clinical features of AD are variable but include memory impairment for recent events with relative preservation of remote recall, language deficit (in verbal fluency, naming, comprehension, and speech content), visuospatial dysfunction, and impairment in executive functions (set shifting, planning, and problem solving). Aphasia and visuospatial dysfunction may be presenting symptoms in some patients. Behavioral symptoms are also common, including depression, agitation, hallucinations, delusions, and anxiety. Results of neurologic examination, other than mental status, are essentially normal, but some patients may have extrapyramidal rigidity, gait disorder, myoclonus, or seizures, particularly in later stages of the disease.

Alzheimer's disease is a diagnosis of exclusion, but standardized diagnostic criteria are in wide use (see Table 1). Definite AD can be diagnosed only by autopsy or biopsy. When strict diagnostic criteria are followed, accuracy of antemortem diagnosis of AD is approximately 80% to 90%. Alzheimer's disease can be mistaken for Pick's disease, which is characterized by early disinhibited behavior and frontal lobe dysfunction. CT or MRI can show asymmetric frontal or temporal lobe atrophy. Rapid forms of AD with myoclonus must be differentiated from Creutzfeldt-Jakob disease. Vascular dementia, the second most common cause of dementia, can be distinguished based on evidence of strokes in neuroimaging. Key clinical differentiating factors include abrupt onset, stepwise deterioration, focal neurologic signs and symptoms, and risk factors for stroke.

TABLE 1
Criteria for Clinical Diagnosis of Alzheimer's Disease

I. The criteria for the clinical diagnosis of PROBABLE Alzheimer's disease include:

Dementia established by clinical examination and documented by the Mini-Mental Test, Blessed Dementia Scale, or some similar examination, and confirmed by neuropsychological tests.

Deficits in two or more areas of cognition.

Progressive worsening of memory and other cognitive functions.

No disturbance of consciousness.

Onset between ages 40 and 90, most often after age 65.

Absence of systemic disorders or other brain diseases that in and of themselves could account for the progressive deficits in memory and cognition.

II. The diagnosis of PROBABLE Alzheimer's disease is supported by:

Progressive deterioration of specific cognitive functions such as language (aphasia), motor skills (apraxia), and perception (agnosia).

Impaired activities of daily living and altered patterns of behavior.

Family history of similar disorders, particularly if confirmed neuropathologically.

Laboratory results of:

Normal lumbar puncture as evaluated by standard techniques.

Normal pattern or nonspecific changes in EEG, such as increased slow-wave activity.

Evidence of cerebral atrophy on CT with progression documented by serial observation.

TABLE 1—cont'd
Criteria for Clinical Diagnosis of Alzheimer's Disease

III. Other clinical features consistent with the diagnosis of PROB-
ABLE Alzheimer's disease, after exclusion of causes of dementia
other than Alzheimer's disease, include:

Plateaus in the course of progression of the illness.

Associated symptoms of depression, insomnia, incontinence,
delusions, illusions, hallucinations, catastrophic verbal, emotional, or physical outbursts, sexual disorders, and weight
loss.

Other neurologic abnormalities in some patients, especially
with more advanced disease and including motor signs such
as increased muscle tone, myoclonus, or gait disorder.

Seizures in advanced disease.

CT normal for age.

IV. Features that make the diagnosis of PROBABLE Alzheimer's
disease uncertain or unlikely include:

Sudden, apoplectic onset.

Focal neurologic findings such as hemiparesis, sensory loss,
visual field deficits, and incoordination early in the course of
the illness.

Seizures or gait disturbances at the onset or very early in the
course of the illness

V. Clinical diagnosis of POSSIBLE Alzheimer's disease:

May be made on the basis of the dementia syndrome in the
absence of other neurologic, psychiatric, or systemic disorders sufficient to cause dementia, and in the presence of
variations in the onset, in the presentation, or in the clinical
course.

May be made in the presence of a second systemic or brain
disorder sufficient to produce dementia, which is not considered to be *the* cause of the dementia.

Continued.

TABLE 1—cont'd
Criteria for Clinical Diagnosis of Alzheimer's Disease

Should be used in research studies when a single, gradually progressive severe cognitive deficit is identified in the absence of other identifiable cause.

VI. Criteria for diagnosis of DEFINITE Alzheimer's disease are:

The clinical criteria for probable Alzheimer's disease and histopathologic evidence obtained from a biopsy or an autopsy.

VII. Classification of Alzheimer's disease for research purposes should specify features that may differentiate subtypes of the disorder, such as:

Familial occurrence.

Onset before age of 65.

Presence of trisomy-21.

Coexistence of other relevant conditions such as Parkinson's disease.

From McKhann G et al: *Neurology* 34:939, 1984.

Tetrahydroaminoacridine (THA) is a reversible acetylcholinesterase inhibitor used for the treatment of mild and moderate AD. The response may be an improvement in memory and attention. Starting dose is 10 mg qid, increasing up to 40 mg qid as tolerated. Liver function tests (particularly ALT) must be monitored weekly for the first 18 weeks of therapy.

Behavioral symptoms may be disruptive and require symptomatic treatment. The new onset of disruptive behavior requires thorough evaluation of possible environmental precipitants and exclusion of physical illness (e.g., urinary tract infection) before a regimen of psychoactive medication is started. Medication with minimal anticholinergic effect should be used: nortriptyline, fluoxetine, sertraline, or trazodone for depression and haloperidol, thioridazine, or other neuroleptics for agitation and symptoms of psychosis. Benzodiazepines are associated with frequent paradoxic effects, although oxazepam is useful for episodic anxiety. Chloral hydrate is useful for insomnia. The intensity of symptoms can fluctuate widely, and close follow-up will dictate need for continued treatment.

REF: Whitehouse PJ, ed: *Dementia*, Philadelphia, 1993, FA Davis.

AMAUROSIS FUGAX

Amaurosis fugax is the symptom of partial or complete "transient monocular blindness (TMB)." It is to be distinguished from "transient visual obscuration" resulting from increased intracranial pressure and from papilledema. TMB is a TIA of the retinal vasculature of sudden onset and short duration (seconds to rarely longer than 5 minutes) and consists usually of negative symptoms (blackness or graying of the visual field) with occasional positive phenomena (scintillating scotomas or points of light). The most common cause is embolization from the internal carotid artery or heart (see Table 2). Recurrent TIA in young persons may have a vasospastic origin and respond to verapamil.

REF: Amaurosis Fugax Study Group: Current management of amaurosis fugax, *Stroke* 21:201–208, 1990.

Winterkonn JM et al: Brief report: treatment of vasospastic amaurosis fugax with calcium-channel blockers, *New Engl J Med* 329:396–398, 1993.

AMNESIA   *(see Memory)*

AMYOTROPHIC LATERAL SCLEROSIS   *(see Motor Neuron Disease)*

ANALGESICS   *(see Pain)*

ANENCEPHALY   *(see Developmental Malformations)*

ANEURYSMS   *(see also Hemorrhage)*

Intracranial aneurysms are classified as saccular (berry), mycotic, arteriosclerotic, traumatic, dissecting, and neoplastic.

Clinical presentations include cranial nerve palsies (especially of nerve III, including the pupil, and nerves IV and VI), headache, mass lesion or "steal" phenomena effect (giant aneurysms), and thrombosis (atherosclerotic aneurysms). Rupture with subarachnoid hemorrhage (SAH) is the primary manifestation. Ruptured saccular aneurysms account for 80% of nontraumatic SAH (most common after age 20); a severe headache of sudden onset is characteristic. The size and location of the bleed and the presence of intraparenchymal and ventricular extension (associated with a significantly higher mortality) affect the level of consciousness (lethargy to coma). Sudden loss of consciousness

TABLE 2
Causes of Transient Monocular Blindness

I. Embolic.
   A. Carotid embolism.
   B. Cardiac embolism.
   C. Embolism related to intravenous drug abuse.
II. Hemodynamic.
   A. Hypoperfusion.
   B. Vasospasm.
   C. Inflammatory arteritides such as temporal arteritis, Takaya-su's syndrome, and polyarteritis nodosa.
   D. Severe atherosclerotic occlusive disease of internal carotid or ophthalmic artery.
   E. Carotid dissection.
   F. Hypertensive crises.
III. Ocular.
   A. Anterior ischemic optic neuropathy.
   B. Central retinal vein occlusion.
   C. Intraocular causes such as hemorrhage, tumor, and glau-coma.
   D. Drusen.
IV. Neurologic disorders.
   A. Disease of the vestibular or oculomotor system.
   B. Optic neuritis (mainly demyelinating diseases).
   C. Optic nerve or optic chiasmal compression.
   D. Increased intracranial pressure.
   E. Migraine.
V. Psychogenic.
VI. Idiopathic.

Adapted from Amaurosis Fugax Study Group: Current management of amaurosis fugax, *Stroke* 21:201–208, 1990.

is the presenting feature in 20% of cases. Meningeal signs, papilledema, retinal hemorrhage, and seizures are common. Focal signs in the first 24 hours usually indicate parenchymal dissection, cerebral edema, or hypoperfusion distal to the ruptured aneurysm. After the first 48 to 72 hours focal signs may be due to vasospasm.

Diagnostic evaluation includes CT (results are negative in approximately 15% of cases) and LP if CT finding is negative. Angiography may locate and define the cause of SAH (aneurysm, AVM) and should be repeated in 5 to 15 days if results are initially negative. Magnetic resonance angiography is a promising alternative to conventional angiography.

The Hunt-Hess grading scale is commonly used for prognosis and timing of aneurysm surgery:

0: Unruptured aneurysm (symptomatic or incidental discovery).
I: Asymptomatic rupture or minimal headache and nuchal rigidity.
Ia: No acute meningeal or brain reaction, but fixed neurologic deficit.
II: Moderate to severe headache, nuchal rigidity, no neurologic deficit other than cranial nerve palsy.
III: Drowsiness, confusion, or mild focal neurologic deficit.
IV: Stupor, moderate to severe hemiparesis, possible early decerebrate rigidity and vegetative disturbances.
V: Deep coma, decerebrate rigidity, moribund appearance.

Complications and sequelae of SAH result from systemic dysfunction (SIADH, cardiac arrhythmias, diabetes insipidus, pulmonary embolism, GI bleeding, respiratory depression, and cardiac arrest), vasospasm, rebleeding, seizures, herniation, and hydrocephalus. Cerebral ischemia or infarction is frequent in the first 4 to 14 days after the initial bleed because of arterial vasospasm. The amount of subarachnoid blood correlates positively with the rate of occurrence of vasospasm. The use of calcium channel blockers like nimodipine (60 mg q 4 hr for 21 days) seems to reduce the occurrence of severe neurologic complications (death, coma, and permanent major motor deficits). The use of other agents such as aminophylline, dopamine, and isoproterenol remains controversial.

Lysis of the clot surrounding the aneurysm after the initial bleed results in rebleeding, which may become evident as apnea, development of new focal signs, or worsened clinical status. Slightly more than 20% of patients rebleed in the first 2 weeks; more than 30% rebleed in the first month. The mortality rate with rebleeding is over 40%, higher than with the initial bleeding. After the first 6 months the annual rebleeding rate is about 5%, with an annual mortality rate of 1% to 3%. Treating hypertension and maintaining the blood pressure in the normal range helps prevent rebleeding. In the acute phase, induced hypotension is associated with significant ischemic complications and should be avoided. The use of antifibrinolytic agents such as epsilon aminocaproic acid (Amicar), which are given by continuous IV infusion (at least 36 g per day) for up to 3 weeks and then tapered gradually, results in a decreased mortality rate for rebleeding. The decrease, however, is offset by an increased mortality rate for vasospasm. Side effects of epsilon aminocaproic acid include diarrhea, reversible myopathy, and thromboembolic disease.

Surgical clipping of the aneurysm, with intraoperatively induced hypotension and controlled ventilation, is the definitive therapy and should be performed as soon as possible, especially in stable patients (Hunt-Hess grades I to III), to avoid the risk of rebleeding. Late occurrence of hydrocephalus may require shunting.

The most common sites for aneurysms in adults are shown in Figure 1. A higher frequency of aneurysm has been reported in some familial cases and in patients with polycystic kidneys, coarctation of the aorta, and fibromuscular dysplasia.

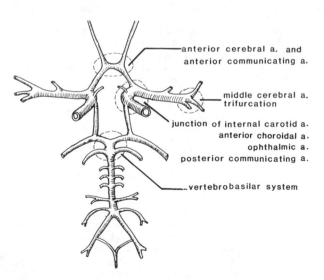

FIGURE 1
Most common sites of aneurysms.

REF: Raps EC et al: The clinical spectrum of unruptured intracranial aneurysms, *Arch Neurol* 50:265–268, 1993.

Weir B: Intracranial aneurysms and SAH: An overview, *Neurosurgery* 159:1308–1329, 1987.

ANGIOGRAPHY

Conventional cerebral angiography combines standard x-ray with injection of radioopaque dyes directly into the arterial system of interest. This is done by threading a catheter (usually through the femoral artery in the groin) to the aortic arch or selectively to the carotid or vertebrobasilar systems. Computerized subtraction techniques improve the resolution of the image. Angiography also provides evaluation of the vessels in a given time frame ("ciné") following the distribution/dispersals of dye through arterial and venous phases.

It is indicated in the evaluation of suspected vascular malformations (aneurysms, angiomas), vasculopathies, and vasculitides; stenotic or ulcerative vascular lesions; and in delineating vascular anatomy and vascular supply to various tumors.

Local complications include puncture site hematomas, intimal tears, pseudoaneurysms, and AV fistulas. Systemic complications include manifestations of anaphylaxis. Many forms of CNS (and ocular) dysfunction have been reported ranging from diffuse encephalopathy to focal ischemia. Most neurologic complications are transient. Complication rate is greater with increasing age and preexisting cerebrovascular disease. Permanent neurologic deficit occurs in approximately 0.5% (series variability).

Angiographic anatomy is depicted in Figures 2 and 3.

ANGIOMAS

Angiomas are congenital vascular lesions resulting from disordered embryogenesis. Histologic subtypes include the following (percentages refer to the frequency at autopsy): (1) *telangiectasias* (16%)—abnormal capillaries; (2) *venous angiomas* (59%)—anomalous veins; (3) *arteriovenous malformations* (AVMs) (14%)—clusters of abnormal vessels composed of arteries and veins without intervening capillaries; (4) *cavernous angiomas* (9%)—sinusoidal vessels without intervening neural tissue; and (5) *varices* (2%)—dilated veins. Angiomas are usually asymptomatic; symptoms usually are due to AVMs or cavernous angiomas. The most common intracranial locations are the cerebral hemispheres (75%) and basal ganglia (18%); posterior fossa angiomas

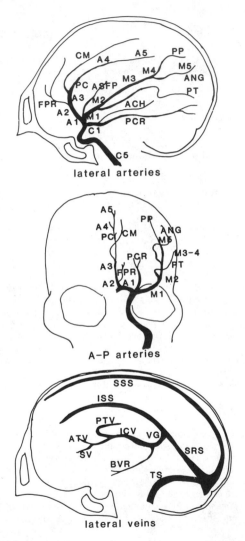

FIGURE 2
Internal carotid circulation.

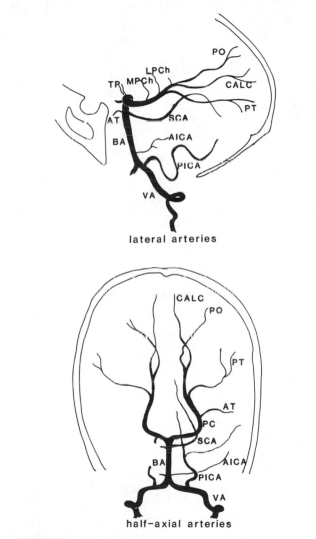

FIGURE 3
Vertebrobasilar circulation.

Angiographic anatomy
Internal carotid circulation

A₁–A₅	Segments of anterior cerebral artery
ACH	Anterior choroidal artery
ANG	Angular artery
ASFP	Ascending frontoparietal artery
ATV	Anterior terminal vein
BVR	Basal vein of Rosenthal
CM	Callosomarginal artery
C₁–C₅	Segments of internal carotid artery
FPR	Frontopolar artery
ICV	Internal cerebral vein
ISS	Inferior sagittal sinus
M₁–M₅	Segments of middle cerebral artery
PC	Pericallosal artery
PCR	Posterior cerebral artery
PP	Posterior parietal artery
PTV	Posterior terminal vein
SRS	Straight sinus
SSS	Superior sagittal sinus
SV	Septal vein
TS	Transverse sinus
VG	Great cerebral vein of Galen

Vertebrobasilar
circulation

AICA	Anterior inferior cerebellar artery
AT	Anterior temporal artery (branch of PC)
BA	Basilar artery
CALC	Calcarine artery (branch of PC)
LPCh	Lateral posterior choroidal artery
MPCh	Medial posterior choroidal artery
PC	Posterior cerebral artery
PICA	Posterior inferior cerebellar artery
PO	Parieto-occipital artery (branch of PC)
PT	Posterior temporal artery (branch of PC)
SCA	Superior cerebellar artery
TP	Thalamoperforate artery
VA	Vertebral artery

are much less frequent (6%), occurring primarily in the pons; the spinal cord is a much rarer location (see Spinal Cord). Angiography detects most angiomas, with the notable exception of cavernous angiomas and telangiectasias. MRI is the preferred noninvasive neuroimaging modality.

AVMs are the most common symptomatic angioma. Eighty percent to 90% are supratentorial. Clinical manifestations include: hemorrhage (30% to 50%), seizures (approximately 30%), migrainelike headaches (20%), and gradually progressive focal neurologic deficits (10%). Hemorrhage occurs at a rate of 1% to 2% per year. Intraparenchymal hemorrhage occurs in two thirds of cases, subarachnoid hemorrhage in one third of cases. The short-term prognosis for patients with ruptured AVMs is better than that for patients with aneurysms, with lower rates of vasospasm (rare), mortality (10%), and rebleeding (6% in the first year, reverting to 1% to 2% subsequently). Recurrent hemorrhage is associated with higher rates of mortality and overall disability. The prognosis for patients with seizures alone is better than that after hemorrhage. Therapeutic modalities include surgical excision, embolization, and radiotherapy.

REF: Caplan LR: *Stroke: A clinical approach*, ed 2, Boston, 1993, Butterworth Heinemann.

Mohr JP et al. In Barnett HJM et al, eds: *Stroke pathophysiology, diagnosis, and management*, ed 2, New York, 1992, Churchill Livingstone.

ANISOCARIA   *(see Aneurysms, Coma, Herniation, Horner's Syndrome, Pupil)*

ANOMIA   *(see Aphasia)*

ANOXIA   *(see Coma)*

ANTERIOR CEREBRAL ARTERY   *(see Aneurysm, Angiography, Ischemia)*

ANTICOAGULATION   *(see Ischemia)*

ANTICONVULSANT DRUGS   *(see Epilepsy)*

TABLE 3
Side Effects of Antidepressant Drugs*

Drug	Sedation	Insomnia	Anticholinergic Effects	Orthostatic Hypotension	Delay in Cardiac Conduction or Arrhythmia	Nausea
Tricyclic drugs						
Amitriptyline	+++	0	+++	+++	Yes	0
Trimipramine	+++	0	+++	++	Yes	0
Desipramine	+	+	++	+	Yes	0
Doxepin	+++	0	++	++	Yes	0
Imipramine	++	0	++	++	Yes	0
Nortriptyline	++	0	++	+	Yes	0
Protriptyline	+	++	++	+	Yes	0
Monoamine oxidase inhibitors						
Phenelzine	+	+	0	+++	Very rare	0
Tranylcypromine	0	++	0	+++	Very rare	+
Isocarboxazid	0	++	0	++	Very rare	0
Newer agents						
Amoxapine	++	0	+	++	Low	0
Fluoxetine	0	++	0	0	Low	++
Maprotiline	++	0	0	++	Yes	0
Trazodone	+++	0	0	++	None	+
Alprazolam	+	0	0	0	Low	0
Bupropion	0	++	0	0	Low	+

*Zero denotes no side effect, + a minor side effect, ++ a moderate side effect, and +++ a major side effect.
From Potter WZ: *New Engl J Med* 325:637, 1991.

ANTIDEPRESSANTS

Antidepressants encompass several groups of compounds, including tricyclic and tetracyclic compounds, selective serotonin reuptake inhibitors, and monoamine oxidase inhibitors. Table 3 summarizes the relative side effects of tricyclic antidepressants. Anticholinergic side effects include blurred vision, dry mouth, constipation, urinary retention, memory dysfunction, and exacerbation of narrow-angle glaucoma. Patients with dementia and concomitant depression may worsen as a result of anticholinergic effects, whereas patients with Parkinson's disease may improve. Patients with migraine or chronic pain may benefit from antidepressants with a relatively high affinity for serotonin receptors. Selective serotonin reuptake inhibitors (fluoxetine, sertraline, and paroxetine) may cause headache. Choice of antidepressant must be based on assessment of the patient's clinical state, especially cardiac conduction and ability to tolerate orthostatic hypotension, as well as the specific drug's side-effect profile. Suicide risk should be assessed in all depressed patients, since tricyclic antidepressant overdose may be fatal.

REF: Kaplan HI, Sadock BJ, eds: *Synopsis of psychiatry*, ed 6, Baltimore, 1991, William & Wilkins.

Potter WZ et al: The pharmacologic treatment of depression, *New Engl J Med* 325:633–642, 1991.

ANTIDIURETIC HORMONE   *(see Syndrome of Inappropriate Antidiuretic Hormone)*

ANTIEPILEPTIC DRUGS   *(see Epilepsy)*

ANTIPLATELET DRUGS   *(see Ischemia)*

ANTIPSYCHOTIC DRUGS   *(see Neuroleptics)*

APHASIA

Aphasia is the acquired disorder of previously intact language ability. As such, it is not interchangeable with failure of language development. Aphasic patients have disturbances of speech, writing, and reading. The most widely used classification of aphasias was developed by Benson and Geschwind. In this classification three aspects of language are used to classify eight aphasias (see Tables 4 and 5). (1) *Fluency*

TABLE 4
Aphasias with Disordered Repetition*

	Type of Speech	Comprehension†	Other Signs	Emotional State	Localization
Broca's	Nonfluent	+	Right hemiparesis worse in arm	Depressed	Lower posterior frontal
Wernicke's	Fluent	−	Often none	Often euphoric and/or paranoid	Posterior superior temporal
Conduction	Fluent	+	Often none; cortical sensory loss in right arm	Depressed	Usually parietal operculum
Global	Nonfluent	−	Right hemiparesis worse in arm	Flat	Massive perisylvian lesion

*From Geschwind N: Used by permission of the Continuing Professional Education Center, Princeton, NJ.
†Plus sign indicates relatively or fully intact; minus sign, definitely impaired.

TABLE 5
Aphasias with Good Repetition*

	Speech	Comprehension†	Localization
Transcortical motor	Nonfluent	+	Anterior to Broca's area or supplementary speech area
Transcortical sensory	Fluent	–	Surrounding Wernicke's area posteriorly
Transcortical mixed ("Isolation syndrome")	Nonfluent	–	Both of the above
Anomic	Fluent	+	Lesion of angular gyrus or second temporal gyrus

*From Geschwind N: Used by permission of the Continuing Professional Education Center, Princeton, NJ.
†Plus sign indicates relatively or fully intact; minus sign, definitely impaired.

refers to several features of spontaneous speech—rhythm, melody, articulation, and word production rate. When testing spontaneous speech, look for verbal (substitution of one word for another, such as *knife* for *spoon*) and phonemic (substitution of incorrect sounds, such as *spork* for *fork*) paraphasic errors. Paraphasic errors (in the fluent aphasias primarily) and naming abnormalities are the hallmarks of aphasia. (2) *Comprehension* abilities vary from following midline commands (such as "stick out your tongue") to performing multistep requests, (such as "take the paper in your left hand, fold it in half, and then put it on the floor"), to understanding relationships (as in "The lion was killed by the tiger. Which animal died?"). (3) *Repetition* of phrases may be impaired to various degrees; the most difficult phrases to repeat are those involving grammatic function or low-frequency words (for instance, "You know how" or "The spy fled to Greece"). Additional testing of reading (out loud and reading comprehension) and writing (to dictation or spontaneously) is often useful in evaluating patients suspected of having aphasia.

Damage to the thalamus, caudate, putamen, and surrounding structures may produce aphasia. Initial muteness improving to a fluent or nonfluent hypophonic aphasia is common. Paraphasic errors in spontaneous speech, which disappear when the patient is asked to repeat phrases, and rapid resolution of deficit are hallmarks of these subcortical aphasias.

Other syndromes related to aphasia but involving only a single language modality include aphemia or pure word dumbness (inferior frontal dominant hemisphere lesions), pure word deafness (lesions of the dominant superior temporal lobe or bilateral middle portion of the superior temporal gyrus), and alexia without agraphia (left occipital lesions, including posterior corpus callosum).

The classification is based on patients with stable deficits; the acutely ill patient may not be easily classified. Spontaneous recovery often occurs in the first month after onset and may continue for several more months. Speech therapy individualized for the form of aphasia may be helpful in recovery of language function.

REF: Benson DF. In Heilman KH, Valenstein E, eds: *Clinical neuropsychology*, ed 3, New York, 1993, Oxford University Press.

        Strub RL, Black FW: *Neurobehavioral disorders: A clinical approach*, ed 2, Philadelphia, 1988, FA Davis.

APRAXIA

Apraxia is the inability to perform a previously learned motor activity in the presence of intact motor, sensory, and comprehension systems. *Ideational apraxia* (apraxia for object use) is the inability to use common objects in a proper manner or inability to perform sequential movements despite retained ability in performing the individual movements. *Ideomotor apraxia* is the inability to voluntarily complete an act in response to a verbal command. The same act, however, can be performed spontaneously. These forms of apraxia are often associated with lesions in the left hemisphere. A lesion in the arcuate fasciculus may result in bilateral apraxia and a conduction aphasia. A lesion in the left frontal area may result in a bilateral apraxia in addition to a Broca's aphasia. A lesion in the corpus callosum may result in left-sided apraxia without right-sided apraxia. "Apraxia" has been used to describe the inability to construct geometric figures (constructional apraxia; right parietal syndrome) and to describe problems with dressing (right parietal syndrome) or gait (frontal lobe syndrome). These latter disorders represent abnormalities of more complex functions than are involved in pure ideational or ideomotor apraxia. Apraxia testing includes asking the patient to follow simple commands (such as "close your eyes" or "lick your lips"), to perform tasks with the left and right extremities (for instance, "comb hair, brush teeth, hammer a nail, or blow a kiss) and to use objects (as in lighting a match, or using the telephone). Mild apraxia may manifest itself in the use of a body part as an object. For example, the patient may use a finger as a toothbrush.

Patients with ideomotor apraxia are usually self-sufficient because they can manipulate objects correctly on their own, whereas patients with ideational apraxia are often unable to care for themselves.

ARNOLD-CHIARI MALFORMATION *(see Craniocervical Junction)*

ARTERIOGRAPHY *(see Angiography)*

ARTERIOVENOUS MALFORMATIONS *(see Angiomas, Hemorrhage)*

ARTERITIS *(see Vasculitis)*

ASEPTIC MENINGITIS   *(see Meningitis)*

ASTERIXIS

Asterixis is an abrupt, dysrhythmic loss of voluntary tone commonly elicited by extending the arms and dorsiflexing the wrists against gravity, although it may be present in any muscle group. Asterixis is preceded by a 50- to 110-millisecond period of EMG silence. In some cases, it may follow a sharp or biphasic EEG wave, indicating a possible cortical origin similar to cortical myoclonus.

Originally described in hepatic encephalopathy, asterixis may occur in any metabolic encephalopathy. Anticonvulsant-induced asterixis may occur in patients with elevated drug levels. Unilateral asterixis has been described contralateral to lesions in the midbrain, thalamus, internal capsule, and frontal or parietal lobe.

REF: Artieda J et al: *Movement Disorders* 7(3):209, 1992.

ATAXIA   *(see also Spinocerebellar Degeneration)*

An abnormality of movement characterized by errors in rate, range, direction, timing, and force ("coordination") of motor activity. Elements of ataxia include:

1. Decomposition of movement into component parts.
2. Dysmetria—overshooting or undershooting a target.
3. Dysdiadochokinesia—impairment of rapid alternating movements.
4. Tremor.

Ataxia may involve limbs, trunk, eyes, or bulbar musculature and may be due to disease of the cerebellum, brainstem, spinal cord, or motor or sensory nerves. Cerebellar hemispheric disease commonly produces limb ataxia, whereas midline cerebellar disease manifests as truncal and gait ataxia. Tremor may be an action or intention tremor (disease of dentate nucleus or superior cerebellar peduncle) or more coarse ("rubral tremor"). Titubation, a nodding-head tremor, is seen with midline cerebellar disease and may involve the trunk. Ataxic speech has abnormal variability of volume, rate, and phonation and may be slow and slurred or have alternating loudness and quietness. Impaired proprioception resulting from tabes dorsalis, hereditary disease, or dorsal root ganglionopathies may lead to sensory ataxia with impaired gait and presence of Romberg's sign. Gait ataxia may accompany vertigo in vestibular dysfunction.

ATHETOSIS *(see also Chorea)*

Athetosis is an involuntary, slow, sinuous, irregular, writhing movement of any muscle group, usually most prominent in the distal extremities. It frequently coexists with other abnormal movements, particularly dystonia and chorea. Like those movements, athetosis is associated with lesions in the basal ganglia. EMG analysis reveals loss of natural reciprocation between agonists and antagonists. Common syndromes include posthemiplegic athetosis, generalized athetosis ("double athetosis" seen in cerebal palsy and postkernicterus), and drug induced athetosis (e.g., levodopa-induced; also, tardive dyskinesias). Athetosis may be seen in many inherited metabolic diseases such as Huntington's disease, Wilson's disease, Lesch-Nyhan syndrome, glutaric acidemia, D-glyceric acidemia, sulfite oxidase deficiency, Niemann-Pick disease, familial calcification of the basal ganglia, and Hallervorden-Spatz disease.

ATTENTION DEFICIT—HYPERACTIVITY DISORDER (ADHD) *(see also Learning Disabilities)*

Behavior disorder of unknown cause characterized by varying degrees of developmentally inappropriate inattention, impulsiveness, and hyperactivity. ADHD affects an estimated 3% of all children, is familial, and is 4 to 6 times more common in boys.

DSM-IV diagnostic criteria: (a) onset before age 7 years; (b) some impairment in two or more settings (e.g. school and home); (c) clinically significant impairment in social, academic or occupational functioning; (d) absence of pervasive developmental disorder, or other mental disorder to account for the symptoms; (e) either six or more symptoms of inattention, or six or more symptoms of hyperactivity-impulsivity.

Inattention
1. Often fails to give close attention to details or is careless.
2. Has difficulty sustaining attention in tasks.
3. Often does not listen when spoken to directly.
4. Often does not follow through on instructions or fails to finish tasks.
5. Has difficulty organizing tasks or activities.
6. Often loses things necessary for tasks.

7. Is easily distracted by extraneous stimuli.
8. Is often forgetful in daily activities.

Hyperactivity
1. Often figits with limbs or squirms in seat.
2. Often leaves seat in classroom or other places where sitting is expected.
3. Often runs or climbs excessively.
4. Has difficulty playing quietly.
5. Is often "on the go" or often acts as if "driven by a motor".
6. Often talks excessively.

Impulsivity
1. Often blurts out answers before questions are completed.
2. Often has difficulty awaiting turn.
3. Often interrupts or intrudes on others.

Educational intervention in the form of special class placement (more structure and individual attention) is sometimes necessary, and behavioral therapy can be helpful. Methylphenidate, 0.3 to 0.6 mg/kg bid-tid, is a CNS stimulant and 70% to 80% effective in increasing attention and decreasing hyperactive motor activity. Common, but usually transient, adverse effects include sleep disturbance, decreased appetite, abdominal pain, and irritability. Growth retardation can occur; the risk is minimized by using the smallest effective dose and by avoiding the drug on weekends, school holidays, and during the summer. As tics and Tourette's syndrome have been associated with methylphenidate, this drug is contraindicated in children with such a history or family history. Pemoline is similar to methylphenidate but is associated with hepatotoxicity. Clonidine can be effective in reducing the impulsive component of behavior. Side effects include orthostatic hypotension. Tricyclic antidepressants are less effective but useful when stimulants are contraindicated.

In most cases, manifestations of the disorder persist throughout childhood. Affected children may develop a conduct disorder later in childhood or adolescence, and one third of children will show symptoms as adults.

REF: American Psychiatric Association: *Diagnostic and statistical manual of mental disorders, third edition, revised*, Washington, DC, 1987.

AUTONOMIC DYSFUNCTION
CLASSIFICATION

Autonomic dysfunction occurs in a large number of diseases affecting either the central or peripheral nervous systems (see Table 6). Progressive autonomic failure (Shy-Drager syndrome) is an idiopathic degenerative disease that may be associated with parkinsonism or spinocerebellar syndromes. Spinal cord lesions above T6 interrupt descending central connections to cells in the intermediolateral cell column, which innervate the splanchnic vascular bed, important in reflex regulation of blood pressure. Acute pandysautonomia may be a variant of Guillain-Barré syndrome. Autonomic dysfunction is most likely in neuropathies that prominently affect small fibers.

DIAGNOSIS

Autonomic dysfunction is suspected in the presence of orthostatic hypotension or other derangements of cardiovascular regulation, loss of sweating, bladder or bowel dysfunction, impotence, or pupillary abnormalities. The following noninvasive screening tests can be performed at the bedside: (1) *Orthostatic blood pressure and heart rate.* An estimate of the time typically required to produce symptoms on standing is made based on the patient's history. Resting supine blood pressure and heart rate are measured. The patient then stands up, and after at least 3 minutes (or after the estimated time interval, whichever is longer), blood pressure and heart rate measurements are repeated. It is important to measure blood pressure with the arm extended horizontally when the patient is standing, to avoid spurious readings resulting from hydrostatic forces in a dependent limb. A fall in systolic blood pressure of 20 to 30 mm Hg or diastolic blood pressure of 10 to 15 mm Hg is abnormal. Heart rate normally increases by 11 to 29 beats per minute immediately on standing. An abnormal fall in blood pressure, in the absence of drugs or hypovolemia, indicates a lesion either in the afferent baroreflex pathways or in efferent sympathetic vasomotor fibers. (2) *Heart rate variation.* Under normal circumstances the heart rate increases during inspiration as a result of decreased cardiac vagal activity (respiratory sinus arrhythmia [RSA]). To quantitate RSA, the patient breathes deeply at 6 breaths per minute while the ECG is recorded, and the times of inspiration and expiration are noted on the ECG tracing. A difference in heart rate between inspiration and expiration of less than 10 beats per mintue or an expiration-to-inspiration ratio of R-R intervals of less than 1:2 is abnormal in individuals under 40 years of age. RSA becomes less prominent with age. (3) *Tests of pupillary function.* Instillation of dilute 0.1% epinephrine into the

TABLE 6
Classification of Autonomic Disorders

I. Diseases affecting the central nervous system.
  A. Progressive autonomic failure ([PAF], idiopathic orthostatic hypotension).
    1. Pure PAF.
    2. PAF with multiple-system atrophy (Shy-Drager syndrome).
      a. With parkinsonian features.
      b. With spinocerebellar degeneration.
  B. Parkinson's disease.
  C. Spinal cord lesions.
  D. Wernicke's encephalopathy.
  E. Miscellaneous diseases.
    1. Cerebrovascular disease.
    2. Brainstem tumors.
    3. Multiple sclerosis.
    4. Adie's syndrome.
    5. Tabes dorsalis.
II. Diseases affecting the peripheral autonomic nervous system.
  A. Disorders with no associated sensory-motor peripheral neuropathy.
    1. Acute and subacute autonomic neuropathy.
      a. Pandysautonomia.
      b. Cholinergic dysautonomia.
    2. Botulism.
  B. Diseases associated with sensory-motor peripheral neuropathy in which autonomic dysfunction is clinically important.
    1. Diabetes.
    2. Amyloidosis.
    3. Acute inflammatory neuropathy.
    4. Acute intermittent porphyria.
    5. Familial dysautonomia (Riley-Day syndrome: HMSN III [Hereditary Motor-Sensory Neuropathy])
    6. Chronic sensory and autonomic neuropathy.
  C. Disorders in which autonomic dysfunction is usually clinically unimportant.
    1. Alcohol-induced neuropathy.
    2. Toxic neuropathies (caused by vincristine sulfate, acrylamide, heavy metals, perhexiline maleate, or organic solvents).

TABLE 6—cont'd
Classification of Autonomic Disorders

    3. HMSNs I, II, and V.
    4. Malignancy.
    5. Vitamin B_{12} deficiency.
    6. Rheumatoid arthritis.
    7. Chronic renal failure.
    8. Systemic lupus erythematosus.
    9. Mixed connective tissue disease.
   10. Fabry's disease.
   11. Chronic inflammatory neuropathy.

Adapted from McLeod JG, Tuck RR: *Ann Neurol* 21:419–430, 1987.

conjunctival sac has no effect on normal pupils but dilates a pupil with a lesion in postganglionic sympathetic innervation because of denervation supersensitivity. Likewise, dilute 0.125% pilocarpine causes little or no contraction in normal pupils but causes miosis in the presence of abnormal parasympathetic innervation. All pharmacologic tests of pupillary function are distorted by corneal trauma (e.g., contact lenses and testing the corneal reflex) within 24 hours of the eye drops. (4) *Other tests.* More extensive autonomic testing includes measurement of plasma norepinephrine levels and determination of denervation supersensitivity, quantitative Valsalva and tilt-table testing, baroreflex sensitivity testing, thermal sweat testing, and skin blood-flow measurements.

TREATMENT

Management of orthostatic hypotension begins with minimizing or avoiding drugs that may contribute to symptoms, including diuretics, antihypertensives, and tricyclic antidepressants. Patients should be told to avoid sudden standing, straining during defecation or urination, excessive heat, large meals, and alcohol. Elevation of the head of the patient's bed reduces nocturnal volume loss and is generally recommended, as is increased salt intake unless there is associated congestive heart failure. Waist-high elastic garments may be helpful but are cumbersome; knee-high or thigh-high stockings offer little benefit. Drinking two cups of coffee after large meals may reduce postprandial hypotension. The mainstay of pharmacologic therapy is fludrocortisone; a start-

TABLE 7
Drugs Used in Treating Orthostatic Hypotension*

Drugs†	Possible Mechanisms of Action
Fludrocortisone (A,b,j)	A Increase sodium and fluid retention
Indomethacin (a,b,f,G)	B Sensitization of vascular α-adrenergic receptors
Propranolol (e,H)	C Indirectly acting sympathomimetic drug
Ephedrine (C,d)	D α-agonist drug
Phenylephrine (D)	E Blockade of neuronal uptake
Amphetamine (C,d,K)	F Block presynaptic inhibitory adrenergic receptor
Methylphenidate (d,K)	G Decrease circulating vasodilator prostaglandins
MAO inhibitors (L)	H Inhibit β-adrenergic activity
Dihydroergotamine (I)	I Nonadrenergic vasoconstrictor
Vasopressin (I)	J Inhibits extraneuronal catecholamine uptake
Metoclopramide (M)	K CNS "stimulant" drug
Clonidine (D)	L Diminish norepinephrine catabolism
Prednisone (A,b,J)	M Blocks dopamine receptors

*Modified from Polinsky RJ: *Neurol Clin* 2:487-498, 1984.
†Mechanism of action is in parentheses; primary mechanism is capitalized.

ing dosage of 0.1 mg per day is increased by 0.1 mg every 3 to 4 days until symptoms are controlled or until a maximum dosage of 1 mg per day is reached. Complications include supine hypertension, peripheral edema, hypokalemia, and congestive heart failure. Other agents (see Table 7) include ephedrine (25 mg tid or qid), dihydroergotamine (5 to 10 mg tid), and indomethacin (starting at 25 mg bid-tid).

REF: Low PA: *Clinical autonomic disorders: Evaluation and management*, Boston, 1993, Little, Brown.

McLeod JG, Tuck RR: *Ann Neurol* 21:419-430, 1987.

BASAL GANGLIA   *(see Athetosis, Chorea, Dystonia, Huntington's Disease, Parkinson's Disease, Parkinsonism, Rigidity, Tremor, Wilson's Disease)*

BASILAR ARTERY   *(see Ischemia)*

BELL's PALSY   *(see Facial Nerve)*

BENIGN INTRACRANIAL HYPERTENSION   *(see Pseudo-tumor Cerebri)*

BENZODIAZEPINES

Benzodiazepines are used in the treatment of anxiety, insomnia, epilepsy, vertigo, and certain movement disorders. They are also used in the management of ethanol withdrawal. Prolonged use of any drug in this class may cause dependence, particularly in patients with a history of alcohol or substance abuse. Therefore only the lowest effective doses should be used for the shortest possible period. Side effects include sedation, amnesia (especially with triazolam), agitation, and gait disorder. Withdrawal symptoms may occur after 1 to 6 weeks of use and include flulike symptoms, insomnia, irritability, seizures, nausea, headache, tremor, and muscle cramps. In those at risk for withdrawal, the dose should be tapered over several weeks. Acute intoxication with depressed mental status may be reversed with the benzodiazepine receptor antagonist flumazenil, starting at 0.2 mg IV over 30 seconds. Failure to respond to a total dose of 5 mg makes it unlikely that sedation is due to benzodiazepines.

BLADDER

Proper lower urinary tract function is immediately controlled by bladder stretch receptors (generating sympathetic input to spinal cord), the bladder wall detrusor muscle (activated by parasympathetic outflow), the internal sphincter (smooth muscle), and the external sphincter (striated muscle under voluntary control). Neural control is mediated by cerebral hemispheric centers, the pontine "micturition" center, the sacral "micturition" center, and the hypogastric, pelvic, and pudendal nerves (Figure 4). These centers and nerves work together to

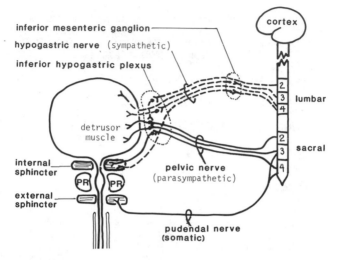

FIGURE 4
Neuroanatomy of bladder control.

achieve (1) storage of urine without leaking; (2) adequate perception of increased intravesical pressure; (3) release of cortical inhibition of emptying in appropriate circumstances; (4) proper synergy of urinary tract muscular structures; and (5) complete bladder emptying. Thus disorders of bladder control can be caused by local factors (such as previous childbirth, pelvic surgery, or urinary tract infection) or disorders of the upper or lower motor neuron (see Table 8).

Detrusor hyperreflexia resulting from cerebral cortical dysfunction is a deficit of normal inhibitory mechanisms in which the micturition reflex itself is intact, since the lesion is above the pontine micturition center. Symptoms include frequency, urgency, and urge incontinence. Common neurologic disorders leading to uninhibited bladder contraction include stroke, mass lesion, and hydrocephalus. Detrusor hyperactivity due to suprasacral spinal cord lesion leads to loss of detrusor-sphincter coordination. Simultaneous contraction of both detrusor and sphincter can lead to increased intravesical pressures and upper urinary tract damage. Multiple sclerosis, spinal cord tumor or trauma, vascular malformation, and herniated intervertebral disk are common causes.

TABLE 8
Bladder Dysfunction

Upper Motor Neuron	Lower Motor Neuron
Characteristic feature	
Decreased capacity for storage	Decreased emptying ability
Cause	
Hemisphere or cord injury above T12 (trauma, multiple sclerosis, stroke, tumor)	1. Sensory: diabetes mellitus, tabes dorsalis 2. Motor: amyotrophic lateral sclerosis 3. Mixed sensory and motor: spinal dysraphism (meningomyelocele), tumor or trauma of lower cord, conus, or cauda
History	
Urge incontinence with dry intervals	Overflow incontinence
Wet at night	Urinary retention Straining to void Wet or dry at night
Bulbocavernous reflex	
Present	Absent
Cystometrogram	
"Hyperreflexic bladder" Small bladder capacity Small residual volumes Vesicoureteral reflux (and upper urinary tract damage) may occur at peak pressures.	"Flaccid bladder" Large bladder capacity Large residual volumes Vesicoureteral reflux and upper urinary tract damage can occur with persisting urinary retention.
Treatment goal	
Increase storage capacity	Increase bladder tone; avoid storage of large urinary volumes; promote bladder emptying

Continued.

TABLE 8—cont'd
Bladder Dysfunction

Upper Motor Neuron	Lower Motor Neuron
Treatment	
Oxybutynin (Ditropan) anticholinergic	Bethanechol (Urecholine) cholinergic
Dose:	Dose:
Child: 2.5 mg PO bid—tid	Child: 5 mg/day, increase as below for adult
Adult: 5 mg PO tid—qid	Adult: 2.5—10 mg SC tid—qid, or 5—50 mg PO tid—qid
Side effects: dry mouth, blurred vision	Contraindicated asthma, hyperthyroidism, coronary artery disease, ulcer disease
Propantheline bromide (Pro-Banthine) anticholinergic	Phenoxybenzamine (Dibenzyline) antiadrenergic
Dose:	Dose:
Child: not currently approved for use	Child: 0.3—0.5 mg/kg/day
Adult: 15—30 mg PO tid—qid	Adult: 10—30 mg/day
Side effects: dry mouth, blurred vision	Side effects: retrograde ejaculation, drowsiness, orthostatic hypotension
Imipramine (Tofranil) mixed anticholinergic and adrenergic	
Dose:	
Child: 1.5—2 mg/kg qid	
Adult: 25 mg PO qid	
Side effects: dry mouth, blurred vision, constipation, tachycardia, sweating fatigue, tremor	
Intermittent self-catheterization	Intermittent self-catheterization or Crédé maneuver

Detrusor areflexia is due to lesions of the sacral micturition center or its connections to the bladder. Sphincter function is preserved, but detrusor contraction is not activated, commonly resulting in overflow incontinence. Causes include myelopathy resulting from herniated disk or tumor and interruption of the reflex arc as a result of pelvic or pudendal nerve injury following trauma or operation.

Autonomic dysreflexia occurs after spinal cord lesion above the region of major sympathetic outflow (T5 to L2). Splanchnic sympathetic outflow is no longer moderated by supraspinal centers, and bladder distention, catheterization, or other manipulation causes an acute syndrome of hypertension, anxiety, sweating, headache, and bradycardia. Prompt recognition and treatment are essential.

REF: Blaivas JG: *J Am Geriatr Soc* 38:306-310, 1990.

Fowler CJ et al: *J Neurol Neurosurg Psychiatry* 55:986-989, 1992.

Gelber et al: *Stroke* 24:378-382, 1993.

Kaplan SA et al: *J Urol* 146:113-117, 1991.

Wein AJ: *J Am Geriatr Soc* 38:317-325, 1990.

BLEPHAROSPASM   *(see Dystonia)*

BRACHIAL PLEXUS

The brachial plexus (Figure 5) comprises the anastomoses derived from the anterior primary rami of vertebral segments C5 to T1. Trauma (penetrating, traction, avulsion, compression, or stretch) is the most common cause of damage. Other causes include radiation, neoplastic infiltration, and infections; damage also may be vaccine induced.

Upper plexus lesions (C5-6, upper trunk, *Duchenne-Erb palsy*) are the most common; they usually result from forceful separation of the head and shoulder but can be due to pressure on the shoulder *(knapsack paralysis)*. The lesions are characterized by weakness of shoulder abduction, external rotation, elbow flexion, and forearm supination as well as variable amounts of triceps weakness. Sensory loss is variable and may involve the deltoid region, the external aspect of the upper arm, and the radial side of the forearm.

Lower plexus lesions (C8-T1, *Dejerine-Klumpke palsy*) are usually due to traction of an already abducted arm or to infiltration or compression resulting from tumors of the lung apex *(Pancoast's syndrome)*. The lesions are characterized by weakness of intrinsic hand muscles,

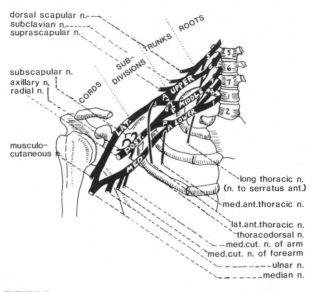

FIGURE 5
Brachial plexus. *(From Haymaker W, Woodhall B: Peripheral nerve injuries: Principles of diagnosis, Philadelphia, 1953, WB Saunders. Used by permission.)*

long finger flexors, and extensors. Sensory loss may involve the medial arm and forearm and the ulnar aspect of the hand. The cords of the brachial plexus are usually injured in variable combinations as a result of humeral head dislocation, direct axillary trauma, and supraclavicular compression.

Radiation brachial plexopathy occurs between 5 months and many years after radiation. In contrast to plexopathy due to tumor infiltration, the upper trunk or entire plexus is affected, pain is less common, lymphedema is frequent, and Horner's syndrome is rare.

Idiopathic brachial plexus neuritis *(Parsonage-Turner syndrome, neuralgic amyotrophy)* develops suddenly; shoulder pain is exacerbated by shoulder or arm movement but not by neck movement or Valsalva maneuver. Pain persists for several weeks, followed by weakness and atrophy. Onset may be preceded by a viral illness or immunization. In one-third of cases the neuritis is bilateral. Prognosis is usually good, and treatment should include range-of-motion exercises to prevent shoulder arthropathy.

REF: Dyck PJ, Thomas PK: *Peripheral neuropathy*, ed 3, Philadelphia, 1993, WB Saunders.

BRAIN DEATH   *(see also Cardiopulmonary Arrest, Coma)*

An irreversible loss of all recognizable brain function (incompatible with continued cardiopulmonary function off mechanical support). Legal criteria for death vary by state. Each institution may also set policy defining more specific requirements for brain death or discontinuation of life-sustaining measures. An interdisciplinary task force developed the following commonly accepted guidelines for the diagnosis of brain death in adults. There are also specific criteria for establishment of brain death in children; a pediatric neurologist should be consulted.

  I. Clinical criteria (*all* are mandatory).
      A. Preceding coma of known cause due to an irreversible cerebral process. Must not be due to CNS depressant or neuromuscular-blocking drugs, shock, hypothermia (<32°C/90°F), metabolic or endocrine disturbances.
      B. No cerebral function. No behavioral or reflex responses involving structures above the cervical spinal cord can be elicited by stimuli to any part of the body. No spontaneous movement or posturing to deep pain. Spinal reflex withdrawal is allowable. Deep tendon (spinal) reflexes may be present if all other criteria are met.
      C. No brainstem function (including reflexes).
          1. Pupils unreactive to light (midposition or dilated).
          2. Corneal reflexes absent.
          3. Vestibular-ocular reflexes absent. No response to oculocephalic maneuvers and 50-ml ice water caloric stimuli in each ear.
          4. Gag reflex absent (move endotracheal tube to elicit).
          5. No other brainstem reflexes (e.g., blink, ciliospinal, cough, snout).
      D. Criteria should be present for 6 hours (minimum).

II. Laboratory criteria (confirmatory).
    A. Negative toxicology screen or specific drug levels.
    B. Isoelectric EEG. Technical standards published by the American Electroencephalographic Society (Guidelines in EEG. Pts. 1-7. *J Clin Neurophysiol* 3:131-168;1986).
    C. Brainstem auditory and somatosensory-evoked potentials can provide additional evidence of absent brainstem functions.
    D. Absence of cerebral circulation *may* be demonstrated by cerebral arteriography, transcranial Doppler, bolus radioisotope angiography, or intracranial pressure (by ICP monitor) exceeding mean systolic pressure for ≥1 hour.
    E. No spontaneous respiration or respiratory effort during apneic oxygenation for 10 minutes or with a PCO_2 >60 (caution in using PCO_2 with chronic lung disease patients). Patients are ventilated for 10 to 30 minutes with 100% O_2 (maintain baseline, PCO_2) and then disconnected from the ventilator while 100% O_2 is supplied by tracheal catheter at ≥6 L/minute. Blood gas levels are measured before the ventilator is disconnected and 5 to 10 minutes after disconnecting the ventilator.

REF: Kaufman H: *Neurosurgery* 19:850, 1986.

    Levy DE et al: *JAMA* 253:1420-1426, 1985.

    Manks SJ, Zisfein J: *Arch Neurol* 47:1066, 1990.

    President's Commission on Guidelines for the Determination of Death: *Neurology* 32:395, 1982.

    Task Force for the Determination of Brain Death in Children: *Neurology* 37:1077, 1987.

BRAIN STEM AUDITORY EVOKED POTENTIALS *(see Evoked Potentials)*

BRAINSTEM SYNDROMES *(see Ischemia)*

BREATHING *(see Coma, Hyperventilation)*

BULBAR PALSY

A syndrome of weakness or paralysis of muscles supplied by cranial nerves IX, X, XI, and XII resulting from lesions of the nuclei or nerves (see Pseudobulbar Palsy for lesions of the supranuclear pathways). Involved muscles include those of the pharynx and larynx, the sterno-cleidomastoid, the upper trapezius, and the tongue. Patients may have dysarthria, dysphagia, hoarseness, nasal voice, palatal deviation, diminished gag reflex, or weakness of the sternocleidomastoid, upper trapezius, or tongue (may have atrophy and fasciculations). Causes include motor neuron disease ("progressive bulbar palsy" is one form), cerebrovascular lesions of the brainstem, intramedullary and extramedullary posterior fossa tumors, syringobulbia (may be associated with syringomyelia), meningitis, encephalitis, herpes zoster, poliomyelitis, diphtheria, aneurysms (uncommon), granulomatous disease, and bone lesions (platybasia, Paget's disease, and foraminal syndromes). Guillain-Barré syndrome, myasthenia gravis, and other neuromuscular disorders affecting bulbar innervated muscles must also be considered.

CALCIFICATION, CEREBRAL

Calcification may be physiologic or pathologic. Physiologic calcification is rare in patients under 10 years of age. Basal ganglia calcification is most often idiopathic (especially in elderly patients), as is calcification in the pineal gland, choroid plexus, falx, tentorium, habenula, dentate nucleus, dura, and large vessels.

Causes of pathologic calcification include the following

Congenital or developmental: Tuberous sclerosis, Sturge-Weber syndrome, Fahr's disease, familial idiopathic (autosomal dominant with basal ganglia and dentate calcifications), Gorlin's syndrome (basal cell nevus), neurofibromatosis, Cockayne's syndrome, and Down's syndrome.

Inflammatory or infectious: "TORCH" (toxoplasmosis, syphilis, rubella, cytomegalovirus, or herpes virus), bacterial, tuberculosis, HIV infection, parasitic (cysticercosis, coccidiomycosis, echinococcosis, or sparganosis), and granuloma.

Metabolic or endocrine: Hyperparathyroidism and hypoparathyroidism, pseudohyperparathyroidism, and celiac disease with low serum folate levels.

Vascular: Cavernous angiomas (50%), AVMs (25%), aneurysms (5%), and infarcts (rare).

Trauma: Chronic subdural hematomas and other hematomas (rare).

Toxic effects: Postradiotherapy (especially when combined with methotrexate), carbon monoxide, lead encephalopathy, and birth anoxia.

Neoplastic: Virtually all types of neoplasms can calcify. Most common are low-grade astrocytoma (10%), oligodendroglioma (50%), medulloblastoma (5%), ependymoma (33% to 66%), craniopharyngioma (70% to 80%), meningioma (10% to 20%, with adjacent bony sclerosis), dermoid, and teratoma. Metastases may rarely calcify.

REF: Osborn AG: *Handbook of neuroradiology*, St. Louis, 1991, Mosby.

CALCIUM   *(see Electrolyte Disorders)*

CALORICS   *(see also Vestibulo-Ocular Reflex, Coma)*

Water that is colder or warmer than body temperature, when applied to the tympanic membrane, changes the firing rate of the ipsilateral vestibular nerve, causing ocular deviation and nystagmus. Cold water normally induces a slow ipsilateral deviation with contralateral "corrective" fast phases. Warm water induces a slow contralateral deviation and ipsilateral fast phases. Since the direction of nystagmus is conventionally described as that of the fast phase, the mnemonic COWS ("cold opposite, warm same") indicates the direction of caloric nystagmus for cold and warm stimuli. Bilateral irrigation induces vertical nystagmus; the mnemonic CUWD ("cold up, warm down") refers to the fast phases.

Caloric testing may be done at the bedside or quantitatively in a laboratory. Quantitative caloric testing is used to evaluate vestibular function. Bedside caloric testing is used (1) to establish the integrity of the ocular motor system in patients with an apparent gaze paresis and (2) to evaluate altered states of consciousness. Caloric stimulation may be used to elicit vestibular eye movements if oculocephalic maneuvers (see Vestibulo-Ocular Reflex) have negative results or when a cervical injury is suspected.

Bedside caloric testing is performed after the external auditory canal has been examined, the impacted cerumen removed, and the tympanic membrane established to be intact. The head is elevated 30 degrees from horizontal, aligning the horizontal semicircular canal in the vertical plane and maximizing lateral horizontal nystagmus. Water is gently injected with a syringe through a soft catheter inserted in the external auditory canal. Usually 1 ml of ice-water is sufficient in alert patients and minimizes discomfort. Up to 100 ml of ice-water can be used in unresponsive patients, and several minutes should be allowed for a response. Irrigation is repeated in the opposite ear after waiting at least 5 minutes for vestibular equilibration. Warm water (44° C) may also be used. Because of the risk of thermal injury, hot water should never be used.

Eye movements elicited by vestibular stimuli, whether passive head rotation (see Vestibulo-Ocular Reflex) or caloric, may allow localization within the ocular motor system. Impaired movement of both eyes to one side occurs with lesions of the ipsilateral paramedian pontine reticular formation. Impaired abduction in one eye suggests a palsy of cranial nerve VI. Impaired adduction is seen in third-nerve palsies and in the eye ipsilateral to a medial longitudinal fasciculus lesion (internuclear ophthalmoplegia). Bilateral internuclear ophthalmoplegias cause, in addition to bilateral adduction weakness, impaired vertical vestibular eye movements. Eye deviation may occur in aberrant directions in patients with drug intoxication or structural disease of central vestibular connections.

As consciousness declines, the caloric stimulus–induced eye movements relate to the integrity of brainstem structures. Tonic eye deviation indicates integrity of brainstem function. Asymmetric horizontal responses are interpreted as previously described and may give localizing information. Lack of any response may result from lesions of vestibulo-ocular reflex pathways in the medulla or pons, the eighth cranial nerve, labyrinth or drug intoxications, such as those resulting from vestibular suppressants (barbiturates, phenytoin, tricyclic antidepressants, or major tranquilizers), and neuromuscular blockers. The presence of caloric-induced nystagmus in an acutely unresponsive patient suggests a psychogenic cause of unresponsiveness.

REF: Plum F, Posner JB: *The diagnosis of stupor and coma*, ed 3, Philadelphia, 1982, FA Davis.

CAPILLARY TELANGECTASIA   *(see Angiomas)*

CARBAMAZEPINE   *(see Epilepsy)*

CARCINOMATOUS MENINGITIS   *(see Cerebrospinal Fluid, Tumor)*

CARDIOPULMONARY ARREST   *(see also Brain Death, Coma)*

Prediction of neurologic outcome following cardiopulmonary arrest requires serial evaluations and is not completely accurate. Most patients with good outcome (independent self-care) emerge from coma within

24 to 48 hours. Conversely, coma duration greater than 48 hours has high likelihood of mortality or permanent neurologic deficit. Deterioration in level of consciousness is indicative of poor prognosis. Absence of pupillary light reflex at initial exam, absence of motor responses at 1 day, and failure to follow commands at 1 week are all strong predictors of poor neurologic outcome.

Prearrest morbidity affects survival. Preexisting pneumonia, hypotension, renal failure, cancer, or home-bound lifestyle are predictive of poor prognosis. Arrest for longer than 15 minutes is associated with an in-hospital mortality rate of 95%.

REF: Bedell SE et al: *New Engl J Med* 309:569-576, 1983.

   Levy DE et al: Predicting outcome from hypoxic-ischemic coma, *JAMA* 253:1420-1426, 1985.

   Longstreth WT, Diehr P, Inui TS: Prediction of awakening after out-of-hospital cardiac arrest, *New Engl J Med* 308:1378-1382, 1983.

CAROTID ARTERY   *(see Angiography, Ischemia)*

CARPAL TUNNEL SYNDROME

Carpal tunnel syndrome occurs as a result of compression of the median nerve as it courses beneath the transverse carpal ligament. Associated conditions include ligamentous or synovial thickening, trauma, pregnancy, obesity, diabetes, scleroderma, thyroid disease, lupus erythematosus, mucopolysaccharidoses, amyloidosis, gout, acromegaly, Paget's disease, tuberculosis, and congestive heart failure.

Patients frequently have intermittent numbness and paresthesias in the median distribution (although the numbness and parasthesias may radiate outside this area), which are worse at night. Weakness and atrophy of the opponens pollicus, the abductor pollicus brevis, and the first two lumbricals are late signs that occur months after onset. The symptoms are reproduced by tapping over the carpal tunnel (Tinel's sign) or by flexion of the wrist (Phalen's sign). Differential diagnosis includes C6 or C7 radiculopathy, brachial plexopathy, peripheral polyneuropathy, and median neuropathies.

Electromyogram (EMG) studies show prolongation of distal median motor and sensory (more sensitive) latencies and a difference between the distal median and ulnar motor latencies. Fibrillation potentials are frequent. Bilateral EMG and nerve-conduction abnormalities are common, even in asymptomatic patients.

Treatment consists of avoiding activities that may precipitate symptoms and wearing a wrist extension splint at night. Local corticosteroid injections may provide limited relief. Indications for surgery are weakness, atrophy, or EMG evidence of denervation. Surgical treatment is usually not necessary during pregnancy, since symptoms resolve spontaneously.

CARPOPEDAL SPASM   (see Cramps, Electrolyte Disorders)

CATAPLEXY   (see Sleep Disorders)

CAUDA EQUINA

Causes of cauda equina and conus medullaris syndromes (see Table 9) include tumors, spinal stenosis, disk disease, arachnoiditis, and trauma.

TABLE 9
Clinical Differentiation of Cauda Equina and Conus Medullaris Syndromes

Conus Medullaris (Lower Sacral Cord)	Cauda Equina (Lumbosacral Roots)
Sensory deficit	
Saddle distribution	Saddle distribution
Bilateral, symmetric	Asymmetric
Sensory dissociation present	Sensory dissociation absent
Presents early	Presents relatively later
Pain	
Uncommon	Prominent, early
Relatively mild	Severe
Bilateral, symmetric	Asymmetric
Perineum and thighs	Radicular
Motor deficit	
Symmetric	Asymmetric
Mild	Moderate to severe
Atrophy absent	Atrophy more prominent

Continued.

TABLE 9—cont'd
**Clinical Differentiation of Cauda Equina and
Conus Medullaris Syndromes**

Conus Medullaris (Lower Sacral Cord)	Cauda Equina (Lumbosacral Roots)
Reflexes	
Achilles reflex absent	Reflexes variably involved
Patellar reflex normal	
Sphincter dysfunction	
Early, severe	Late, less severe
Absent anal and bulbo cavernosus reflex	Reflex abnormalities less common
Sexual dysfunction	
Erection and ejaculation impaired	Less common

Modified from DeJong RN: *The neurologic examination,* ed 4, New York, 1979. Harper & Row.

CAVERNOUS ANGIOMA   *(see Angiomas)*

CENTRAL CORE DISEASE   *(see Myopathy)*

CENTRAL PONTINE MYELINOLYSIS   *(see Alcohol, Electrolyte Disorders, Syndrome of Inappropriate Antidiuretic Hormone)*

CEREBELLUM   *(see Alcohol, Ataxia, Spinocerebellar Degeneration)*

CEREBRAL CORTEX   *(see also Frontal Lobe, Occipital Lobe, Temporal Lobe, Parietal Lobe)*

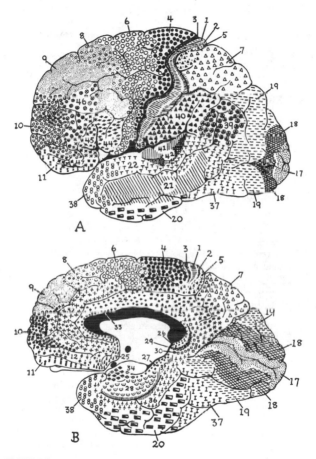

FIGURE 6

Brodmann's cytoarchitectural map of cerebral cortex, indicating major functional areas. *4*, Primary motor strip; *3, 1,* and *2*, sensory strip; *17*, primary visual cortex; *18* and *19*, visual association cortex; *8*, frontal eye fields; *6*, premotor cortex; *41* and *42*, auditory cortex; *5* and *7*, somaesthetic association cortex. Areas *13* to *16* (not shown) make up the insula. Labeling is from anterior to posterior. *(From Carpenter MB:* Core text of neuroanatomy, *ed 4, Baltimore, 1991, Williams & Wilkins.)*

REF: Carpenter MB. *Core text of neuroanatomy*, ed 4, Baltimore, Williams & Wilkins.

Gorman DG, Unuetzer J: Brodmann's "missing" numbers, *Neurology* 43:226–227, 1993.

CEREBRAL EDEMA   *(see Intracranial Pressure)*

CEREBRAL EMBOLISM   *(see Ischemia)*

CEREBRAL INFARCTION   *(see Ischemia)*

CEREBRAL PALSY

An early-onset nonprogressive disorder of tone, movement, and posture. There are four main categories.

1. *Pyramidal or spastic form* includes spastic quadriplegia—arms more severely affected than legs, commonly associated with severe mental retardation, pseudobulbar signs, optic atrophy, and generalized seizures; spastic diplegia—greater motor involvement of legs than arms ("scissored" position) often associated with generalized seizures, mental retardation, and periventricular leukomalacia; and spastic hemiparesis—unilateral involvement, usually of arm more than leg, and often not diagnosed until several months of age.
2. *Extrapyramidal form* is thought to result from direct damage to the extrapyramidal system and has two main groups. The hyperkinetic type is characterized by choreiform and choreoathetoid movements. In the dystonic type, postures are abnormal. These movements and postures commonly occur in the second and third years of life.
3. *Hypotonic or atonic form* with generalized hypotonia persisting beyond two years of age can include cerebellar deficits and mental retardation.
4. A *mixed form* is marked by both spasticity and extrapyramidal movements.

Most cases of cerebral palsy are related to intrapartum or peripartum events or are idiopathic. Factors associated with increased risk of cerebral palsy include maternal mental retardation, low birth weight, prematurity, fetal malformation, and neonatal factors such as asphyxia and seizures.

REF: Menkes JH: *Textbook of child neurology*, ed 4, Philadelphia, 1990, Lea & Febiger.

CEREBRAL VASCULAR ACCIDENT   *(see Ischemia)*

CEREBRAL VASCULAR DISEASE   *(see Aneurysms, Hemorrhage, Ischemia)*

CEREBRAL VEIN THROMBOSIS   *(see Venous Thrombosis)*

CEREBROSPINAL FLUID
FORMATION

The rate of cerebrospinal fluid (CSF) formation is about 500 ml per day. The primary site of production is the choroid plexus. Secretion is an energy requiring a process related to ion exchange (Na/K). Production also depends on the cytosolic enzyme carbonic anhydrase. Therefore a carbonic acid inhibitor (acetazolamide) substantially reduces CSF formation.

APPEARANCE

CSF is clear and colorless until white blood cell counts (WBCs) reach approximately 200/mm³ or red blood cell counts (RBCs) reach approximately 400/mm³; then it becomes turbid or cloudy. Lower cell counts can be detected by observing for *Tyndall's effect*. This phenomenon refers to a snowy or sparkling quality of CSF when viewed in direct sunlight and results from suspended particles scattering ambient light. Viscous CSF can result from large numbers of cryptococci within the CSF, due to their polysaccharide capsules. *Clot* or pellicle formation occurs with elevated protein levels. *Froin's syndrome* refers to clot formation in the setting of complete spinal block and very high protein levels, usually resulting from a cord tumor. CSF is perceived as grossly bloody with RBCs greater than 6000/mm³, and at RBCs between 500/mm³ and 6000/mm³ *xanthochromia* appears. Xanthochromia refers to the yellow, pink, or orange coloration of the CSF corresponding to the breakdown products of RBCs. Oxyhemoglobin released from red blood cells can be detected within the supernatant fluid within 2 to 4 hours after the release of blood into the subarachnoid space; it reaches a maximum level at about 36 hours and disappears in about 7 to 10 days. Supernatant fluid may, however, remain clear for as long as to 12 hours after a subarachnoid bleed.

CYTOLOGY

Cytologic analysis should occur soon after lumbar puncture is performed, since significant cell lysis may occur within about an hour. Prompt refrigeration is also necessary. Lymphocytes are the predominant leucocyte forms in normal CSF. An occasional granulocyte is seen in normal fluid and is not necessarily pathologic if the total WBC is normal. A few or moderate numbers of granulocytes may occur after spinal anesthesia, myelography, or other intrathecal injections or with trauma, hemorrhage, or infarct in the absence of infection. Table 10-1 gives a formula for correction of abnormal numbers of WBCs in the presence of a traumatic tap or significant anemia. Detection of tumor cells is enhanced by collection of large volumes of fluid (more than 20 ml) or lumbar or cisternal taps.

PROTEINS

Protein levels serve as a nonspecific indicator of disease. Normally the blood-CSF barrier keeps serum protein out of the CSF. Most CNS diseases disrupt the barrier, allowing entrance of serum protein and consequent elevation of CSF protein levels. Increases greater than 500 mg/dl are infrequent and occur mainly in spinal block, meningitis, arachnoiditis, and subarachnoid hemorrhage. Certain metabolic conditions such as myxedema and evident diabetic neuropathy may cause increases in protein levels. The major immunoglobulin in normal CSF is IgG. The IgG/albumin index and synthesis rate (Table 10-1 and 10-2) correct for elevated levels of serum IgG. Elevated levels may result from production within the CNS in various immune response disorders. Oligoclonal bands indicate the presence of immune-mediated pathologic processes such as multiple sclerosis and Subacute Sclerosing Panencephalitis (SSPE). Oligoclonal bands occur in 80% to 90% of patients with clinically definite multiple sclerosis. Myelin basic protein, a product of oligodendroglia, may be increased by various processes that result in myelin breakdown, such as stroke or anoxia, and elevated levels are not a specific marker of demyelinating disease. Low CSF protein levels may occur with dural leaks and in benign intracranial hypertension. Normally the protein value in cisternal CSF is 50% of the lumbar value and is even lower (25%) within the lateral ventricles.

GLUCOSE

Glucose is derived from serum and is a reflection of the previous 4 hours of systemic glucose levels. Normal CSF-to-blood glucose ratio is 0.6. A simultaneous measurement of serum glucose should be obtained. Hypoglycorrhachia occurs in bacterial, fungal or tubercular

TABLE 10-1
Normal Values for Lumbar Fluid

Age	Protein mg/dl	Glucose mg/dl	Cell Count/mm³	Lymph/PMN Ratio	Opening Pressure (mm CSF)
Preterm	115	50	9	40/60	
Term	90	52	8	40/60	80–100
Child	5–40	40–80	0–5		60–200
Adult	20–40	50–70	0–5	100/0	60–200
Ventricular	6–15				
Cervical	20–30				

IgG/albumin ratio (CSF IgG/Alb) upper limit: 0.27
IgG/albumin Index (CSF IgG/Alb)/(serum IgG/Alb) upper limit: 0.60
Myelin basic protein upper limit: 4 ng/ml
Corrections
WBC: Reduce WBC by one cell for every 700 RBC (if hematocrit is normal)
OR
$$WBC (corr) = WBC(csf) - WBC(blood) \times RBC(csf)/RBC(blood)$$
Protein: Subtract 1 mg/ml for every 1000 RBC

TABLE 10-2
CSF Profiles in Various Diseases

	Pressure	Cell Count/mm³	Protein	Glucose
Purulent meningitis	Increased (inc) in 90% 200–1500	100–10,000 90%–95% PMN	N1–2200	Decreased (dec)
Aseptic meningitis	May be inc	10–1000 L+M (PMN early)	N1 to 400	N1
Fungal meningitis	N1 Need to check india ink and cryptococcal antigen.	inc PMN+L+M	N1 or inc	Dec
Tuberculous meningitis	Inc	50–500	100–1000	Dec
Sarcoidosis	N1 or inc	10–100 L+M	50–200	N1 or dec
Neoplastic meningitis	N1 or inc	0–500 PMN+L+M Cytology may show atypical cells, and cell surface markers may be helpful.	N1 or inc	N1 or dec

Condition	Pressure	Cells	Protein	Glucose	Comments
Subarachnoid hemorrhage	Inc	N1 or inc	N1 or inc	N1 or dec	Lysis of RBC begins after 2 to 4 hours. Xanthochromia is visible after 8 to 10 hours and may persist for weeks.
Herpes encephalitis	N1	50–100 L+M	N1	N1	RBC and xanthochromia are often present (which distinguishes this disease from other viral meningitides).
SSPE	N1	N1	N1 or inc	N1	Gammaglobulins are markedly inc and may account for 50% of the total protein. Oligoclonal bands are present.
Guillain-Barré	N1	0–25 L+M	N1 or inc	N1	Protein values peak between day 4 and day 18. Oligoclonal bands are often present.
Migraine	N1 or inc	5–15 L+M	N1	N1	A migrainous syndrome with white blood cell counts greater than 200/mm³ has been described.
Optic neuritis	N1	Less than 25 L+M	N1 or inc	N1	

Continued.

TABLE 10-2—cont'd
CSF Profiles in Various Diseases

	Pressure	Cell Count/mm³	Protein	Glucose
Multiple sclerosis	N1	N1 or inc Less than 25 L+M	N1 or inc	N1
	Oligoclonal bands, IgG/albumin index and ratio elevated, indicating intra-CNS antibody production. Myelin basic protein may increase with an exacerbation.			
Acute disseminated encephalomyelitis	N1 or inc	5–150 L+M+PMN	N1 or inc	N1
Spinal block	Dec	N1 or inc	Markedly increased	N1
	Clotting (Froin's syndrome) occurs when the protein value is greater than 1000.			
Seizure	N1	N1 or inc Up to 25 L+M rarely PMN	N1 or inc	N1
	Pleocytosis is usually associated with prolonged or frequent seizures.			
CNS Lyme disease	N1 or inc	Inc L+M Up to 20% plasma cells	Inc	N1 or dec
	Oligoclonal bands, IgG/Albumin index and ratio may be elevated, indicating intrathecal anti-Borrelia antibody production.			

HIV and AIDS				
Encephalopathy	N1	N1	N1 or inc	N1
Toxoplasmosis	N1 or increased	Inc Positive Toxo. Antibody	Inc	N1
Cryptococcosis	N1 or inc	N1 or inc Positive cryptococcal antigen	N1 or inc	N1 or dec
Polyneuropathy				
Distal, symmetric	N1	N1	N1 or inc	N1
Chronic inflammatory	N1 or inc	Inc	Inc	N1

meningitis, inflammatory processes such as sarcoid, carcinomatous meningitis, and subarachnoid hemorrhage. The mechanism of hypoglycorrhchia in meningeal disorders is related to an increase in anaerobic glycolysis in contiguous brain and spinal cord and, to a variable degree, PMNs, as well as to an inhibition of glucose entry resulting from altered glucose membrane transport.

COMPLICATIONS OF LUMBAR PUNCTURE
Headache

Incidence 10%. Onset is 5 minutes to 4 days after lumbar puncture (LP). Pain is worse when upright and better when lying flat. Post–lumbar puncture headaches usually resolve spontaneously, the majority within 1 week, but may persist up to several months. Preventive measures include use of the smallest practical spinal needle, insertion of the needle bevel parallel to the dural fibers of the posterior longitudinal ligament, and the use of short bevel needles. These headaches are more common in younger patients, particularly women. The headaches also correlate with needle size and the amount of CSF removed. Treatment of an established post–LP headache involves bed rest, adequate hydration (particularly if nausea and vomiting occur), and analgesics. Caffeine, 300 to 500 mg PO, and theophylline may be used. For persistent cases, epidural blood patching, with the injection of 10 ml of the patient's freshly drawn blood into the epidural space where it can clot, is usually curative.

Brain herniation

May occur immediately or up to 12 hours after LP. Occurs in patients with supratentorial mass lesions and midline shift or obstructing posterior fossa tumors.

Spinal subdural, epidural, and subarachnoid hemorrhage

May occur in patients treated with anticoagulants or those with thrombocytopenia or bleeding diathesis.

Diplopia

Rare transient unilateral or bilateral abducens palsy.

Others

Radicular irritation, meningitis, implantation of epidermoid tumor. Contraindications to LP include infection over the site of entry, bleeding disorder, and presence of a posterior fossa mass or supratentorial mass with midline shift.

REF: Fishman RA: *Cerebrospinal fluid in diseases of the nervous system*, ed 2, Philadelphia, 1992, WB Saunders.

CHEMOTHERAPY, NEUROLOGIC COMPLICATIONS OF

Agents	Possible effects
Antimetabolites	
Methotrexate	High dose—strokelike encephalopathy; leukoencephalopathy.
	Intrathecal—chemical meningitis; myelopathy.
5-fluorouracil (5-FU)	Pancerebellar dysfunction; encephalopathy.
Cytarabine (ARA-C)	High dose—cerebellar syndrome; encephalopathy; peripheral neuropathy; leukoencephalopathy.
	Intrathecal—demyelinating myelopathy.
Alkylating agents	
Cisplatin (Platinol, DDP)	Sensorineural hearing loss; peripheral large-fiber symmetric sensory polyneuropathy; Lhermitte's symptoms; encephalopathy; retinopathy; cranial neuropathy; intracarotid-stroke-like syndrome.
Ifosfamide	Encephalopathy.
Nitrosoureas (incl. BCNU)	High dose—encephalopathy.
	Intracarotid—ipsilateral encephalopathy; local pain; retinopathy; ocular necrosis.
Vinca alkaloids	
Vincristine (Oncovin)	Peripheral neuropathy almost 100%; cranial neuropathy; seizures; SIADH.
Podophyllotoxins	
Etiposide (VP-16)	Encephalopathy.
Taxol	Symmetric distal polyneuropathy.
Biologic response modifiers	
Alpha-interferon	Acute reversible encephalopathy; mild distal sensorimotor polyneuropathy; neuropsychiatric disturbances.
Interleukin-2	Mild encephalopathy; transient focal deficits.

Agents	Possible effects
Miscellaneous agents	
L-asparaginase	Encephalopathy; coagulopathy with hemorrhage or thrombosis.
Corticosteroids	Proximal myopathy; action tremor; psychosis; mood alteration.
Procarbazine	Encephalopathy; peripheral neuropathy; cerebellar symptoms.
Tamoxifen	Encephalopathy; retinopathy.

Thiamine may help prevent the neurotoxic effects of 5-FU. Oral glutamic acid may reduce the peripheral neuropathy produced by vincristine. These preventative measures are investigational.

(*References:* Aminoff MJ: *Neurology and general medicine*, Edinburgh, 1989, Churchill Livingstone.

Macdonald DR: Neurologic complications of chemotherapy, *Neurol Clin* 9(4):955–967, 1991.)

CHIARI MALFORMATION *(see Craniocervical Junction)*

CHIASM *(see Pituitary, Visual Fields)*

CHILD NEUROLOGY *(see also Cerebral Palsy, Chromosomal Syndromes, Craniosynostosis, Degenerative Disease of Childhood, Developmental Malformations, Encephalopathy, Fontanel, Hyperactive Child, Hypotonic Infant, Immunization, Learning Disorders, Macrocephaly, Metabolic Disorders of Childhood, Microcephaly, Neurocutaneous Syndromes, and other individual subject headings)*

I. *History:* Include assessment of pregnancy, labor, delivery (drugs, illnesses, complications, etc.) and reasons for cesarean delivery;

weeks of gestation, Apgar scores or ask the parent if newborn cried at birth or required help to breathe; birth weight; length of neonate's hospital stay (reasons for any stay longer than 3 days); developmental milestones (see Denver Developmental Screening Test, Figure 7). Girls generally achieve developmental milestones earlier than boys.

A. *School-aged children:* Include assessment of school performance. Do not forget a drug and alcohol history, especially if there has been a change in behavior (questions preferably asked when parent is out of room).

B. *Adolescents:* If accompanied by a parent, allow the adolescent to decide whether the parent should leave or remain in the room. Drug history, contraceptive history, and the like are best elicited during casual history taking when the parent is out of the room.

II. *General exam:* Measure head circumference and check age-specific norms (Figures 8 to 10). Pay particular attention to skin, morphology of the face and extremities, and cardiovascular exam. In *neonates:* Look for external trauma such as cephalohematoma or subgaleal hematoma. Retinal hemorrhages resulting from the birth process may be seen. Measure the size of the anterior and posterior fontanels, and note whether they are bulging. Auscultate head for bruits. Transilluminate head.

III. *Neurologic exam:*

A. *Infants:* Much of the information regarding the neonate is obtained through simple observation of level of alertness, posture, spontaneous movements (symmetry), and so forth. Assess pitch and volume of cry. Assess tone in trunk by holding infant by the chest in ventral suspension. Arching of the neck and back may be an early sign of increased tone. Assess tone in extremities by passive range-of-motion and by holding infant at the shoulders in vertical suspension. Hypotonic infants "slip through your fingers" at the shoulders, and their legs will flop apart in a frog-leg posture; hypertonic infants' legs will scissor. Assess head control (head "lag") as infant is pulled from supine to sitting by gentle traction on both arms. Contractures are always abnormal. Assess primitive reflexes (Table 11). Look for grimace or cry in response to noxious stimuli rather than just withdrawal of the extremity.

1. *Premature infants* normally are hypotonic and have head lag. Prematures will not be able to turn the head from side to side when placed face down. Arms and legs are held in extension until 35 weeks' gestation.

FIGURE 7
Denver Developmental Screening Test.

DENVER DEVELOPMENTAL SCREENING TEST

REVISED DDST-R

PERCENT OF CHILDREN PASSING

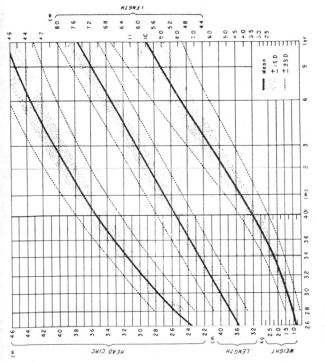

FIGURE 8
Fetal and infant norms: weight, length, and head circumference.

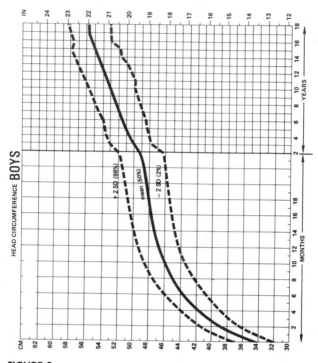

FIGURE 9
Head circumference, boys. *(From Nellhaus G: Pediatrics 41:106, 1968. Used by permission.)*

   2. *Full-term infants* should be able to lift their heads for short
      periods and turn them from a central face-down position
      to one side. When held at the axillae, facing the examiner,
      the normal full-term infant should flex arms and legs and
      hold head erect.
B. *Older Children:* For the young child, do as much as the exam
   as possible with the child on the parent's lap. Examining the
   hands and feet for tone and reflexes is often a nonthreatening

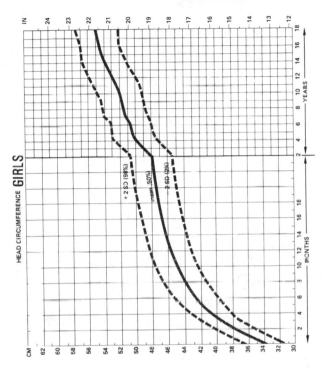

FIGURE 10
Head circumference, girls. *(From Nellhaus G: Pediatrics 41:106, 1968. Used by permission.)*

way to begin. For a toddler, much motor information can be obtained while the child is playing with toys on the floor. Older children are typically quite cooperative and the exam is much the same as in adults.

REF: Behrman RE, Kliegman RM, eds: *Nelson's essentials of Pediatrics*, Philadelphia, 1994, WB Saunders.

TABLE 11
Primitive Reflexes

Reflex	Appears (age)	Disappears (age)
Suck: Place pacifier or clean finger in infant's mouth. Bursts of upward pressure of tongue with contraction of buccinators should be felt.	32–34 wk	Awake 4 mo
Gag: Place feeding tube in hypopharynx.	32 wk	Persists
Grasp: Place finger under fingers (palmar) or toes (plantar).	32–34 wk	Palmar 6 mo Plantar 10 mo
Tonic neck: With infant in supine position turn head to one side. Extension of arm (and leg) on the side to which face is turned, and flexion of opposite arm (and leg), "fencing posture" should be seen.	Incomplete 34 wk Complete 2 mo	6 mo
Ventral suspension (Landau): Infant is supported on examiner's hand in prone position. Should extend head, trunk, and hips. Legs should be flexed at knees.	3 mo	24 mo
Moro: Infant is placed in the supine position. Examiner lifts infant's head by placing hand under it, then suddenly releases the head toward the bed, keeping hand under the head to protect it. The full reflex consists of opening of hands, extension and abduction of arms, and extension of legs, followed by flexion of the upper extremities and an audible cry.	34 wk	3 mo

Reflex	Appears	Disappears
Placing: Infant is held upright, and the dorsal edge of the foot is brushed to the lower surface of a bed or table. The baby should flex the knee and lift the foot.	35 wk	6 wk
Stepping: Infant is held vertically, feet making firm contact with exam table. Initially, cocontraction of opposing muscles will fix joints of lower extremities, followed by automatic walking movement, the infant placing one foot in front of the other.	35 wk	
Crossed adductor response: Contraction of opposite adductor group with percussion of ipsilateral adductor group.	35 wk	7 mo
Parachute: Infant is held suspended in prone position, then suddenly thrust toward floor. Arms extend and adduct and the fingers spread, as if to break the fall.	9 mo	Persists
Extensor plantar response (Babinski): Lateral aspect of foot is stroked. Great toe dorsiflexes.	Birth (unilateral response may indicate corticospinal (tract dysfunction)	10 mo (plantar flexor response established)
Neck Righting: When head is turned, infant will roll trunk in the same direction.	4–6 mo	2 yr

CHOREA

Chorea is involuntary, rapid, jerky, arrhythmic movements of muscle groups. It can involve the upper or lower extremities, trunk, neck, or face and may be generalized, symmetric, asymmetric, or unilateral. Chorea is distinguished from other movement disorders by the random timing and distribution. The movements are often incorporated into deliberate movements by the patient to camouflage the disorder. Grimacing and respiratory grunts may be manifestations.

Following are the most common causes of chorea.

1. Huntington's disease.
2. Drug-induced (see below).
3. Systemic lupus erythematosus.
4. Polycythemia vera.
5. Hyperthyroidism.
6. Pregnancy (chorea gravidarum) or oral contraceptive use.
7. Neuroacanthocytosis, a multisystem neurologic disease characterized by dementia, psychiatric disturbances, seizures, chorea, dystonia, tics, akinetic-rigid features, diminished deep tendon reflexes, muscle atrophy and weakness, and acanthocytes in peripheral blood.

Other causes by group include the following.

Age-Related.
  Physiologic chorea of infancy.
  Kernicterus.
  Cerebral palsy.
  Buccal-oral-lingual chorea of aging.
  "Senile" chorea.
Hereditary.
  "Benign" familial.
  Amino acid, carbohydrate, and lipid disorders.
  Lesch-Nyhan syndrome.
  Wilson's disease.
  Hallervorden-Spatz disease.
  Ataxia-telangiectasia.
  Tuberous sclerosis.
  Sturge-Weber syndrome.
  Myoclonus epilepsy.
  Pelizaeus-Merzbacher disease.

Sickle-cell disease.
Leigh's disease.
Porphyria.
Paroxysmal kinesiogenic and dystonic choreas.
Familial basal ganglia calcification.
Olivopontocerebellar atrophy.

Drug-induced and toxic.
  Neuroleptics.
  Antiparkinsonian agents: Dopaminergic, amantadine, anticho-
    linergics.
  Anticonvulsants: Carbamazepine, phenytoin, phenobarbital.
  Noradrenergic stimulants: Amphetamine, methylphenidate,
    pemoline, aminophylline, theophylline, caffeine.
  Anabolic steroids and oral contraceptives.
  Opiates: Methadone, heroin.
  Others: Antihistamines, lithium, tricyclics, isoniazid, reserpine,
    metoclopramide, digoxin, methyldopa, diazoxide, triazolam.
  Toxins: Ethanol intoxication and withdrawal, carbon monoxide,
    mercury, manganese, thallium, toluene.

Metabolic.
  Hyponatremia and hypernatremia.
  Hypocalcemia.
  Hypomagnesemia.
  Hypoglycemia and hyperglycemia.
  Hypoparathyroidism.
  Addison's disease.
  Pregnancy.
  Hepatic encephalopathy.
  Renal failure.
  Vitamin deficiencies: thiamine (beriberi), niacin (pellagra), B_{12}.

Infectious or Immunologic.
  Sydenham's chorea (St. Vitus' dance) post–rheumatic fever.
  Diphtheria, pertussis, 2nd typhoid fever, including postvaccinal.
  Viral encephalitis.
  Neurosyphilis.
  Lyme disease.
  Legionnaires' disease.
  Sarcoidosis.
  Systemic lupus erythematosus, Henoch-Schönlein purpura,
    Behçet's syndrome, periarteritis nodosa; antiphospholipid an-
    tibody syndrome.
  Multiple sclerosis.

Cerebrovascular.
  Basal ganglionic infarction or hemorrhage.
  Arteriovenous malformation.
  Migraine.
Miscellaneous.
  Posttraumatic.
  Brain tumors: Primary, metastatic, lymphoma.
  Epidural and subdural hematomas.
  Electrical injury.

REF: Hardie RJ et al: *Brain* 114:13, 1991.

Joseph AB, Young RR, eds: *Movement disorders in neurology and neuropsychiatry*, Boston, 1992, Blackwell Scientific Publications.

CHROMOSOMAL DISORDERS

Mental retardation (MR), often with microcephaly, is a characteristic of most chromosomal disorders. Partial deletions and partial trisomies have been described for almost every chromosome, but only trisomies 21, 18, and 13 and several sex chromosome anomalies have a recognizable clinical syndrome likely to be diagnosed prior to karyotyping. Therefore, karyotype analysis is indicated in the evaluation of most children with mental retardation, especially if there are associated dysmorphic features.

Trisomy 21 (Down's syndrome): (1 in 660 births) MR, hypotonia, infantile spasms, oblique palpebral fissures, median epicanthal fold, Brushfield spots (accumulation of fibrous tissue appearing as light-colored spots encircling the periphery of the iris), low-set ears, thick protruding tongue, bilateral simian creases, short extremities and digits, heart anomalies, GI anomalies (duodenal atresia), and upper cervical spine malformations. In later life, these patients also have progressive cognitive decline with pathologic findings of neuritic plaques, neurofibrillary tangles, and reduced cortical choline acetyltransferase activity as seen in Alzheimer's disease.

Trisomy 13: (1 in 5000 births) Severe MR; microcephaly; microphthalmos; arhinencephaly spectrum; median facial anomalies; low-set, dysplastic ears; heart anomalies; polycystic kidneys.

Trisomy 18 (Edward's syndrome): (1 in 4500 births) Severe MR; brain grossly and microscopically normal in 50%; long, narrow skull; low-set, dysplastic ears, second finger overlies third; thumbs distally implanted and retroflexible; heart anomalies; polycystic kidneys.

XXY (Klinefelter's syndrome): (1 in 500 males) Mild MR, learning disabilities, language disorder, behavior disorders, intention tremor, tall with long limbs, hypogonadism, hypogenitalism, increased FSH levels, gynecomastia.

XYY: Borderline MR, learning disabilities, behavior disorders, tall stature.

Fragile X: (1 in 2000 males) MR, long face, large floppy ears, macroorchidism. May have macrocephaly. Usually X-linked recessive pattern of inheritance, but some heterozygous females may also be MR along with having developmental Gerstmann's syndrome. To demonstrate the fragile X chromosome, cells (lymphocytes or fibroblasts) must be cultured in folate-deficient medium; patients should receive folate-deficient diet and avoid multivitamins for 1 week before testing. Direct testing with genetic probes and polymerase chain reaction is being developed, which can assay the mutant gene (trinucleotide repeat sequence).

XXX: MR without other specific findings.

XO (Turner's syndrome): Usually *normal* intelligence, short stature, broad chest with widely spaced nipples, low posterior hairline, webbed neck, congenital lymphedema, cubitus valgus, ovarian dysgenesis.

REF: Smith DW. *Recognizable patterns of human malformation,* ed 3, Philadelphia, 1982, WB Saunders.

CLUSTER HEADACHE *(see Headache)*

COCHLEAR NERVE *(see Cranial Nerves, Hearing)*

COGWHEEL RIGIDITY *(see Parkinson's Disease, Rigidity)*

COMA *(see also Brain Death, Cardiopulmonary Arrest)*

Consciousness is the state of awareness of self and surroundings. Loss of awareness with concomitant defects in arousal constitutes coma, and when less pronounced, lethargy, stupor, and obtundation. Coma is neither a unitary state nor an etiologic diagnosis. Its presence suggests specific dysfunction of both hemispheres or dysfunction of the brainstem reticular activating system, or both. The mechanism of dysfunction may be a structural lesion (supratentorial or subtentorial), a metabolic disturbance, or psychogenic.

Evaluation of coma requires a detailed medical history (from others) and general physical examination to establish potential causes. In addition to complete chemistry tests, blood cell count, and coagulation panels, blood gas levels (observe color and request CO level), toxicology screens (on blood, urine, and gastric contents), thyroid function tests, cortisol level, and cultures should be obtained at the time of initial evaluation of coma of unknown cause. Emergency management is outlined in Table 12.

The neurologic examination is focused toward determining the

TABLE 12
Emergency Management of Coma of Unknown Cause

1. Ensure oxygenation. Clear airway, suction, perform bag-valve-mask ventilation, and use intubation as needed. Immobilize cervical spine prior to neck extension until C-spine injury is excluded radiographically. Atropine, 1 mg IV, may prevent vagally mediated bradyarrhythmias during intubation.
2. Maintain circulation with fluids and pressors to keep mean arterial pressure above 100 mm Hg. Continuous ECG monitoring is necessary.
3. Thiamine, 100 mg IV, followed by glucose 25 g (50 ml D50) IV, immediately after blood is drawn (large volume) for diagnostics.
4. Treat intracranial hypertension if suspected (see Intracranial Pressure).
5. Stop seizures when present (see Epilepsy).
6. Restore acid-base balance.
7. Treat drug overdose. For suspected narcotics give naloxone (Narcan) 0.4 mg IV, repeat as necessary if effective (short half-life) or in 5 min. For suspected anticholinergics (e.g., tricyclics), give physostigmine, 1 mg IV. For suspected benzodiazepine overdose, give Flumazenil starting at 0.2 mg IV over 30 seconds. Failure to respond to a total dose of 5 mg makes it unlikely that coma is due to benzodiazepines.
8. Exclude intracranial masses by CT (uncontrasted).
9. Normalize body temperature.
10. Treat infection if suspected (see Meningitis).
11. Specific therapy should be instituted as soon as a diagnosis is established.

pathophysiologic features by distinguishing the location and degree of CNS dysfunction, including the following.

I. Level of consciousness: Response to voice, shaking, or pain. Consider status epilepticus, akinetic mutism, vegetative state, locked-in (de-efferented) syndrome, and psychogenic states (see below).

II. Brainstem function.

    A. Pupils: Light reflex tests for cranial nerves II and III (midbrain).

        1. Anisocoria: With Horner's syndrome, suggests hypothalamic or lateral medullary dysfunction; without Horner's, suggests transtentorial herniation.

        2. Miosis: Common in toxic or metabolic encephalopathy (preserved light reflex is a hallmark of metabolic coma) and central herniation with supratentorial mass lesion. Pinpoint, barely reactive pupils suggest acute pontine lesion or presence of opioids.

        3. Mydriasis: In association with absent light reflex and (sometimes) irregular pupils, suggests dorsal midbrain dysfunction. Beware of atropine or sympathomimetics commonly given during resuscitation.

        4. Fixed, midposition pupils suggest midbrain nuclear (third nerve) dysfunction.

    B. Eye movements: Assess conjugacy, gaze deviation or preference, nystagmus, and spontaneous movements. Oculocephalic responses and vestibulo-ocular testing with ice-water evaluate brainstem connections of cranial nerves III, IV, VI, and VIII. Presence of nystagmus without ocular deviation to the irrigated ear on caloric testing suggests psychogenic coma, since it indicates integrity of brainstem and hemispheric pathways. Roving eye movements suggest intact brainstem. Ocular bobbing and its variants suggest pontine lesions.

    C. Corneal or sternutatory reflexes test cranial nerves V and VII (pons).

    D. Gag (pharynx) or cough (larynx-trachea) reflexes test cranial nerves IX and X (medulla).

III. Breathing patterns.

    A. *Cheyne-Stokes respiration* consists of cyclically increasing, then decreasing respiratory depth and rate, separated by apneic phases. It results from the interaction of an increased ventilatory drive to pCO_2 and a decreased forebrain stimulus for respiration when pCO_2 is decreased. It suggests bilateral deep cerebral hemispheric or diencephalic dysfunction but may be produced by any encephalopathic state.

B. *Central neurogenic hyperventilation* is attributed to brainstem injury. *Tachypnea* is more common and is usually associated with hypocapnia and hypoxemia. It often resolves with correction of the metabolic abnormalities, whereas central neurogenic hyperventilation does not. Tachypnea with brainstem disease may be associated with neurogenic pulmonary edema.

C. *Apneustic breathing* consists of prolonged "jamming" of respiration in inspiratory and expiratory phases. Although rare, it is seen with dorsolateral pontine lesions at the level of the sensory trigeminal nucleus.

D. *Ataxic breathing* consists of generally slow, irregular respirations with variable amplitude and can progress rapidly to complete apnea. It is due to bilateral lesions of the reticular formation in the caudal dorsomedial medulla, where the respiratory rhythm is generated. Medullary compression, usually caused by acute lesions, may result in respiratory arrest, which typically occurs before cardiovascular collapse.

These breathing patterns may be a false localizing sign in cases of coexisting metabolic derangement. For example, metabolic acidosis and hypoxia cause reactive hyperventilation, simulating neurogenic hyperventilation.

IV. Sensorimotor.

A. Spontaneous activity. Assess for volitional movement, choreoathetosis, posturing (arms decorticate or flexor vs. decerebrate or extensor), asterixis, myoclonus, and seizures.

B. Response to noxious stimuli (listed in order of increasing severity of coma). Lateralizing features of response should be noted.

1. Purposeful.
2. Flexion withdrawal.
3. Abnormal flexion (decorticate posturing): Usually slow, stereotyped flexion of arm, wrist, and fingers with shoulder adduction and variable leg extension.
4. Abnormal extension (decerebrate posturing): Extension of wrist and arm with adduction and internal rotation of shoulder; extension and internal rotation of leg with plantar flexion of foot.
5. No response.

C. Tone: Assess for flaccidity, rigidity, spasticity, clonus, and paratonia.

V. Tendon reflexes: Assess for asymmetry, increase, or decrease in response.

The Glasgow coma scale quantitates level of consciousness. It is easy to use and reliable, with low interobserver variability (see Table 13). Since the scale does not assess brainstem reflexes, it does not communicate a complete neurologic assessment but is useful for rapid identification, reliable communication, serial quantitation, and aid in assessing prognosis, particularly when used in evaluation of posttraumatic coma.

CAUSES OF COMA

I. Accurate localization can identify likely causes of altered consciousness.
   A. Supratentorial lesion.
      1. Subcortical destructive lesion: Thalamic infarct.
      2. Hemorrhage: Epidural, subdural, subarachnoid, intracerebral; hypertensive, vascular malformation.

TABLE 13
Glasgow Coma Scale

			Score
Eye opening	Open	Spontaneously	4
		To verbal command	3
		To pain	2
	Do not open		1
Best motor response	To verbal command	Obeys	6
	To painful stimulus	Localizes pain	5
		Flexion withdrawal	4
		Flexion-abnormal (decorticate)	3
		Extension-abnormal (decerebrate)	2
		No response	1
Best verbal response		Oriented and converses	5
		Disoriented and converses	4
		Verbalizes	3
		Vocalizes	2
		No response	1
	Total: (Range, 3 to 15)		-

      3. Infarction: Thrombotic or embolic arterial occlusion, venous thrombosis.
      4. Tumor: Primary, metastatic.
      5. Abscess: Intracerebral, subdural.
      6. Closed head injury.
  B. Infratentorial lesion.
      1. Compressive: Cerebellar hemorrhage, infarct, tumor, or abscess; posterior fossa subdural, extradural hemorrhages, basilar aneurysm.
      2. Destructive: Brainstem hemorrhage, infarction, tumor, demyelination, or abscess; basilar migraine.
  C. Diffuse brain dysfunction.
      1. Intrinsic: Encephalitis, progressive multifocal leukencephalopathy, meningitis, concussion, ictal or postictal state, herniation.
      2. Hypoxic or metabolic: Anoxia, ischemia, nutritional (e.g., Wernicke's syndrome), hepatic encephalopathy, uremia, dialysis, pulmonary disease.
      3. Endocrine: Nonketotic hyperglycemic hyperosmolar coma, ketoacidosis, DIC, hypoglycemia, Addison's disease, myxedema, thyrotoxicosis, panhypopituitarism.
      4. Toxic, drug-induced: Amphetamines, cocaine, psychedelics, tricyclics, phenothiazines, lithium, benzodiazepines, methaqualone, glutethimide, barbiturates, alcohol, opiates, ibuprofen, aspirin.
      5. Ionic and acid-base disorders: Hypo-osmolarity or hyperosmolarity; hyponatremia or hypernatremia, hypocalcemia or hypercalcemia, hypophosphatemia, lactic acidosis, cerebral edema.
      6. Hypothermia, hyperthermia.
      7. Remote effects of cancer (paraneoplastic): Limbic encephalitis, thalamic degeneration.
  D. Psychogenic coma.
      1. Conversion reaction, catatonic stupor, malingering.
II. The clinical course may also suggest localization and cause.
  A. Supratentorial mass with diencephalic or brainstem compression.
      1. Early focal cerebral dysfunction.
      2. Rostral to caudal progression with signs referrable to one area at a time.
      3. Asymmetric motor signs.
      4. Third-nerve palsy preceding coma (early herniation).

B. Infratentorial mass or destruction.
    1. Early brainstem dysfunction or sudden onset of coma with accompanying brainstem signs.
    2. Vestibulo-ocular abnormalities present.
    3. Cranial nerve palsies usually present.
    4. Abnormal respirations common, appear early.
C. Metabolic causes.
    1. Confusion and stupor precede motor signs.
    2. Motor signs usually symmetric.
    3. Pupillary reactions usually preserved (except with certain drugs and toxins; see Pupil).
    4. Asterixis, myoclonus, tremor, and seizures are common.
    5. Acid-base disturbance with hypoventilation or hyperventilation is common.
D. Psychogenic unresponsiveness.
    1. Lids tightly closed.
    2. Pupils reactive or dilated (factitious mydriatics).
    3. Oculocephalic responses highly variable; nystagmus and arousal occur with caloric stimuli.
    4. Motor tone normal or inconsistent.
    5. Breathing normal or rapid.
    6. Reflexes nonpathologic.
    7. Normal EEG.

III. Other states that may resemble coma.
    A. Vegetative state: Subacute or chronic condition after severe brain injury characterized by wakefulness, sleep-wake cycles, and eye opening to auditory stimuli, without evidence of consistent cognitive function or response to stimuli. Blood pressure and respirations are maintained. Can follow coma and persist for years (a duration longer than 1 month is persistent vegetative state). About one third of patients eventually become more responsive (more common in traumatic than in hypoxic cases). May occur with forebrain, occipital, hippocampal, or diffuse cerebral or cerebellar destruction.
    B. Akinetic mutism: Subacute or chronic condition characterized by seeming alertness, yet minimal vocalization or movement even with noxious stimuli. May occur with cingulate, limbic, corpus striatum, globus pallidus, thalamic, or reticular formation damage.
    C. Locked-in syndrome: Intact consciousness plus quadraplegia and lower cranial nerve dysfunction. Voluntary vertical, and sometimes horizontal, eye movements are preserved. Usually

occurs with ventral pontine infarcts, tumors, hemorrhages, and myelinolysis; ventral midbrain infarction; head injury; or severe neuromuscular disease. May be transient or chronic.

IV. Prognosis in coma, excluding traumatic and drug-related causes, is usually poor. Prediction is less reliable in cases of intoxications and trauma but more precise after cardiopulmonary arrest (see Cardiopulmonary Arrest). In general, the longer coma lasts, the lower the chance for regaining independent function (i.e., "good recovery").

   A. Prediction: Data obtained from 500 patients, excluding known trauma or drug intoxication (Levy et al., 1985).
      1. At 6 hours after onset of coma, absence of any of the following was associated with less than 5% chance of good recovery.
         a. Pupillary light reflex.
         b. Corneal reflexes.
         c. Oculocephalic reflexes.
         d. Vestibulo-ocular reflexes (calorics).
      2. At 1 day after onset, none of the patients with absent corneal reflexes had satisfactory recovery.
      3. At 3 days after onset, no patient with absence of any of the following had satisfactory recovery.
         a. Pupillary reflexes.
         b. Corneal reflexes.
         c. Motor function.
      4. Predictors of good outcome are less reliable than negative predictors.
         a. At 6 hours after onset, with moaning or better verbal response *plus* pupillary, corneal, *or* oculovestibular responses: 41% of patients had good recovery.
         b. At 1 day after onset, with inappropriate or better words *plus* any three of pupillary, corneal, oculovestibular, or motor responses: 67% had good recovery.
         c. At 3 days after onset, with inappropriate or better words *plus* corneal *and* motor responses: 74% had good recovery.
         d. At 7 days after onset, with eye opening to pain *plus* localizing motor response: 75% had good recovery.
   B. Overall outcome.
      1. 16% of patients were back to independent life in 1 year.
      2. 11% were severely disabled.

3. 12% were in vegetative state.
4. 61% died without recovery.

REF: American Neurological Association committee on ethical affairs. *Ann Neurol* 33:386-390, 1993.

Levy D et al: *JAMA* 253:1420-1426, 1985.

Plum F, Posner JB: *The diagnosis of stupor and coma*, ed 3, Philadelphia, 1982, FA Davis.

COMPUTED TOMOGRAPHY (CT)

Computed tomography (CT) combines conventional x-ray with a digitized, computerized reconstruction technique that yields multiple two-dimensional images of the body. Tissues are assigned absorption coefficients by the computer (CT or Hounsfield numbers) and are displayed as shades of gray (see Table 14). The range of CT numbers displayed can be manipulated to focus on certain structures (e.g., bony structures or intracranial contents) by "windowing." The *window width* (WW) determines the range of CT numbers displayed, and the *window level* (WL) determines the center of the window width. Large windows,

TABLE 14
CT Density

Moiety	Hounsfield Units
Bone	1000
Calcification	100
Acute blood	85
Tumor	30-60
Gray matter	35-40
White matter	25-30
CSF	0
Adipose	−100
Air	−1000

From Woodruff WW: *Fundamentals of neuroimaging*, Philadelphia, 1993, WB Saunders.

TABLE 15
CT Findings in Stroke

Duration	Infarct Without Contrast	With Contrast
Hyperacute (< 1 day)	Normal or blurring of gray-white junction and/or effacement of gyri	No enhancement
Acute (1-7 days)	Vaguely defined hypodensity, best seen after 3-4 days; maximal edema and mass effect	No enhancement
Subacute enhancement (8-21 days)	Hypodensity less evident; decreased mass effect and edema	Gyral (peaks at week 3)
Chronic (> 21 days)	Hypodensity sharply defined and isodense to CSF	Enhancement usually in 6-7 weeks

In evaluating stroke a negative initial CT should be repeated in 2 to 3 days, when edema (and hypodensity) is maximal, as appropriate.

Duration	Intraparenchymal Hemorrhage Appearance	Mass Effect
Acute	Homogeneous hyperdensity	Mass effect
Subacute		
Early (3 days to 3 weeks)	Enlarging hypodense periphery with hyperdense center	Mass effect
Late (3-5 weeks)	Hypodense periphery; isodense center	Mass effect
Chronic (> 5 weeks)	Hypodense periphery; hypodense center	Mass effect resolves after several months

Ring enhancement is present from week 1 to week 7.

From Woodruff WW: *Fundamentals of neuroimaging,* Philadelphia, 1993, WB Saunders.

for example, one with a WW of less than 400, are used for evaluating bone, whereas smaller windows, such as when WW = 200, are used for evaluating brain tissue.

Iodinated IV contrast material enhances (brightens) many normal vascular structures (large vessels, choroid plexus, tentorium, and falx) as well as highly vascular pathologic structures (meningiomas, pituitary adenomas, chordomas, medulloblastomas, lymphomas, sarcomas, metastases, optic nerve gliomas, acoustic neurinomas, and late infarcts) (see Table 15). "Ring" enhancement (white rim or dark core) is seen with abscess capsules, glioblastomas, metastases, dermoid cysts, and other lesions. Little or no enhancement is usually seen in normal brain tissue, oligodendrogliomas, astrocytomas, ependymomas, fresh infarcts, or edema. Variable degrees of enhancement may be seen in glioblastomas, craniopharyngiomas, basilar meningitis, encephalitis, and metastases.

CT is preferred to MRI for imaging *acute* hemorrhage. However, CT is generally less sensitive than MRI, especially in visualizing the posterior fossa and the temporal lobes, where bony artifact degrades CT images. CT combined with myelography is an alternative for spinal imaging, albeit with less resolution of neural structures than with MRI.

REF: Woodruff WW. *Fundamentals of neuroimaging*, Philadelphia, 1993, WB Saunders.

CONFUSIONAL STATE

A disturbance of attention with three primary features: (1) disturbance of vigilance, (2) inability to maintain a stream of thought, and (3) inability to carry out goal-directed movements. Mild anomia, dysgraphia, dyscalculia, and constructional deficits may be seen. Perceptual distortions may lead to illusions and hallucinations. Tremor, myoclonus, or asterixis may accompany acute confusional states.

Metabolic disturbances, toxic exposure, drugs, infection (systemic and CNS), head trauma, and seizures are common causes of confusional states. Unilateral or bilateral damage to the fusiform and lingual gyri as well as lesions of the nondominant posterior parietal and inferior prefrontal regions may produce a confusional state.

REF: Mesulam MM. *Principles of behavioral neurology*, Philadelphia, 1985, FA Davis.

CONGENITAL MALFORMATIONS *(see Chromosomal Syndromes, Craniocervical Junction, Developmental Malformations)*

CONUS MEDULLARIS *(see Cauda Equina)*

CONVULSIONS *(see Epilepsy)*

COPPER *(see Wilson's Disease)*

CORTEX *(see Cerebral Cortex)*

CRAMPS

Cramps are painful muscle spasms. When pathologic, they may represent abnormalities of muscle, nerve, or CNS. Although the following disorders do not have true cramps, patients with myotonia, neuromyotonia, tetany, tetanus, and stiff-man syndrome often complain of "cramps"; therefore they are included in the differential diagnosis.

I. Myopathic disorders.
   A. The painful muscle spasms associated with glycogenoses (most commonly phosphorylase or phosphofructokinase deficiency), disorders of lipid metabolism, and carnitine palmityltransferase (CPT) deficiency are designated *contractures*, and there is severe, intermittent, sharp muscle pain with palpable shortening and hardening of the affected muscles. Contractures may be precipitated by exercise (glycogenoses and CPT deficiency) or fasting (CPT deficiency); they are associated with increased weakness and are unaffected by curare or nerve block. The EMG is electrically silent during contractures. Treatment includes a high-carbohydrate diet for phosphorylase deficiency and a high-carbohydrate, low-fat diet for CPT deficiency.
   B. The "cramps" associated with myotonic disorders are painless (see Myotonia).
II. Disorders of peripheral nerves.
   A. *Tetany* results from hypocalcemia and alkalosis. Hypomagnesemia and hyperkalemia may cause carpopedal spasm. Severe tonic spasms are painful only during prolonged attacks.

They may be provoked by hyperventilation or limb ischemia causing a lowered depolarization threshold of motor nerve fibers. EMG reveals asynchronous, grouped motor unit potentials discharging at a rate of 5 to 15 per second and separated by periods of electrical silence. Treatment is the correction of the underlying cause.

B. *Neuromyotonia* (generalized myokymia, continuous muscle fiber activity, and Isaac's syndrome) manifests as muscle stiffness. In severe cases stiffness is present at rest and impedes movement. Neuromyotonia occurs at any age and is usually sporadic. The defect is in the distal portion of the nerve, and the motor activity is not altered by spinal or proximal nerve block. The EMG shows short bursts of motor unit activity at 10 to 100 Hz. Treatment is with phenytoin, carbamazepine, or dantrolene.

C. *Motor neuron disease* and *muscle denervation* of any cause may be associated with cramps.

III. Central disorders.

A. *Stiff-man syndrome* is characterized by the adult onset of rigid, uncontrolled proximal and axial muscle contractions that are present only during wakefulness. Proximal muscle contractions are usually greater than distal contractions. The cramps are extremely painful and may be precipitated by movement, noise, or other sensory stimuli; they are blocked by curare, general anesthesia, and nerve block. The EMG shows continuous activity in agonist and antagonist muscles with normal motor unit morphology. Treatment is with diazepam, clonazepam or other muscle relaxants. Stiff-man syndrome appears to be an autoimmune disease resulting from antibodies directed at basal ganglia.

B. *Tetanus* is characterized by acute, rapidly progressive, generalized, continuous tonic contractures with superimposed painful spasms caused by loss of inhibitory postsynaptic potentials in the spinal cord. Tonic spasms of the masticatory muscles (trismus or lockjaw) are common. The spasms may be stopped with curare and during sleep. EMG is similar to that in stiff-man syndrome. Treatment includes ventilatory support, tetanus antitoxin, diazepam, chlorpromazine, phenobarbital, or curare.

IV. Physiologic Cramps. Painful muscle cramps may occur in normal individuals, usually at rest or after extreme exercise. EMG shows a high-voltage, high frequency burst of motor unit potentials. Passive stretching of the muscle usually stops the cramp. Occasionally quinine, phenytoin, carbamazepine, or diazepam is helpful.

REF: Darnell RB et al: *Neurology* 43:114–121, 1993.

Layzer RB, Rowland LP: *N Engl J Med* 285:31–40, 1971.

CRANIAL NERVES

Nerve	CNS Nucleus	Function and Innervation
I	Olfactory bulb	Smell
II	Lateral geniculate	Vision
III	Oculomotor	Extraocular muscles except superior oblique and lateral rectus
	Edinger-Westphal	Sphincter pupillae and ciliary muscle
IV	Trochlear	Superior oblique muscle
V	Spinal and main sensory	Sensory from face, deep tissues of head and neck, dura mater, and tympanic membrane
	Mesencephalic	Muscle spindles; mechanoreceptors of face and mouth
	Trigeminal motor	Muscles of mastication and tensor tympani
VI	Abducens	Lateral rectus muscle
VII	Facial motor	Muscles of facial expression and stapedius
	Spinal trigeminal	Sensory from external ear and tympanic membrane
	Solitary	Taste from anterior two thirds of tongue
	Superior salivatory	Salivary and lacrimal glands
VIII	Cochlear and vestibular	Balance and hearing
IX	Ambiguous	Muscles of pharynx
	Spinal trigeminal	Sensory from external ear, tympanic membrane, and posterior third of tongue
	Solitary	Taste from posterior third of tongue

	Solitary and spinal trigeminal	Carotid body and sinus; sensation from nasal nuclei and oral pharynx
	Inferior salivatory	Parotid gland
X	Nucleus ambiguous	Muscles of larynx and pharynx
	Spinal trigeminal	Sensory from external ear
	Solitary	Taste buds of epiglottis
	Solitary and spinal trigeminal	Parasympathetics from thoracic and abdominal viscera, sensory from larynx and pharynx
	Dorsal motor	Parasympathetics to thoracic and abdominal viscera
XI	Ambiguous	Muscles of larynx and pharynx
	Accessory	Sternocleidomastoid and trapezius
XII	Hypoglossal	Intrinsic tongue muscles

REF: Haines DE: *Neuroanatomy: An atlas of structures, sections, and systems,* ed 3, Baltimore, 1991, Urban and Schwarzenberg.

Kandel ER et al: *Principles of neural science,* ed 2, New York, 1985, Elsevier.

CRANIOCERVICAL JUNCTION

Dysfunction resulting from lesions at the foramen magnum or craniocervical junction is usually produced by compression or shearing. Signs and symptoms are usually chronic, since acute lesions usually become evident with respiratory arrest, and may include various combinations of the following: spastic quadriparesis; cranial nerve palsies such as dysphagia, dysarthria, absent gag, hearing loss, vocal cord paralysis, nystagmus (downbeat and periodic alternating) vertigo, facial weakness or diplopia; hydrocephalus; head and neck pain; extremity weakness or paresthesias; facial pain; drop attacks; syringomyelia; ataxia; papilledema; dorsal column signs; and recurrent apnea or stridor. Some individuals with abnormalities of the craniocervical junction may be asymptomatic. Abnormalities causing symptoms at the craniocervical junction include the following.

BONY DEFORMITIES

Platybasia (flattening of the base of the skull). *Congenital:* Down's syndrome, achondroplasia, mucopolysaccharidosis, Arnold-Chiari malformation, cleidocranial dysplasia, and osteogenesis imperfecta. *Acquired:* Rickets, osteomalacia, Paget's disease, fibrous dysplasia, hypothyroidism, neoplasia, infection, or trauma.

Basilar invagination (impression). Upward extension of the skull base around the foramen magnum. The dens may protrude into the cranium. *Congenital:* May be associated with tonsillar herniation, syringomyelia, high arched palate, syndactyly, pes cavus, iris heterochromia, Sprengel's deformity, scoliosis, torticollis, short neck, skull deformities, and Arnold-Chiari malformation, type 1. *Acquired:* Paget's disease.

Atlantoaxial subluxation (chronic or acute cord compression syndrome). *Congenital:* Down's syndrome or Morquio syndrome. *Acquired:* Trauma or rheumatoid arthritis.

Fusion of atlas and foramen magnum (congenital). The most common of the bony abnormalities at the craniocervical junction; symptoms may also occur if the dens is high, long, or posteriorly angulated.

MALFORMATIONS OF THE NEURAXIS

Arnold-Chiari malformations: Congenital anomalies of the hindbrain with caudal displacement of pons, medulla, and cerebellar vermis.

Type 1: Cerebellar tonsils are displaced into spinal canal, and medulla elongated. Syringomyelia and bony deformities may be present. Myelomeningocele is rare. Symptoms develop during adolescence or adulthood.

Type 2: Medulla and cerebellum are displaced inferiorly and deformed. An elongated medulla overlies the cervical cord, which may be small, with upward-directed cervical roots. Spina bifida with meningomyelocele is invariably present. Symptoms usually begin in infancy or early childhood. Hydrocephalus is the most common presentation. Associated findings include polymicrogyria, heterotopias, syringomyelia, hydromyelia, enlargement of the foramen magnum, elongation of the cervical arches, platybasia, basilar invagination, assimilation of the atlas, and Klippel-Feil anomaly.

Type 3: Includes cervical spina bifida, cerebellar herniation through the defect, and an open, dystrophic posterior fossa. Rarely compatible with postnatal life.

Type 4: Cerebellar hypoplasia. May be related to or the equivalent of the Dandy-Walker malformation (hydrocephalus, incomplete vermian fusion, and enlarged fourth ventricle).

Tumors of the brainstem, cerebellum, spinal cord, and bone, including brainstem gliomas, medulloblastomas, ependymomas, meningiomas, acoustic neuromas, teratomas, dermoids, neurofibromas, bony tumors, granulomas, hemangioblastomas, and metastatic lesions.

The differential diagnosis of dysfunction at the craniocervical junction also includes multiple sclerosis, cervical dislocation, cervical degenerative joint disease, spinocerebellar degeneration and other multiple-system atrophies, myelitis, amyotrophic lateral sclerosis, and bulbar and pseudobulbar palsy.

Magnetic resonance imaging is the diagnostic procedure of choice for evaluating the craniocervical junction.

REF: Critchley E et al: *Diseases of the spinal cord*, London, 1992, Springer-Verlag.

CRANIOSYNOSTOSIS

Premature closure of one or more cranial sutures. Fetal head constraint is thought to be an important cause of isolated craniosynostosis. Craniosynostosis may also occur in association with other anomalies as part of sporadic or genetic syndromes or diseases (Crouzon's, Apert's, Saethre-Chotzen, Pfeiffer's, and Carpenter's), metabolic disorders (hyperthyroidism, rickets, and hypophosphatasia), and hematologic disorders with bone marrow hyperplasia. Primary failure of brain development (microcephaly) or shunting for hydrocephalus may result in craniosynostosis, but the skull is usually not misshapen.

Craniosynostosis produces characteristic cranial deformities depending on the suture(s) involved (see Table 16).

Evaluation of suspected craniosynostosis includes palpation of the calvarial bones (palpable ridging) and skull x-rays (hyperostotic bony fusion and obliteration of the suture). Multiple-suture synostosis may have associated increased intracranial pressure, so correction should be undertaken at age 1 to 2 months to prevent neurologic damage. For sagittal synostosis, surgical correction is simply cosmetic. Surgery is not indicated for secondary synostosis due to microcephaly.

REF: David R, ed: *Pediatric neurology for the clinician*, Norwalk, CT, 1992, Appleton-Lange.

Jacobson RI: *Neurol Clin* 3:117–145, 1985.

TABLE 16
Types of Craniosynostosis

Suture Closed	Skull Deformity	Characteristics
Sagittal	Scaphocephaly (boathead)	60% of all types; may be familial, boys > girls, neurologically normal
Coronal	Brachycephaly (short head)	20% of all types; girls > boys; *if untreated, may have neurologic abnormalities*
Single coronal or lambdoidal	Plagiocephaly (oblique head)	Similar head shape occurs in congenital torticollis without synostosis
Metopic (forehead)	Trigonocephaly (triangle head)	May have related neurologic abnormalities, including mental retardation
Multiple	Oxycephaly (pointed head)	*May cause increased intracranial pressure*

CREUTZFELDT-JAKOB DISEASE (see also Dementia)

Creutzfeldt-Jakob disease (CJD) is a rare disorder with peak incidence in the sixth and seventh decades, although it has been described in patients from 20 to 80 years of age and older. Men and women are affected equally. CJD frequently has a stereotypic clinical presentation, but some atypical forms may occur. Initial symptoms are often subtle and overlooked, including vague physical discomfort, difficulties with sleep and concentration, and changes in appetite. Typically within several weeks progressive dementia and myoclonus are obvious. Signs of cerebellar, pyramidal, and extrapyramidal involvement (rigidity, tremor, or choreoathetosis) develop in most patients; less common are amyotrophic features, cortical blindness, seizures, and cranial nerve palsies. Average duration before death is 8 to 12 months, but some patients survive for years. Laboratory and imaging studies are nonspecific with the exception of the EEG. In early stages of the disease the

EEG shows gradual slowing of the background rhythm; with disease progression periodic EEG complexes develop—either triphasic sharp waves or a burst-suppression pattern—in most patients. These EEG changes are not pathognomic for CJD, but together with rapid dementia and myoclonus they are suggestive of the diagnosis. Results of brain biopsy are usually definitive. There is no therapy.

CJD is regarded as both a genetic and a transmissible infectious disorder. It can be transmitted to several animal species, and in some patients iatrogenic transmission has been reported after treatment with cadaver-derived human growth hormone, dura mater graft, corneal transplants, and contaminated depth electrodes for epilepsy monitoring. However, the infectious agent, called a *prion*, is unique: it is an altered form of the normally occurring cellular prion protein that is somehow capable of self-replication. There is no evidence that blood, saliva, stool, or urine is infectious. Familial CJD, comprising 10% of cases, is associated with specific mutations of the cellular prion protein. *Kuru* was an endemic form of prion disease associated with cannibalism in the Fore tribe of New Guinea. *Gerstmann-Straussler-Scheinker disease* is another prion disease similar to CJD. Most cases are familial with autosomal dominant inheritance. Ataxia is prominent, and other symptoms include dementia, supranuclear gaze palsy, aphasia, and parkinsonism. The course is slower than for CJD, leading to death in 4 to 10 years. *Familial fatal insomnia* also belongs to the group of human prion diseases.

Atypical CJD with prominent amyotrophic or ataxic features and longer duration or absence of typical EEG changes can cause diagnostic uncertainty. These cases may be misdiagnosed as amyotrophic lateral sclerosis, multiple sclerosis, or paraneoplastic cerebellar degeneration. CJD must be also distinguished from other rapidly progressing forms of dementia, including Alzheimer's disease with myoclonus or HIV infection, particularly in younger patients.

REF: Brown P et al: *Ann Neurol* 20:597–602, 1986.

Palmer MS, Collinge J: *Curr Opin Neurol Neurosurg* 5:895–901, 1992.

Prusiner SB: *Curr Opin Neurobiol* 2:638–647, 1992.

CRYPTOCOCCAL MENINGITIS   *(see Meningitis)*

DANDY-WALKER-SYNDROME   *(see Craniocervical Junction)*

DEGENERATIVE DISEASES OF CHILDHOOD

These disorders can be classified on a pathoanatomic basis wherein clinical phenomena and pathologic features suggest the maximum or most obvious site of involvement. This classification scheme results in five major categories.

Polioencephalopathies (cortical gray-matter diseases) have myoclonus, seizures, and cognitive decline as prominent early manifestations. Common hereditary polioencephalopathies ("poliodystrophies") include neuronal ceroid lipofuscinosis, GM2 gangliosidosis (Tay-Sachs disease), mucopolysaccharidoses, Gaucher's disease, and Niemann-Pick disease. Nongenetic causes include hypoxia, Lennox-Gastaux syndrome, and postvaccinal encephalopathy.

Leukoencephalopathies (white-matter diseases) have long-tract signs (spasticity, hyperreflexia, and Babinski's sign), optic atrophy, and cortical blindness or deafness. Seizures may occur late in the course, but myoclonus is rare. Common hereditary leukoencephalopathies ("leukodystrophies") include adrenoleukodystrophy (ALD), metachromatic leukodystrophy (MLD), Pelizaeus-Merzbacher disease, globoid-cell leukodystrohy (Krabbe's disease), and phenylketonuria with dysmyelination. Nongenetic causes include acute disseminated encephalomyelitis (ADEM) and multiple sclerosis.

Corencephalopathies (deep telencephalic, diencephalic, or mesencephalic diseases, including both gray and white matter) have movement disorders (chorea, parkinsonism, and dystonia). Common corencephalopathies include Huntington's disease, dystonia musculorum deformans, Hallervorden-Spatz disease, and Leigh's subacute necrotizing encephalomyelitis.

Spinocerebellopathies (diseases of the pons, medulla, cerebellum, and spinal cord) usually manifest with ataxia or spinal cord signs. Common spinocerebellopathies include hereditary spastic paraparesis, Friedreich's ataxia, and olivopontocerebellar degeneration.

Diffuse encephalopathies include degeneration resulting from subacute sclerosing panencephalitis (SSPE), neurocutaneous diseases, metabolic disorders (hyperammonemias, lactic acidemias, and homocystinuria), and hypoxia.

Laboratory evaluation includes the following tests when appropriate (see Metabolic Diseases of Childhood).

Urine levels: Dermatan and heparan sulfate (increased in mucopolysaccharidoses), arylsulfatase A (decreased in MLD), and copper (increased in Wilson's disease).

Serum levels: Hexosaminidase A (decreased in Tay-Sachs' disease), acid phosphatase (increased in Gaucher's disease), pyruvate and lactate (elevated in Leigh's disease), measles titer (elevated in SSPE), and copper and ceruloplasmin (decreased in Wilson's disease).

WBC count: Arylsulfatase A (decreased in MLD), galactocerebrosidase (decreased in Krabbe's disease), sphingomyelinase (decreased in Niemann-Pick disease), and beta-glucosidase (decreased in Gaucher's disease).

CSF levels: Protein (elevated in MLD, Krabbe's disease, SSPE, and the like), gammaglobulin (elevated in SSPE, ADEM, and multiple sclerosis), and measles titer (elevated in SSPE).

EEG: Helpful in many polioencephalopathies (SSPE, ceroid lipofuscinosis, and Lennox-Gastaux syndrome).

MRI (or CT): Particularly helpful in leukoencephalopathies.

EMG and nerve conduction study: Useful in degenerative diseases with neuropathy (MLD and Krabbe's disease).

Tissue studies: Bone marrow aspirate (characteristic cells in Gaucher's disease and Niemann-Pick disease), liver or muscle biopsy (glycogen storage disease), and electron microscopic examination of leukocytes or fibroblasts (characteristic abnormalities in many conditions, especially lysosomal storage disorders). C26: C22 fatty acid ratio is increased in cultured fibroblasts in ALD.

REF: David R, ed: *Pediatric neurology for the clinician,* Norwalk, CT, 1992, Appleton-Lange.

Dyken P, Krawiecki N: *Ann Neurol* 13:351–364, 1983.

DEGENERATIVE DISEASES—OTHER *(see Individual Listings)*

DELIRIUM *(see Confusional State)*

DELIRIUM TREMENS *(see Alcohol)*

DEMENTIA *(see also Alzheimer's Disease, Creutzfeldt-Jakob Disease, Mental Status Testing)*

Dementia is a clinical syndrome characterized by loss of function in multiple cognitive abilities in an individual with previously normal (or at least higher) intellectual level and occurring in clear consciousness (i.e., in the absence of delirium). *DSM IV-R* diagnostic criteria require memory impairment and abnormalities in at least one of these areas: language, judgment, abstract thinking, praxis, constructional abilities, or visual recognition. This deficit must be sufficient to interfere with activities of daily living, work duties, or other social activities. The term "dementia" does not imply a specific underlying cause, a progressive course, or irreversibility. The definition also excludes patients with isolated deficits such as aphasia or apraxia, or if symptoms are occurring exclusively during a delirium.

Examination for suspected dementia should include assessment of multiple areas of cognitive performance, including memory, language, perception, praxis, attention, judgment, calculation, and visuospatial functions. The presence of psychiatric features (affective disorder, hallucinations, delusions, and anxiety) must be also sought. Questions about the patient's activities and self-care capabilities should be obtained from collateral sources of information (caregiver). Short, standardized mental status tests such as Mini-Mental Status Examination and the Short Blessed Dementia Scale are widely used. Mild cognitive deficit may require more extensive neuropsychologic testing.

The differential diagnosis requires not only history and physical examination but also laboratory screening tests for potentially treatable causes of dementia. Laboratory tests should include electrolyte and screening metabolic panel, complete blood cell count and differential, urinanalysis, thyroid function tests, syphilis serology, vitamin B_{12} and folate levels, CT or MRI scan, ECG, and chest x-ray. Other tests (EEG, lumbar puncture, HIV titer, serologic testing for vasculitis, heavy metal screening, angiography, brain biopsy, and formal psychiatric assessment) are not routinely indicated unless suggested by the history or physical examination. In younger adults dementia can be caused by late onset of childhood metabolic diseases, and additional special studies may be required.

Conditions causing dementia can be divided into the following groups: degenerative disorders (Alzheimer's disease [AD], Pick's disease, Huntington's disease, Parkinson's disease, and diffuse Lewy body disease); metabolic and deficiency disorders (hypothyroidism, hepatic encephalopathy, Cushing's syndrome, porphyria, Wilson's disease, and vitamin B_{12} deficiency); cerebrovascular disease and infections (syphilis, viral and postviral encephalitic syndromes, chronic meningitis of various origins, progressive multifocal encephalopathy, HIV infection, and Creutzfeldt-Jakob disease); systemic disorders (lupus erythematosus, sarcoidosis, and Sjögren's syndrome); toxins and drugs (heavy metals, carbon monoxide, and anticholinergic, psychoactive, and other medications); head trauma; brain tumors; psychiatric disorders (depression); multiple sclerosis; and normal-pressure hydrocephalus. The most common cause of dementia in adults is AD (50% to 60%), followed by vascular dementias (20%); in another 15% to 20% of patients vascular dementias coexist with AD. Potentially treatable causes account for about 10% of cases.

The modified Hachinski scale (see Table 17) may help differentiate multi-infarct dementia from Alzheimer's disease.

New diagnostic criteria for vascular dementias include dementia with evidence of cerebrovascular disease demonstrated by history, clinical examination, or brain imaging; the two disorders must be reasonably related, with onset of dementia within 3 months after a recognized vascular event. Vascular dementias can be divided in several types. Multiinfarct dementia (MID) is caused by multiple, complete infarcts involving both cortical and subcortical areas. Small vessel disease with dementia includes bilateral lacunae in the white matter; Binswanger's

TABLE 17
Clinical Features of the Ischemic Score (Modified Hachinski Scale)

Feature	Point Value
Abrupt onset	2
Stepwise deterioration	1
Fluctuating course	2
Nocturnal confusion	1
Relative preservation of personality	1
Depression	1
Somatic complaints	1
Emotional incontinence	1
History of presence of hypertension	1
History of strokes	2
Evidence of associated atherosclerosis	1
Focal neurologic symptoms	2
Focal neurologic signs	2

Adapted from Rosen WG et al: *Ann Neurol* 7:486-8, 1980.
Score ≤4 suggests primary degenerative dementia; score >7 suggests dementia.

disease (subacute arteriolar encephalopathy) is one subtype of small vessel disease. Dementia can also be caused by a single infarct involving an area with important cognitive function (e.g., angular gyrus syndrome). Hypoperfusion resulting from cardiac arrest can also cause global cognitive decline. Treatment is directed at prevention of further vascular events.

REF: Coker BS: *Neurology* 41:794–798, 1991.

Consensus Development Panel of the National Institutes of Health: *JAMA* 258:3411, 1987.

Cummings JL, Benson DF: *Dementia: a clinical approach*, ed 2, Boston, 1992, Butterworth-Heinemann.

Roman et al: *Neurology* 43:250–260, 1993.

DEMYELINATING DISEASE *(see also Neuropathy, Multiple Sclerosis)*

These CNS disorders—demyelinating disease, neuropathy, and multiple sclerosis (MS)—involve destruction of normally formed myelin and oligodendroglia, in contrast to the dysmyelinating diseases (e.g., leukodystrophies) in which myelin is abnormally formed. Multiple sclerosis is the most common. MS and the related acute disseminated encephalomyelitis (ADEM) appear to be immune mediated, although etiopathogenesis remains an enigma.

CLASSIFICATION

I. Autoimmune.
   A. Primary diseases of myelin.
      1. Multiple sclerosis (MS).
      2. Devic's disease, a variant of MS, consists of optic neuritis and transverse myelitis.
      3. Schilder's disease, a rapidly progressive sporadic disease, results in bilateral, massive hemispheric demyelination and is seen mainly in children and adolescents.
      4. Balo's sclerosis, also a possible variant of MS, results in acute demyelination in a concentric pattern.
   B. Parainfectious or postvaccination.
      1. ADEM, a uniphasic, inflammatory demyelinating disorder, occurs shortly after measles, varicella, rubella, or other viral illnesses, after vaccination, or after immunizations.
      2. Acute hemorrhagic leukoencephalitis, a hyperacute nec-

rotizing form of ADEM, occurs usually after upper-respiratory tract infections, and pathologic features are more tissue-destructive.

3. Site-restricted, uniphasic, acute inflammatory demyelinating disorders include transverse myelitis, optic neuritis, cerebellitis, and Bickerstaff's brainstem encephalitis.

4. Chronic or recurrent parainfectious or postvaccination encephalomyelitis (possibly related to MS).

II. Infectious.
   A. Progressive multifocal leukoencephalopathy.
   B. Subacute sclerosing panencephalitis.
III. Nutritional.
   A. Alcohol or tobacco amblyopia.
   B. Central pontine myelinolysis.
   C. Marchiafava-Bignami syndrome.
   D. Vitamin B_{12} deficiency.
IV. Toxic or metabolic.
   A. Anoxia or hypoxia.
   B. Carbon monoxide poisoning.
   C. Mercury intoxication (Minamata disease).
   D. Radiation therapy.
   E. Methotrexate, especially with radiation therapy.
V. Hereditary.
   A. Familial spastic paraplegia.
   B. Hereditary ataxias.
   C. Leber's disease.

REF: Baker D, Davison AN: *Neurochem Res* 16:1067–1072, 1991.

Francis GS, Antel JP, Duquette P: Inflammatory demyelinating diseases of the central nervous system. In Bradley WG et al: *Neurology in clinical practice*, Boston, 1991, Butterworth-Heinemann.

DERMATOMES   *(see Inside Front Cover and Figures 11 to 14)*

DERMATOMYOSITIS   *(see Muscle Disorders, Myopathy)*

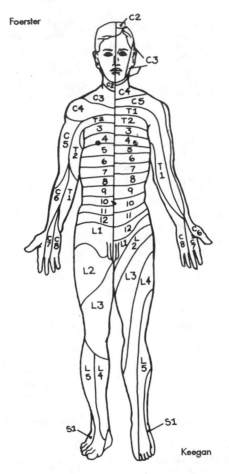

FIGURE 11
Cutaneous sensory distribution of spinal roots (anterior). *(From Kopell HP, Thompson WAL: Peripheral entrapment neuropathies, Huntington, NY, 1973, Robert E Krieger.)*

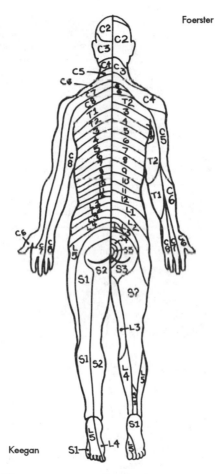

FIGURE 12
Cutaneous sensory distribution of spinal roots (posterior). *(From Kopell HP, Thompson WAL: Peripheral entrapment neuropathies, Huntington, NY, 1973, Robert E Krieger.)*

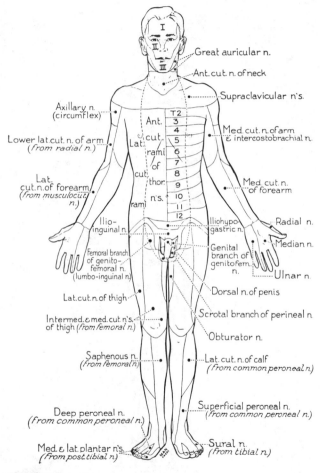

FIGURE 13

Cutaneous sensory distribution of peripheral nerves (anterior). *(From Haymaker W, Woodhall B: Peripheral nerve injuries: Principles of diagnosis, Philadelphia, 1953, WB Saunders.)*

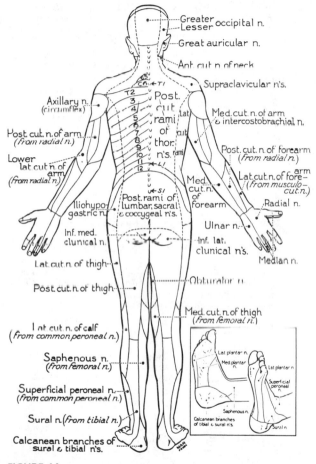

FIGURE 14

Cutaneous sensory distribution of peripheral nerves (posterior). (From Haymaker W, Woodhall B: Peripheral nerve injuries: Principles of diagnosis, Philadelphia, 1953, WB Saunders.)

DEVELOPMENTAL MALFORMATIONS *(see also Craniocervical Junction)*

I. Neural tube defects (dysraphism).
   A. Rachischisis: General term describing any failure of closure of the neural tube; used loosely to describe any failure of closure of the vertebral arches.
   B. Congenital dural sinus: Communication between meninges and dermis via incompletely closed vertebral arch.
   C. Spina bifida occulta: Closure defect of vertebral arch only, usually at L5-S1. May have overlying tuft of hair, discoloration, dimple, or dural sinus. Clinically asymptomatic; common incidental radiographic finding.
   D. Meningocele: Leptomeninges protrude through defect in vertebral arch or skull.
   E. Myelomeningocele: Meninges and spinal cord protrude through defect in vertebral arch. Arnold-Chiari malformation (Chiari, type 2) and hydrocephalus are frequently associated. Meningitis and recurrent urinary tract infections are frequent complications.
   F. Spina bifida cystica: General term for spinal meningocele or myelomeningocele.
   G. Diastematomyelia: Splitting of the spinal cord by intervening mesodermal band, which may have a bony component. Often becomes symptomatic during growth because of the abnormal fixation of the cord in the canal.
   H. Encephalocele: Meninges and brain parenchyma protrude through skull defect. Usually (75% to 80%) occurs in occipital region.
   I. Anencephaly: Absent or hypoplastic calvaria and absent cerebrum. Brainstem and cerebellum may be present but are abnormal. The primary defect is thought to be failure of skull development, exposing the cerebrum to destruction.
II. Defective cleavage, proliferation, and migration.
   A. Holoprosencephaly (unicameral brain): Failure of cleavage of embryonic forebrain into paired cerebral hemispheres, resulting in absence of interhemispheric fissure, large single ventricle, and marked absence of cerebral parenchyma. Frequently associated with chromosomal abnormalities.
   B. Arhinencephaly: Term originally used interchangeably with holoprosencephaly; now describes olfactory bulb and tract aplasia. ("Olfactory aplasia" is more precise.)

C. Porencephaly: Originally used to describe congenital cerebral defects with complete communication between subarachnoid space and ventricles; currently used loosely to describe any abnormal CSF-filled cavity in brain parenchyma.

D. Schizencephaly: Lateral clefts through both cerebral hemispheres extending from cortical surface to the ventricles, considered by some to be due to failure of development of the cerebral mantle in zones of cleavage of the primary cerebral fissures. Others believe that it is due to a destructive process and is a form of porencephaly.

E. Hydranencephaly: Destructive lesion in which the only remnant of the cerebral hemisphere is a paper-thin membrane sac composed of glial tissue filled with CSF and covered by intact leptomeninges. Parts of frontal and temporal lobes may be preserved. Brainstem and cerebellum are present.

F. Lissencephaly (agyria): Absence of gyri.

G. Pachygyria: Abnormally wide and thick gyri with abnormal lamination.

H. Microgyria, polymicrogyria: Areas of small gyri, usually markedly increased in number, with abnormal lamination.

I. Heterotopias: Ectopic collections of gray matter. Frequently associated with mental retardation and other neurologic signs.

REF: Barth PG: *Can J Neurol Sci* 14:1-16, 1987.

Friede RL: *Developmental neuropathology*, ed 2, Berlin, 1989, Springer-Verlag.

Leech RW, Payne GG: *J Child Neurol* 6:286-287, 1991.

DEVELOPMENTAL MILESTONES *(see Child Neurology)*

DIABETES INSIPIDUS *(see Electrolyte Disorders)*

DIABETES MELLITUS *(see Glucose, Ischemia, Neuropathy)*

DIALYSIS *(see also Uremia)*

Two neurologic syndromes are related to dialysis. The *dialysis disequilibrium syndrome* is the acute onset of neurologic manifestations during or after hemodialysis or peritoneal dialysis. These include seizures (generalized more often than focal), headache, anorexia, nausea, disorientation, cramps, and coma. The cause is probably an accumulation of urea and idiogenic osmoles in the brain during renal failure. With dialysis, plasma osmolality decreases and the subsequent osmotic gradient results in obligatory retention of water by the brain and subsequent brain edema. Slower dialysis may offer the brain more time to rid itself of the idiogenic osmoles. The syndrome is usually self-limited, and recovery usually occurs in a few days.

The *dialysis dementia syndrome* is less common than dialysis disequilibrium syndrome and consists of the subacute development of personality changes, memory difficulties, dysarthria, myoclonus, and seizures. The origin may relate to elevated aluminum levels in the dialysate fluid. Removal of aluminum from dialysis baths by deionization has markedly reduced the frequency of this syndrome. Treatment is with desferrioxamine. Dialysis encephalopathy may be part of a multisystem disease that includes vitamin D–resistant osteomalacia, myopathy, and anemia.

Dialysis patients have an increased frequency of subdural hematomas and confusional states resulting from hyperosmolarity, hypercalcemia, hypophosphatemia, drug intoxication, and Wernicke's encephalopathy.

DIPHENYLHYDANTOIN   *(see Epilepsy)*

DIPLOPIA   *(see Eye Muscles, Ophthalmoplegia)*

DISK DISEASE   *(see Radiculopathy, Spinal Cord)*

DISORIENTATION   *(see Dementia, Mental Status Testing)*

DISSEMINATED INTRAVASCULAR COAGULATION (DIC)

Disseminated intravascular coagulation (DIC) is a clotting disorder complicating many diseases, such as infections (meningitis, sepsis, endocarditis, and the like), immunologic disturbances, obstetric complications, diabetic ketoacidosis, neoplasms, malignancy, tissue damage (stroke, brain hemorrhage, and so forth), or shock. In each case potent thrombogenic stimuli such as tissue factor or an endotoxin trigger the coagulation cascade and activate platelets. Fibrin then deposits in the microcirculation, causing ischemia, red blood cell damage, hemolysis, and secondary fibrinolysis.

The clinical presentation varies with stage and severity of the syndrome. Most often, patients have hemorrhagic or thrombotic complications in venipuncture sites or distal extremities. Any portion of the brain or spinal cord may be affected by hemorrhage or thrombosis, producing a fluctuating encephalopathy, commonly with focal findings. Confusion, delirium, stupor, and coma may occur with hemiparesis, hemianopsia, ataxia, aphasia, seizures, and focal brainstem disease. Patients with severe deficits may completely recover. Laboratory manifestations include elevated prothombin and partial thromboplastin times, low platelet counts, falling levels of fibrinogen (consumptive), and elevated levels of fibrin split products and D-dimer (due to fibrinolysis). Anemia, fragmented red blood cells, and schistocytes may be found.

Treatment consists of correcting the underlying cause. Fresh frozen plasma and cryoprecipitate to replenish clotting factors and platelet concentrates to correct thrombocytopenia are necessary in cases of active bleeding. Thrombotic complications may be treated with heparin. When platelets and plasma fail, heparin is sometimes used to treat hemorrhage.

REF: Aminoff MJ, ed: *Neurology and general medicine*, ed 2, Edinburgh, 1994, Churchill Livingstone.

DIVALPROEX SODIUM   *(see Epilepsy)*

DIZZINESS   *(see also Syncope, Vertigo)*

Dizziness is a nonspecific term commonly used to describe a variety of subjective experiences. An accurate description of what the patient means, a detailed medical history, and reproduction of the patient's symptoms by means of provocative maneuvers such as hyperventilation, Barany's maneuver, and stooping over, as well as measuring orthostatic blood pressures, help suggest the following more specific etiologic categories:

I. *Vertigo:* The illusion of self-motion or environmental motion (see Vertigo).
II. *Syncope or presyncope:* The sensation of impending faint or loss of consciousness. Causes include cardiac arrhythmia, carotid sinus hypersensitivity, postural hypotension (diabetic autonomic neuropathy or side effect of antihypertensive, diuretic, dopaminergic, or other drugs), anemia, and Addison's disease (see Syncope).

III. *Disequilibrium:* Loss of balance without various subjective movement sensations of head. May occur with cerebellar or proprioceptive disturbances or with muscle weakness.

IV. Dizziness that is due to causes other than those previously mentioned may be described as lightheadedness, floating, wooziness, faintness, or some other sense of altered consciousness. Causes include the following.

   A. Hyperventilation syndrome. One of the most common causes of dizziness or lightheadedness. Circumoral and digital paresthesias are frequently associated. Symptoms may be reproduced during hyperventilation. Occasionally a patient has positional vertigo with hyperventilation (see Hyperventilation, Vertigo).

   B. Multiple sensory deficits. Two or more of the following are usually present: visual impairment (often caused by cataracts), neuropathy, vestibular dysfunction (see Vertigo), cervical spondylosis, and orthopedic disorders that interfere with ambulation. Patients may complain of lightheadedness when walking and turning. Holding the examiner's finger lightly may provide enough additional sensory input to relieve the symptoms. Patients are often elderly or diabetic, or both.

   C. Psychogenic dizziness (not associated with hyperventilation). Patients complain of vague lightheadedness, mental fuzziness, or difficulty thinking. They may be depressed or anxious. Dizziness is usually continuous rather than episodic. Patients may state that all or none of the maneuvers performed during physical examination produce dizziness.

   D. Severe anemia or polycythemia may cause symptoms of lightheadedness or dizziness.

   E. Drugs may produce symptoms of dizziness that are not necessarily related to orthostatic changes in blood pressure or presyncope. These include antiarrhythmics, anticonvulsants, antidepressants, antihistamines, antihypertensives, antiparkinsonian agents, hypnotics, hypoglycemics, phenothiazines, alcohol, and tobacco.

   F. Endocrinologic disorders (hypoglycemia, Addison's disease, hypopituitarism, and insulinoma).

Treatment of dizziness depends on the underlying cause. For evaluation and management of vertigo, see Vertigo.

REF: Tusa RJ, Herdman SJ: Vertigo and dysequilibrium. In Johnson RT, Griffin JW, eds: *Current therapy in neurologic disease,* ed 4, St Louis, 1993, Mosby.

DOLL'S HEAD MANEUVER *(see Vestibulo-ocular Reflex)*

DOUBLE VISION *(see Eye Muscles, Ophthalmoplegia)*

DOWN'S SYNDROME *(see Chromosomal, Alzheimer's Disease)*

DYSARTHRIA *(see also Bulbar Palsy, Pseudobulbar Palsy)*

A disorder of speech produced by disturbances of the muscles of articulation. Six patterns of dysfunction have been distinguished: flaccid, spastic, ataxic, hypokinetic, hyperkinetic, and mixed. Although each has differing sound characteristics to the trained ear, most clinicians rely on associated neurologic signs such as limb ataxia, involvement of cranial nerve VII, IX, X, or XII, or brisk jaw jerk or gag reflex to distinguish the speech patterns (ataxic, flaccid, and spastic, respectively).

DYSKINESIA

A descriptive term encompassing all abnormal involuntary movements (exclusive of epilepsy). They are classified according to the following characteristics: rhythmic vs. arrhythmic, sustained vs. nonsustained, present during sleep vs. when awake, paroxysmal vs. continuous, at rest vs. during action, slow vs. fast, ballistic vs. nonballistic, powerful (painful) vs. easy to overcome, suppressible, complex, and associated with vocalization, self-mutilation, and a combination of various movements. By itself, "dyskinesia" is a nonspecific term and should be related to one or more of the elementary movement disorder types (See Asterixis, Chorea, Choreoathetosis, Dystonia, Myoclonus, Neuroleptics, Parkinson's Disease, Parkinsonism, Rigidity, and Tremor). The dyskinesias most commonly seen in practice relate to the use of neuroleptics (tardive dyskinesia) and dopaminergic drugs used to treat Parkinson's disease (dopa dyskinesia).

DYSPHAGIA

Difficulty in swallowing primarily liquids is typical of neurologic disorders, whereas dysphagia associated mainly with solids is typical of mechanical obstruction. Dysphagia may be diagnosed by obtaining a simple history of symptoms and by bedside testing. Food remaining in the mouth or pooling of oropharyngeal secretions may be due to swallowing akinesia or to facial or bulbar weakness; coughing or choking on swallowing suggests laryngeal weakness; nasal regurgitation of liquids suggests palatal weakness.

Local structural lesions of the upper GI tract frequently cause dysphagia by mechanical obstruction. Neurologic causes of dysphagia involve lesions anywhere along the pathways subserving swallowing; the coordination of swallowing depends on sensation from the tongue, mouth, pharynx, and larynx and on voluntary and reflex motor activity of cranial nerves V, VII, IX, X, and XII. The "swallowing center" is in the medulla, near the respiratory center. Lesions of the inferior precentral gyrus and posteroinferior frontal gyrus both cause severe dysphagia without buccolingual apraxia, speech impairment, or weakness. Bilateral upper motor neuron disease manifesting as pseudobulbar palsy is usually associated with dysphagia. Lesions of cerebellar and extrapyramidal pathways may also cause dysphagia. Dysphagia is seen in peripheral nervous system diseases such as Guillain-Barré syndrome, myasthenia, polymyositis, and oculopharyngeal dystrophy. Thus dysphagia is nonlocalizing and is associated with lesions from muscle to cerebral cortex.

Swallowing evaluation by a speech therapist should be obtained in cases of suspected aspiration. Preventive treatment is aimed primarily at the underlying disorder. For patients in whom oral feeding is unsafe, nasogastric tube, percutaneous gastrostomy tube, or cervical esophagostomy can be used. If the cricopharyngeal sphincter fails to relax, cricopharyngeal myotomy may be helpful. Total parenteral nutrition may be useful for short periods of time.

REF: Wiles CM: Neurogenic dysphagia. *J Neurol Neurosurg Psych* 54:1037-1039, 1991.

DYSPHASIA   *(see Aphasia)*

DYSTONIA

Dystonia is a purposeless, involuntary movement affecting muscle groups of the face, neck, limbs, or trunk and manifested as an extreme attitude or abnormal sustained posture. Dystonia may be phasic and reversible (torsion dystonia) or fixed. It may be generalized (entire body), segmental (one or more limbs or the neck), or focal (as in writer's cramp). Dystonia may be triggered by voluntary movements (action myoclonus) or specific motor acts (such as playing a piano or chewing). It is worsened by stress and fatigue and improved by rest, relaxation, or touching the affected body part ("sensory tricks"). It may be primary (familial or idiopathic) or secondary (symptomatic); in the latter case it may occur with other abnormal movements (tremor, chorea, or athetosis).

CLASSIFICATION

I. Primary dystonia.
  A. Dystonia musculorum deformans or idiopathic torsion dystonia.
    1. Hereditary: The recessive form begins in early childhood, progresses over years, and is restricted to Jewish patients; the dominant form is not limited to Jews, begins in late childhood and adolescence, and progresses more slowly; there also is an X-linked form. Dystonia may begin in one limb or cranial muscle but eventually involve trunk, spine, pelvis, and shoulder. Initially the spasms are intermittent, but they become more frequent and continuous until the body is grotesquely contorted. Dystonia is worsened by excitement and improved by sleep. Deep tendon reflexes are normal, and corticospinal tract signs are absent. The defective gene is located in the q32-q34 region of chromosome 9.
    2. Sporadic.
  B. Periodic dystonia.
    1. Hereditary (familial paroxysmal choreoathetosis): Paroxysmal attacks of dystonic spasms (autosomal recessive) and choreoathetosis (autosomal dominant) of limbs and trunk that last from minutes to hours and occur in children and young adults. The attacks may be precipitated by sudden movement or startling (paroxysmal kinesiogenic choreoathetosis) with brief multiple movements or may be nonkinesiogenic with more prolonged spontaneous movements.
    2. Sporadic.
  C. Focal, segmental, and multifocal.
    1. Meige's syndrome (cranial dystonia): Symmetric, focal oromandibular dystonia, laryngeal dystonia, and blepharospasm (presenting symptom in two thirds of patients); becomes evident as grimacing, blinking, chewing, lip smacking and pursing, mouth opening, tongue protrusion, a hoarse, strained voice, dysphagia, and deviation of the jaw.

Meige's syndrome is exacerbated by stress and fatigue and relieved by rest, sleep, and in some instances, neck pinching, talking, or singing. Fifty years of age is the peak age of onset, and it occurs more frequently in women. The cause is unknown.

   a. Blepharospasm: An involuntary, spasmodic closure of the eyelids preceded by increasing frequency and force of blinking. It is usually bilateral and occurs in middle or older age, more frequently in women. It may increase with noise, sunlight, wind, stress, or head movement. Some patients become functionally blind because of the severity of the spasms. Disorders associated with blepharospasm include tardive dyskinesia, Parkinson's disease, Wilson's disease, progressive supranuclear palsy, Schwartz-Jampel syndrome, myotonia, tetany, tetanus, ocular disorders (anterior chamber disease), midbrain disease, drugs (levodopa, antihistamines, and sympathomimetics), reflex blepharospasm, Sjögren's syndrome, systemic lupus erythematosus, myasthenia gravis, and functional disorder.

   b. Oromandibular dystonia (lingual dystonia): Jaw clenching, forced jaw opening, or tongue protrusion.

   c. Spasmodic dysphonia (laryngeal dystonia): Spasm of laryngeal muscles that produces a harsh, strained, hoarse, and sometimes breathy voice.

2. Spasmodic torticollis: Dystonia limited to the neck muscles (primarily trapezius and sternocleidomastoid) that results in head flexion (anterocollis), extension (retrocollis), or lateral rotation. It begins in early to middle adulthood, progresses slowly, and may remit after a few months. The spasms may be painful, may worsen when the patient is erect, and may be reduced by direct physical stimulus. This condition is associated with antipsychotic drugs, dystonia musculorum deformans, and extrapyramidal disease. Similar head postures may be seen in cervical spine disease, posterior fossa masses, and eye muscle imbalance. Grisel's syndrome is painful torticollis associated with nasopharyngeal infection.

3. Occupational dystonias (e.g., writer's cramp or graphospasm): Focal dystonia of the hand precipitated by writing; it may spread to the arm and shoulder and disappears on

cessation of writing). Also includes dystonias such as lip dystonia seen in musicians who play wind instruments.

4. Axial dystonia: Spasms of the trunk that compromise gait, posture, standing, sitting, or lying.

D. Possibly seizure-related dystonias: A spectrum of sleep-related dystonias, probably secondary to seizures arising during non rapid eye movement sleep.

1. Nocturnal paroxysmal dystonia: Sudden nocturnal arousal with dystonic posturing and motor activity, recurring throughout the night. Seizure focus is likely in mesial frontal lobe.

2. Episodic nocturnal wanderings: Episodes of ambulation, unintelligible speech, screaming, and occasionally violent behavior.

3. Paroxysmal arousals: Brief spells of awakening with dystonic posturing.

E. Hereditary progressive dystonia with marked diurnal fluctuation: An autosomal dominantly inherited, generalized dystonia that begins in childhood, is least severe in the morning, and increases throughout the day. Impairment progresses over several years and plateaus in young adulthood. The leg is typically involved first, and involvement may become evident with falls. Genetic penetrance and phenotypic expression are quite variable.

F. Other conditions associated with hereditary dystonia.

1. Neural deafness and intellectual impairment.

2. Amyotrophy (see section II, C).

3. Parkinsonism (see section II, C).

II. Secondary dystonia.

A. Diseases with established metabolic defect: e.g., Wilson's disease, GM1 gangliosidosis, GM2 gangliosidosis, metachromatic leukodystrophy, Lesch–nyhan syndrome, glutaric acidemia, methylmalonic acidemia, homocystinuria, hexosaminidase A deficiency, biopterin deficiency, hypoparathyroidism, and hyperthyroidism.

B. Diseases with undefined metabolic defect: e.g., Hallervorden-Spatz disease, calcification of basal ganglia, Leigh disease, bilateral necrosis of basal ganglia with or without Leber's optic neuropathy, hereditary spastic dystonia associated with Leber's optic neuropathy, Niemann-Pick disease or dystonic lipidosis, ataxia telangiectasia, neuroacanthocytosis, juvenile neuronal ceroid lipofuscinosis, and Hartnup disease.

C. Degenerative CNS diseases: Parkinson's disease, juvenile-onset parkinsonism with dystonia, levodopa–responsive dystonia, amyotrophy, progressive supranuclear palsy, multiple system atrophy, Huntington's disease, pallidal degenerations, olivopontocerebellar atrophy, Machado-Joseph or Azorean disease.

D. Nondegenerative CNS diseases: perinatal anoxia or kernicterus; head trauma; cerebral infarction or hemorrhage; chronic subdural hematoma; arteriovenous malformation; tumor; intracranial mass such as toxoplasmosis, encephalitis and postinfectious syndromes; hemidystonia, usually resulting from contralateral basal ganglial lesion; toxins such as manganese, carbon monoxide, methanol, carbon disulfide, and cyanide; paraneoplastic postoperative thalamotomy; multiple sclerosis; and drugs such as neuroleptics, levodopa or dopamine agonists, amitriptyline, ergotamine, phenobarbital, flecainide, alfentanil, midazolam, buspirone, sulpiride, calcium channel blockers, and anticonvulsants. *Note:* Tardive dystonia or acute dystonic reaction may occur after exposure to a dopamine receptor-blocking agent.

The pathophysiologic basis of dystonia remains a mystery. Dystonic patients with focal brain injury often have disease in the brainstem, caudate nucleus, putamen, or thalamus. Noradrenergic system disturbances may mediate the disorder in some patients.

Treatment of dystonia is best approached by basing it on a specific diagnosis. For the treatment of primary dystonias, levodopa-responsive dystonias (such as diurnal dystonia) respond to 200 to 300 mg/day of levodopa, starting with 100 mg/day, then slowly increasing the dose.

Focal dystonias often dramatically improve with injections of botulinum toxin, type A (Botox). Injections can reduce dystonic contractions for 3 to 6 months. Doses range from 2.5 to 3.75 units of Botox activity for spastic dysphonia to 25 units per eye divided in five or six sites around each eye for blepharospasm, up to 450 units for torticollis and empirical doses for writer's cramp, with repeated injections of tiny amounts of Botox. Injections require EMG guidance in spastic dysphonia, oromandibular and lower facial dystonias, and brachial dystonias but not in blepharospasm. Botox appears safe and effective for focal dystonias, although its safety for chronic use in children has not yet been established.

Segmental, multifocal, and generalized dystonias may respond to low-dose levodopa and high-dose anticholinergics. Trihexyphenidyl is started at 2.5 mg/day and increased by 2.5 mg weekly or even more slowly, up to 100 mg/day or more, until response is seen or toxicity is reached. Trihexyphenidyl is better tolerated in children than in adults. For adults, doses of ethopropazine ranging from 25 mg/day up to 100 mg/day may be better tolerated. About 40% to 60% of patients respond to these medications. Baclofen, clonazepam, carbamazepine or dopamine-depleting agents such as reserpine or metyrosine can also be used, but their response rates are lower. Tetrabenazine, an agent with both dopamine-depleting and dopamine receptor-blocking activity, administered alone or with lithium, may be effective.

Hemidystonia, especially when idiopathic, and refractory bilateral dystonia or severe axial dystonia may subside with thalamotomy. Selective sensory or cervical cord stimulation for cervical dystonias has produced variable results and is a last resort. Paroxysmal dystonias (kinesiogenic more often than nonkinesiogenic) may respond to carbamazepine, phenytoin, clonazepam, or acetazolamide. Nocturnal paroxysmal dystonia seems particularly responsive to carbamazepine.

Secondary dystonias in general respond less impressively to treatment than do primary dystonias. Acute dystonic reactions often respond to anticholinergics. Tardive dystonia may resolve with high-dose anticholinergics, dopamine depletors, antihistamines, or benzodiazepines. Often, treatments must be tried empirically and sequentially before benefit is achieved, and side effects must always be weighed against potential benefits of treatment.

REF: Bressman SB, Greene PE: Treatment of hyperkinetic movement disorders, *Neurol Clin* 8:51-56, 1990.

Lang AE: Movement disorder symptomatology. In Bradley WG et al, eds: *Neurology in clinical practice*, Boston, 1991, Butterworth-Heinemann.

EATON-LAMBERT MYASTHENIC SYNDROME   *(see Lambert-Eaton Myasthenic Syndrome)*

ECLAMPSIA   *(see Pregnancy)*

EDEMA   *(see Intracranial Pressure)*

EDROPHONIUM TEST   *(see Myasthenia Gravis)*

EIGHTH CRANIAL NERVE *(see Cranial Nerves, Hearing Vertigo, Evoked Potentials)*

ELECTROCARDIOGRAM (ECG)

Changes in electrocardiographic rhythm and morphologic characteristics may occur with acute CNS disease in the absence of other causes. Although most frequently reported in subarachnoid hemorrhage (SAH), electrocardiogram (ECG) changes can be seen in migraine, brain tumor, head injury, and stroke. In patients with epilepsy, cortical stimulation of the left insula leads to bradycardia and depressor effects; the opposite effect occurs on stimulation of the right insula.

CNS disease is associated with both ventricular and supraventricular arrhythmias, the former occurring more frequently in the presence of elevated levels of cardiac enzymes. Morphologic changes include Q waves, ST elevation or depression, and U waves. In SAH, large upright or deeply inverted T waves and prolonged QT intervals are characteristic. These changes may be mediated by increased sympathetic tone associated with hypothalamic involvement and are often associated with elevations in creatine kinase levels and regional wall motion abnormalities. Both ischemic and hemorrhagic myocardial damage have been noted in association with SAH.

REF: Oppenheimer MB et al: *Neurology* 42:1727, 1992.

Vingerhoets F et al: *Stroke* 24:26-30, 1993.

ELECTROENCEPHALOGRAPHY (EEG)

Electroencephalography (EEG) provides a recording of electrical activity originating from extracellular current flow in the superficial layers of cerebral cortex. This activity reflects the major influence of subcortical structures, especially the brainstem reticular formation and intralaminar and reticular nuclei of the thalamus, in generating the three normal states of consciousness: waking, nonrapid eye movement sleep (NREM), and rapid eye movement sleep (REM). EEG is useful in clinical practice in large part because it provides real-time information regarding the physiologic rather than structural characteristics of the brain.

I. The normal adult waking EEG may contain the following.

A. Alpha rhythm (8 to 13 Hz): Alpha rhythm is maximally present occipitally in nearly all adults. It appears during relaxed wakefulness with eyes closed and attenuates with eye opening or mental effort; these characteristics distinguish it from *alpha activity*, which merely satisfies the frequency criterion (see mention of alpha coma in section D below). The alpha rhythm reaches a frequency of 8 Hz by about age 3, and stays at or above that frequency in most normal elderly individuals.

B. Beta activity (> 13 Hz): A normal finding unless its amplitude consistently exceeds 25 mV, which may suggest the presence of benzodiazepines, barbiturates, or chloral hydrate. Beta activity is enhanced over skull defects (breach rhythm), sometimes appears quite "spiky" and depressed in areas of focal brain injury and over subdural, epidural, or subgaleal fluid collections.

C. Theta activity (4 to 7 Hz): Admixed and of low voltage in normal records, theta activity becomes more sustained and prominent during drowsiness. Normal elderly individuals may have a limited amount of shifting temporal theta activity. Activity at frequencies slower than 4 Hz *(delta)* should not be present in the waking adult record.

D. Mu rhythm: A rhythm of alpha frequency that is located centrally, appears with eyes open, and blocks with contralateral extremity movement. It originates from sensorimotor cortex.

E. Lambda waves: These sharp, surface negative transients appear over occipital regions, only with eyes open, especially upon looking at a strong visual pattern.

F. Other benign patterns appearing during waking or drowsiness: These include rhythmic temporal theta bursts of drowsiness (psychomotor variant), subclinical rhythmic electrographic discharge of adults (SREDA), benign epileptiform transients of sleep (BETS), positive occipital sharp transients of sleep (POSTS), 14- and 6-Hz positive bursts, 6-Hz phantom spike and wave, and wicket spikes.

G. Hyperventilation (HV) response: A physiologic increase in generalized slowing occurs with prolonged HV, particularly in children, and is accentuated with hypoglycemia. Abnormalities during HV include focal slowing or epileptiform discharges.

H. Photic stimulation response: Normal photomyoclonic responses consist of muscular contractions, typically orbicularis oculi, elicited by each flash. Abnormal photoparoxysmal responses, bursts of generalized epileptiform discharges that may outlast the flash stimuli, are indicative of generalized epilepsy or an inherited EEG trait.

II. The normal adult sleep EEG may contain the following.

  A. Stage 1 sleep (drowsiness) is defined by dropout of the waking alpha rhythm, accentuation of frontocentral theta activity, and slow, rolling eye movements. *Vertex waves*, large-amplitude, sharp, surface-negative transients maximal at the central vertex, may occur.

  B. Stage 2 sleep is marked by the appearance of sleep spindles, rhythmic 12- to 15-Hz waves with morphologic waxing and waning; and K complexes, large, biphasic, sharp transients maximal over the vertex, often precipitated by external stimuli.

  C. Stages 3 and 4 sleep are defined by the presence of delta waves at a frequency of more than 50% 2 Hz or slower and an amplitude greater than 75 μv, which occur during 20% to 50% or during more than 50% of a 30-second epoch (stages 3 and 4, respectively).

  D. REM sleep is defined by relatively low-voltage desynchronized EEG activity, muscular atonia, and bursts of rapid eye movements.

III. EEG abnormalities include the following.

  A. Epilepsy: Interictal epileptiform activity consisting of spikes, sharp waves, or spike-wave complexes is strongly but not absolutely correlated with epilepsy. Thus the presence of spikes, sharp waves, or spike-wave complexes does not unequivocally indicate a diagnosis of epilepsy, nor does their absence exclude it. Nevertheless, their presence, in combination with clinical information, frequently allows one to make a diagnosis in terms of recognized electroclinical syndromes (see Epilepsy). Ictal discharges or electrographic seizures provide irrefutable evidence of an epileptic seizure disorder. In generalized epilepsies electrographic seizures may consist of a pronged run of otherwise typical interictal discharges, but in partial epilepsies this is rarely the case and the ictal patterns have their own morphologic features. The absence of an ictal EEG pattern during a typical generalized convulsion provides strong evidence of a nonpileptic seizure (See Epilepsy), but this is less true for auras, focal motor or sensory seizures, or complex partial seizures.

  B. Focal brain lesions: The presence of continuous, focal, polymorphic delta activity, especially in combination with depression of ipsilateral background rhythms, strongly suggests a focal lesion. However, an area of focal dysfunction, as may be seen after complicated migraine or a focal seizure, should also be considered. Periodic lateralized epileptiform discharges (PLEDs) are frequently associated with irritative lesions such as acute cerebral infarcts or herpes simplex encephalitis.

C. Diffuse encephalopathies: The EEG has a high sensitivity for detecting globally disturbed cerebral function but is nonspecific as to origin. Exceptions include Alzheimer's disease and HIV encephalopathy, in which the EEG may remain normal until late in the course of the disease. Early changes include slowing of the alpha rhythm and the appearance of generalized theta activity, more severe cases show generalized polymorphic delta activity, frontal intermittent rhythmic delta activity (FIRDA), and lack of normal reactivity. Triphasic waves are seen in hepatic or other metabolic encephalopathies and may be periodic. Other conditions associated with periodic discharges include Creutzfeldt-Jakob disease (in which most patients have periodic sharp discharges that occur at intervals of about 1 second, within 12 weeks of diagnosis) and subacute sclerosing panencephalitis (periodic, generalized slow waves or sharp, slow complexes at intervals of about 5 to 10 seconds).

D. Coma: Findings include lack of normal background, reactivity, or state changes in combination with continuous generalized polymorphic delta activity, FIRDA, low-voltage patterns, periodic discharges that include PLEDS or triphasic waves, or burst-suppression pattern (bursts of electrical activity separated by periods of diffuse voltage suppression, indicative of severe diffuse cerebral dysfunction). In patients with coma following seizures, electrographic status epilepticus should be ruled out. Alpha coma with generalized, invariant, unreactive alpha-frequency activity is associated with toxic or metabolic insults and cerebral anoxia and must be distinguished from normal alpha rhythms present in those with a "locked-in state."

E. Brain death: Confirmatory evidence includes the demonstration of electrocerebral silence (ECS) under proper technical conditions in the appropriate clinical context. Conditions associated with reversible ECS include overdose of CNS depressants, hypothermia, cardiovascular shock, metabolic and endocrine disorders, and very young age.

REF: Daly DD, Pedley TA, eds: *Current practice of clinical electroencephalography*, ed 2, New York, 1990, Raven.

ELECTROLYTE DISORDERS

Symptoms are usually more severe with acute changes in electrolyte levels. Occasionally, chronic disturbances may produce signs and symptoms opposite from those in the acute state. In general, central nervous system dysfunction occurs with abnormalities of sodium, peripheral nervous system dysfunction with abnormal potassium levels, and combinations of both with abnormalities calcium, magnesium, and phosphate. Management is directed at treatment of the primary disorder and correction of the electrolyte abnormality. Neurologic findings usually disappear with appropriate therapy (see Table 18 for signs and symptoms).

SODIUM (Na⁺)

Sodium is the main determinant of serum osmolality (Osm) and extracellular fluid volume. Therefore, neurologic symptoms are dependent on the time lag necessary for the brain to compensate for rapid changes in serum Na^+ concentration, and thus, Osm.

Hyponatremia: Acute decreases of Na^+ levels to 130 mEq/L may produce symptoms. Chronic changes to 115 mEq/L may be asymptomatic. EEG abnormalities are common but nonspecific, with slowing that correlates with decreased Na^+ levels. Acute hyponatremia (< 115 mEq/L) with seizures carries a high mortality rate and necessitates rapid (over a 6-hour period) correction to 120 to 125 mEq/L (with hypertonic saline or normal saline and furosemide). *Rapid correction to levels greater than 120 to 125 mEq/L may result in central pontine myelinolysis (CPM),* a disorder primarily affecting alcoholics but also occurring in children and adults with liver disease, severe electrolyte imbalances, malnutrition, anorexia, burns, cancer, Addison's disease, and sepsis. There is symmetric focal myelin destruction predominantly involving the basal central pons.

Asymptomatic chronic hyponatremia usually requires no immediate intervention and is managed by correction of the underlying condition.

Hypernatremia: Neurologic symptoms develop when the serum Na^+ level rises above 160 mEq/L or the serum Osm is greater than 350 mOsm/Kg. Level of consciousness correlates well with the degree of hyperosmolality. Sudden increases in serum Osm may produce decreased brain cell volume, with mechanical traction on cerebral vessels causing subcortical, subdural, or subarachnoid hemorrhage. CSF protein levels may be high without pleocytosis, and the EEG is normal or mildly slowed.

TABLE 18
Neurological Signs and Symptoms of Electrolyte Disturbances

	↓Na⁺	↑Na⁺	↓K⁺	↑K⁺	↓Ca⁺⁺	↑Ca⁺⁺	↓Mg⁺⁺	↑Mg⁺⁺	Acute ↓PO₄⁼	Chronic ↓PO₄⁼
Muscle weakness	–	–	+(1)	+/–	–	+/–	+/–	+(2)	+	+(1)
Reflexes	0	0	0	0	0→↑	↓	↑(4)	↓(3)	→(4)	0→↑
Cognitive changes	+(3)	+(3)	–	–	+(3)	+(3)	+(4)	+(3)	+(4)	–
Seizures	+	+	–	–	+	+/–	+	–	+/–	–
Tetany	–	–	+(5)	–	+	+/–	+	–	–	–
Focal signs	+/–	–	–	–	+	+/–	+/–	–	+(6)	–
Abnormal movements	–	+(7,8,9)	–	–	–	–	+(8,9)	–	–	–
Other	A,B	B(10)	C	C	D	E				

(1) Proximal > distal.
(2) May be severe.
(3) Lethargy to coma.
(4) Variable or unpredictable.
(5) When associated with alkalosis.
(6) Cranial nerve palsies.
(7) Rigidity.
(8) Tremor.
(9) Myoclonus.
(10) May occur with rehydration.

(A) Cramps.
(B) Cerebral edema.
(C) Cardiac toxicity.
(D) Pseudotumor cerebri.
(E) Headache.

– Usually present.
– Usually absent.
+/– Occasionally present
↑ Usually increased
↓ Usually decreased.
0 Usually normal.

Hypernatremia resulting from diabetes insipidus may occur with tumors involving the hypothalamus or pineal region, as well as with basilar meningitis, encephalitis, ruptured aneurysms, sarcoidosis, trauma, or surgery.

Treatment with *isotonic solutions* should be given to reduce the serum Na^+ level by no more than 1 mEq/L every 2 hours during the first 2 days of treatment. Rapid infusion of hypotonic solutions may cause cerebral edema and seizures.

POTASSIUM (K^+)

Almost 60% of total body K^+ is located within muscle; therefore predominantly muscular symptoms occur with altered K^+ levels.

Hypokalemia most commonly occurs with diuretic use but also occurs with GI losses, certain antibiotics, mineralocorticoid excess, and rarely, thyrotoxicosis. Muscle weakness usually develops with serum levels of 2.5 to 3.0 mEq/L, with structural muscle damage occurring at levels below 2.0 mEq/L. Hypokalemia and hypocalcemia frequently coexist, with cancellation of neuromuscular manifestations. Treatment of one condition in isolation may produce symptoms of the other.

ECG and cardiac abnormalities are common and may require ICU monitoring and treatment.

Treatment involves increasing dietary K^+, supplements of KCl, and the use of K^+-sparing diuretics. K^+ infusions are occasionally necessary.

Hyperkalemia is relatively uncommon, but may occur in familial hyperkalemic periodic paralysis (see Periodic Paralysis). Quadriparesis may develop with levels greater than 6.8 mEq/L, and levels greater than 7.0 mEq/L are life-threatening and require ICU monitoring with immediate therapy, which may include administration of glucose and insulin, cation exchange resins, or calcium gluconate.

CALCIUM (Ca^{++})

Plasma Ca^{++} is a stabilizer of excitable membranes in the central and peripheral nervous systems and in muscle. Ca^{++} concentrations are closely controlled through the combined effects of parathyroid hormone, calciferol, and calcitonin on intestine, kidney, and bone.

Hypocalcemia is relatively rare, except in neonates, in patients with renal failure, and after thyroid or parathyroid surgery. The "tetany syndrome" originates in the peripheral nerve axon and initially becomes evident with distal and perioral tingling. Distal tonic spasms (carpopedal spasms) may progress to laryngeal stridor and opisthotonus if severe.

The EEG is diffusely slow with an exaggerated response to photic stimulation. ECG abnormalities are also common.

Treatment of mild cases is accomplished with oral calcium supplements. Tetany or seizures may require 10% IV solutions of calcium gluconate or CaCl. Underlying disorders should be corrected, if possible. Hypocalcemia often coexists with hypomagnesemia. In such cases, total serum calcium levels may be normal, but ionized calcium levels may be low.

Hypercalcemia: Malignant neoplasms are the most common cause of increased serum Ca^{++} levels. Mental status alterations occur with total serum levels greater than 14 mg/dl. Myopathy or carpal tunnel syndrome may occur in association with hyperparathyroidism.

Treatment of symptomatic patients consists of saline hydration and furosemide. Occasionally, mithramycin (suppresses bone resorption) or calcitonin (suppresses bone resorption and increases urinary Ca^{++} excretion) is required.

MAGNESIUM (Mg^{++})

Ninety-eight percent of Mg^{++} is intracellular. It is necessary for the activation of various enzymes. Extracellular Mg^{++} affects central and peripheral synaptic transmission. Changes in serum levels may not reflect total body stores.

Hypomagnesemia occurs most commonly as a result of excess renal loss (chronic alcoholism, diuretics), but may also be the result of decreased intake or absorption. Neurologic symptoms usually develop at levels below 0.8 mEq/L.

The presence of seizures requires treatment with parenteral $MgSo_4$. Oral Mg^{++} supplements may suffice in less severe cases. Calcium gluconate should be available when giving IV $MgSo_4$, as transient hypermagnesemia may cause respiratory muscle paralysis (see also hypocalcemia, above).

Hypermagnesemia, an uncommon disorder, usually occurs with increased intake and renal failure. Deep tendon reflexes may be lost at levels of 5 to 6 mEq/L, and CNS depression occurs at levels above 8 to 10 mEq/L. Muscular paralysis is due to neuromuscular blockade. Treatment of paralysis may be accomplished by small amounts of parenteral calcium gluconate and hydration. Otherwise, discontinuation of Mg^{++}-containing preparations is indicated. If renal function is severely impaired, dialysis may be necessary.

PHOSPHATE (PO$_4^=$)

Hypophosphatemia is often complicated by multiple abnormalities of electrolytes, nutrition, and acid-base balance. The syndrome commonly occurs in malnutrition and chronic alcoholism, especially after the infusion of glucose or hyperalimentation solutions.

Acute hypophosphatemia may not reflect decreased total body stores and may produce neurologic symptoms if severe (< 1.5 mEq/L). Chronic hypophosphatemia is usually moderate (1.5 to 2.5 mEq/L) and may not be symptomatic unless acute stresses (alcohol withdrawal, burns, binding of $PO_4^=$ in the gut) cause sudden decreases below the moderate level.

REF: Riggs JE. In Aminoff MJ, ed: *Neurology and general medicine.*
        New York, 1989, Churchill Livingstone.

RESPIRATORY ALKALOSIS

This condition is frequently observed in patients with bronchial asthma, hepatic cirrhosis, salicylate intoxication, hypoxia, sepsis, pneumonia, and acute anxiety (hyperventilation syndrome). Acute respiratory alkalosis constricts the cerebral arterioles and decreases the cerebral blood flow. Confusion accompanied by a slow EEG may develop.

More severe alkalosis (pH 7.52 to 7.65) in patients with respiratory insufficiency and hypoxia may result in a symptom complex of hypotension, seizures, asterixis, myoclonus, and coma. Other neurologic manifestations include paresthesias, dizziness, cramps as a result of coexistent tetany, hyperreflexia, and muscle weakness.

RESPIRATORY ACIDOSIS

Acute respiratory acidosis is a condition of low pH and high pCO_2, occurring as a result of impairment of the rate of alveolar ventilation. Lethargy and confusion occur as the pCO_2 rises above 55 mm Hg. Seizures, stupor, or coma may occur with levels greater than 70 mm Hg. The serum bicarbonate level is either normal or high, depending on how rapidly the respiratory failure developed.

Neurologic manifestations resulting from cerebral vasodilation include headache, increased intracranial pressure, and papilledema. Hyperreflexia or hyporeflexia and myoclonus may also occur. Causes of acute respiratory acidosis include sedative drugs, brainstem injury, neuromuscular disorders, chest injury, airway obstruction, and acute pulmonary disease. Chronic respiratory acidosis generally occurs in patients with chronic bronchitis, emphysema, extreme kyphoscoliosis, or extreme obesity (pickwickian syndrome). It is most often symptomatic with acute exacerbations of disease. Compensatory polycythemia often results from chronic hypercapneic states.

Therapy involves ventilatory support and treating the underlying disorder. The possibility of sedative or narcotic drug ingestion must be suspected in otherwise healthy patients who suddenly develop acute respiratory depression.

METABOLIC ALKALOSIS

Metabolic alkalosis may result from either excessive ingestion of base or excessive loss of acid. Delirium and stupor owing to this condition are rarely severe and never life-threatening; there is time for a careful diagnostic search. Severe metabolic alkalosis produces a blunted confusional state rather than stupor or coma and may result in cardiac arrhythmias and severe compensatory hypoventilation.

Neurologic manifestations include paresthesias, cramps (due to tetany), muscle weakness (due to associated hypokalemia), and hyporeflexia. Causes of hypokalemic metabolic alkalosis include Cushing's syndrome, vomiting or gastric drainage, diuretic therapy, and primary aldosteronism. Treatment depends on the underlying cause.

METABOLIC ACIDOSIS

Metabolic acidosis occurs when a decrease in plasma bicarbonate level lowers pH. Cardinal features are hyperventilation and, when severe, "Kussmaul's respiration." In chronic metabolic acidosis, hyperventilation may be difficult to detect on clinical examination. The presence of neurologic symptoms depends on various factors, including the type of systemic metabolic defect, whether the fall in systemic pH affects the pH of the brain and CSF, the rate at which acidosis develops, and the specific anion causing the metabolic disorder. All metabolic acidoses produce hyperpnea as the first neurologic symptom. Other manifestations include lethargy, drowsiness, confusion, and mild, diffuse skeletal muscle hypertonus. Extensor plantar responses occur at a later stage. Stupor, coma, or seizures generally develop only preterminally.

The most common causes of metabolic acidosis sufficient to produce coma and hyperpnea include uremia, diabetes, lactic acidosis, and ingestion of acidic poisons. Ketoacidosis occasionally develops in severe alcoholics after prolonged drinking episodes. In diabetics treated with oral hypoglycemic agents, lactic acidosis and diabetic ketoacidosis must be considered.

Since metabolic acidosis is a manifestation of a variety of different diseases, the treatment varies depending on the underlying process and on the acuteness and severity of the acidosis.

REF: Layzer RB: *Neuromuscular manifestations of systemic disease*, Philadelphia, 1985, FA Davis.

Plum F, Posner JB: *The diagnosis of stupor and coma*, ed 3, Philadelphia, 1982, FA Davis.

ELECTROMYOGRAPHY (EMG) AND NERVE CONDUCTION STUDIES (NCS)

Nerve conduction studies (NCSs) provide objective evidence of motor unit dysfunction in patients with weakness; localize and characterize

TABLE 19
Routine Nerve Conduction Studies in Neuromuscular Disorders

Disorder	Amplitude	Distal Latency	Conduction Velocity	F- and H-Wave Latencies
Polyneuropathy				
Axonal	↓	NL	>70%	Mild ↑
Demyelinating	NL or ↓	NL or ↑	<50%	↑
Myopathy	NL or ↓ motor	NL	NL	NL
Radiculopathy	NL or ↓ motor NL sensory	NL	>80%	NL or ↑
Neuromuscular transmission defect				
Presynaptic type	NL or ↓ motor NL sensory	NL	NL	NL
Postsynaptic type	NL	NL	NL	NL
Motor neuron disease	↓ motor N1 sensory	NL	>70%	NL or ↑
Upper motor neuron disease	NL	NL	NL	NL

lesions of peripheral nerves; differentiate peripheral neuropathies from myopathies, neuromuscular junction transmission defects, and motor neuron diseases; detect subclinically abnormal nerves; provide early detection of peripheral diseases (e.g., in familial disorders); and identify and characterize patterns of anomalous innervation (see Table 19).

Motor nerve conduction studies involve stimulating a peripheral nerve and recording from a muscle innervated by that nerve. Sensory nerve conduction studies are made by stimulating a mixed motor-sensory nerve and recording from a cutaneous sensory nerve, or vice versa. The amplitude, duration, shape, and latency of compound muscle action potentials (CMAPs) and sensory nerve action potentials (SNAPs) are noted; responses at two or more recording sites are compared; and distal latencies and conduction velocities are determined. The effect of repetitive stimulation, exercise and rest, and drugs (e.g., edrophonium) may also be studied. Nerve conduction norms vary with body temperature and age.

The *F wave* is a muscle action potential resulting from a supramaximal stimulus of a motor nerve that leads to an antidromic action potential that reaches the alpha motor neuron and then to generation of a second, orthodromic action potential. An F wave is recorded as a low-amplitude muscle action potential occurring after the initial CMAP (M wave) and is a means of evaluating proximal motor nerves. The F-wave latency is prolonged in neuropathies with proximal involvement such as Guillain-Barré syndrome and diabetic neuropathy. It is also prolonged in radiculopathy, some hereditary neuropathies, and motor neuron disease.

The *H wave* is a muscle action potential resulting from submaximal stimulation of a monosynaptic reflex arc with the large-diameter sensory nerves as afferents. Because of practical and anatomic considerations, the tibial H reflex (dorsal and ventral roots of the first sacral nerve [S1]) is the only one typically recorded. Thus the H reflex is the electrical equivalent of the ankle reflex, and the response disappears in peripheral neuropathies or S1 radiculopathy. The H reflex can be normally absent in persons over age 60.

Repetitive stimulation is used to confirm and differentiate defects of neuromuscular transmission. With slow repetitive stimulation (2 to 5 Hz), a CMAP amplitude decrement of more than 10% is seen in myasthenia and Lambert-Eaton syndrome. This decrement improves immediately after exercise (posttetanic facilitation) and worsens 2 to 4 minutes later (posttetanic exhaustion). With fast repetitive stimulation (30 to 50 Hz), a CMAP amplitude increment of more than 100% can be seen in presynaptic disorders such as Lambert-Eaton syndrome and botulism.

The *electromyographic needle examination* records electrical activity in muscle, yielding information on the nature and location of motor unit disorders. Changes in insertional, spontaneous, and voluntary activity may help in differential diagnosis. Abnormalities on needle examination may occur in many combinations; no single abnormality is specific for a given disease. Myopathic processes, especially inflammatory myopathies, are generally associated with increased insertional and spontaneous activity. Motor unit potential amplitude and duration are decreased, and the percentage of polyphasic potentials is increased. Recruitment may be early. In severe myopathies recruitment may be decreased. In some endocrine and metabolic myopathies EMG abnormalities may be minimal or absent (e.g., steroid myopathy).

During the first week, neurogenic lesions are associated with normal insertional and spontaneous activity. Motor unit potentials have a normal appearance, but recruitment is decreased. Within 2 to 3 weeks insertional activity and then fibrillation potentials appear. With reinnervation, spontaneous activity decreases, short-duration polyphasic motor unit potentials appear, and recruitment improves; variation in motor unit potentials may be noted. In chronic neurogenic disorders motor unit potential amplitude and duration are increased, and the percentage of polyphasic potentials is increased.

The following disorders are associated with specific abnormalities found on the needle examination.

INSERTIONAL ACTIVITY

Associated with needle insertion, insertional activity is increased in denervated muscle, myotonic disorders, and some myopathies, especially inflammatory myopathies. It is decreased in periodic paralysis during paralytic phases and when normal muscle tissue is replaced by fibrous tissue.

SPONTANEOUS ACTIVITY

Fibrillation potentials (brief, regular, single-fiber action potentials) and *positive sharp waves* (longer-duration, regular, single-fiber action potentials) occur 2 to 3 weeks after denervation in lower motor neuron disease (diseases of the anterior horn cell, root, plexus, and nerve, especially axonal), myositis, certain dystrophies, hyperkalemic periodic paralysis, acid maltase deficiency, rhabdomyolysis, trichinosis, and muscle trauma and rarely in neuromuscular junction disorders.

Fasciculation potentials are random discharges of an entire motor unit. They are most common in chronic neurogenic disorders (motor neuron disease, peripheral neuropathies, and root compression). They are also seen in normal individuals with fatigue or cramps and in many other disorders including tetany, thyrotoxicosis, and use of anticholinesterases.

Myotonic discharges (crescendo and decrescendo, "dive bomber" discharges) are seen in myotonic disorders, periodic paralysis, acid maltase deficiency, diazocholesterol toxicity, clofibrate toxicity and rarely in polymyositis and colchicine toxicity.

Complex repetitive discharges (bizarre, high-frequency potentials) occur in a wide variety of chronic neurogenic disorders (poliomyelitis, motor neuron disease, radiculopathies, and neuropathies) and myopathic disorders (Duchenne type and limb-girdle muscular dystrophy, polymyositis, hypothyroidism, and Schwartz-Jampel syndrome). Complex repetitive discharges should be distinguished from other repetitive discharges.

Myokymic discharges (regular bursts of normal unit potentials) may be recorded in facial muscle in multiple sclerosis, brainstem neoplasm, polyradiculopathy, or facial palsy. Appendicular myokymia is associated with radiation plexopathy, chronic nerve compression, and gold toxicity.

Neuromyotonia (continuous muscle fiber activity or "pseudo myotonia") can be seen in Isaac's syndrome.

Cramp potentials occur commonly in normal individuals and in many disorders, including electrolyte imbalances, neurogenic atrophy, hypothyroidism, and uremia, as well as during pregnancy.

VOLUNTARY MOTOR UNIT POTENTIALS

Short-duration motor unit potentials occur in disorders with atrophy or loss of muscle fibers in the motor unit. Thus they are present in all muscular dystrophies, many congenital myopathies, toxic myopathies, polymyositis, periodic paralysis, neuromuscular transmission defects, early reinnervation, and late neurogenic atrophy.

Long-duration potentials occur with increased number or density of muscle fibers or with a loss of synchrony of fiber firing within a motor unit, such as in motor neuron disease, chronic radiculopathies, chronic axonal neuropathies with sprouting, and polymyositis.

Polyphasic motor unit potentials (five or more phases) may occur in both myopathic and neurogenic disorders.

Fluctuations in amplitude, duration, or shape of a given motor unit potential from moment to moment are usually due to blocking of individual muscle fiber action potentials in the motor unit and may be seen in disorders of neuromuscular transmission, myositis, muscle trauma, reinnervation, and rapidly progressive neurogenic atrophy.

Recruitment refers to the relation of firing rate of individual potentials to the total number of motor units firing. *Decreased recruitment* (small number of units firing with a high frequency) occurs when there is a loss of whole motor units, as in any neurogenic disorder or in severe myopathies. *Early recruitment* (an excess of motor units for a given force) occurs in myopathies when the force generated by individual motor units is decreased.

Poor activation of motor units (small number of units firing slowly) can be due to upper motor neuron lesions or lack of effort.

REF: Kimura J: *Electrodiagnosis of diseases of nerve and muscle: principles and practice*, ed 2, Philadelphia, 1989, FA Davis.

ELECTRORETINOGRAM *(see Evoked Potentials)*

EMBOLISM *(see Ischemia)*

ENCEPHALITIS

An inflammation of brain related to infectious, postinfectious, or demyelinating states. It can occur as an acute febrile illness associated with headache, seizures, lethargy, confusion, coma, ocular motor palsies, ataxia, abnormal movements, and myoclonus. Alternatively it may become evident as a slowly progressive afebrile disease. With viral infections the meninges (in meningoencephalitis) or the spinal cord (in encephalomyelitis) is often involved. Compared to the high incidence of systemic viral infection, encephalitis is an uncommon complication. Prognosis of viral encephalitis depends on the causative agent (e.g., herpes simplex virus) and the use of antiviral agents. Variable degrees of residua include impaired cognition and memory, behavioral changes, hemiparesis, or seizures.

Transmission of viruses can be from humans (e.g., HIV), animals (e.g., rabies), mosquitos (e.g., St. Louis and Japanese encephalitides), ticks (e.g., central European encephalitis), or other arthropods. Endemic causes in the United States are herpes simplex virus and rabies. Japaneses type B encephalitis is the most common epidemic infection outside North America. Arthropod-borne viruses (arboviruses) tend to be sporadic or epidemic. Viruses enter the central nervous system by one of two routes, hematogenous (most common) or neuronal.

Diagnosis may be difficult and can sometimes be made by the history alone. The season may help determine the causative agent. Examination of the CSF shows a pleocytosis (mostly mononuclear cells), and mildly elevated protein levels are usually seen. Glucose levels tend to be normal. Red blood cells can be found in certain encephalitides (e.g., those caused by herpes simplex virus). Determinations of antibody levels in serum and CSF during acute and convalescent stages typically are only useful retrospectively.

VIRAL CAUSES

Herpes simplex virus encephalitis (HSV type 1): Most common cause of fatal viral encephalitis in the United States. Most cases represent reactivation of endogenous infection. Onset is usually subacute, and fever, headache, behavioral changes, seizures, and focal signs are common. Stupor and coma may result. The EEG is typically abnormal, often showing periodic lateralizing epileptiform discharges (PLEDs) or other focal abnormalities. Spike and slow waves are common and are often localized to the temporal lobe. CT scan, although less sensitive than EEG, may show temporal or insular low densities and focal hemorrhages or enhancement. MRI may show increased medial temporal lobe signal intensity on T2-weighted sequences. CSF is rarely normal; it usually contains 50 to 100 cells per mm^3, elevated protein levels, normal glucose levels, and elevated opening pressure. Red blood cells may be seen. A fourfold rise in titer HSV antibody in CSF is 90% sensitive and 80% specific, peaking at 4 to 6 weeks. Serum: CSF HSV antibody ratio of 20 or less is diagnostic but is usually not positive until day 4. Untreated, HSV type 1 has a mortality rate of about 70%; severe neurologic sequela occur in most of the survivors. Acyclovir, 10 mg per kg q8h for 10 days, significantly reduces morbidity and mortality rates, especially if started early. Brain biopsy should be considered in those who do not respond to therapy or in patients for whom other diagnoses (such as tuberculosis, and the like) are possible.

Rabies: Carriers include skunks, foxes, dogs, bats, and raccoons. The virus is in the saliva and is transmitted by bite. Incubation is from days to months. Not everyone bitten by rabid animals contracts the disease. However, once the infection is established, death almost invariably occurs (usually within 18 days). The prodrome usually consists of headache, malaise, agitation, mental changes, seizures, dysphagia (causing hydrophobia), dysarthria, facial numbness, and spasm. The medulla and pons are most frequently and extensively involved, and paralysis may occur as a result of spinal cord involvement. Treatment consists of mechanically scrubbing wound sites with soap and benzalkonium solution and administering human rabies immunoglobulin or human diploid cell line rabies vaccine. Death invariably results once CNS manifestations occur.

Epidemic encephalitis: Primarily arthropod-transmitted viral diseases with a peak incidence in later summer and fall. In the United States, St. Louis encephalitis is the most common; it occurs in the Ohio–Mississippi River basin and has a mortality rate of 10% to 20%. Venezuelan equine encephalitis is found in the southeastern United States and has a very low mortality rate; most infections result in flulike illnesses. Eastern equine encephalitis occurs along the Gulf of Mexico and the Atlantic seaboard, usually affects horses and birds, and is rare among humans. It has a mortality rate of 25% to 75% and attacks the young and very old with a fulminant, severe course. Western equine encephalitis occurs in the west and southwest and in central North America, and California virus encephalitis, with a low incidence of overt disease and low mortality rates, occurs in the midwestern states. Treatment is aimed at controlling brain edema and seizures.

Nonepidemic viral encephalitis: Enterovirus, enteric cytopathic human orphan virus (ECHO), coxsackie virus, polio, measles, mumps, Epstein-Barr virus, rubella, varicella zoster, and lymphocytic choriomeningitis virus can all cause sporadic encephalitis.

Slow latent viral infections: Cause slowly progressive disease with insidious onset and lack of fever. These include subacute sclerosing panencephalitis (SSPE), a form of chronic measles virus infection, progressive multifocal leukoencephalopathy (PML) (see the discussion below, "Associated with AIDS and immunodeficiency states"), and progressive rubella panencephalitis.

SSPE has had dramatically decreased prevalence in countries with widespread use of the measles vaccine, but prevalence has increased with the occurrence of AIDS. Onset is insidious and becomes evident with changes in cognition, vision, and behavior. Malaise and lethargy are common. Myoclonus can occur. Deterioration progresses over weeks to months; patients become markedly demented. CSF shows a mild pleocytosis, increased protein levels, and occasionally decreased glucose levels. Neuroimaging shows generalized cortical atrophy. The EEG pattern of periodic discharges is characteristic. Pathologic studies show changes suggestive of viral invasion of gray and white matter, and the hypothalamus and brainstem are usually not involved.

Associated with AIDS and immunodeficiency states: PML is caused by a papovavirus designated JC virus (not associated with Creutzfeldt-Jacob disease) usually occurs in patients with lymphoproliferative (leukemia or lymphoma) or granulomatous disease or during immunosuppression. It is characterized by multifocal white matter signs such as impaired speech, vision, and cognition and progresses to death in 1 to 18 months. MRI shows multifocal white matter lesions. Arabinoside C has been used but usually without dramatic results.

NONVIRAL CAUSES OF ENCEPHALITIS OR ENCEPHALOMYELITIS

Prion infections: Prion (proteinaceous infectious particle) diseases are sometimes confused with encephalitides but are slowly progressive with insidious onset and absence of fever. They include Creutzfeldt-Jakob disease, Gerstmann-Straussler-Scheinker syndrome, fatal familial insomnia, and kuru (see Creutzfeldt-Jakob disease).

Rickettsia: Epidemic, murine and scrub typhus, Rocky Mountain spotted fever, Q fever.

Bacteria: Brucellosis, pertussis, legionnaires' disease, tuberculosis, tularemia, typhoid fever, bubonic plague, dysentery, cholera, melioidosis, psittacosis, leprosy, scarlet fever, rheumatic fever.

Spirochetes: Relapsing fever, syphilis (meningovascular), rat bite fever, leptospirosis, Lyme disease.

Protozoa and Metazoa: Entamoeba and Naegleria organisms, trypanosomiasis, leishmaniasis, malaria, toxoplasmosis.

Helminthic: Ancylostomiasis, angiostrongyliasis, ascariasis, cysticercosis, echinococcosis, filariasis, schistosomiasis, toxocariasis, trichinosis.

Miscellaneous: Behçet's disease, Whipple's disease of the CNS, vasculitis, Rasmussen's syndrome (chronic focal encephalitis).

Postinfectious encephalomyelitis: May follow a CNS or systemic viral infection, nonviral infection, or immunization. In the United States, associated most commonly with varicella and upper respiratory infections (especially influenza), whereas worldwide it most commonly follows measles infection. A disturbance of the immune system is the presumed cause; an irreversible monophasic, demyelinating syndrome results. Limited CNS forms include acute transverse myelitis, acute cerebellitis, and postinfectious optic neuritis. Acute hemorrhagic encephalitis (Hurst's disease) is a severe and usually fatal form. The clinical symptoms and CSF profile are similar to those seen during direct viral infections. The role of steroids and other forms of immunosuppression in the treatment of this syndrome has not been determined.

REF: Gorbach SL, Bartlett JG, Blacklow NR: *Infectious disease*, Philadelphia, 1992, WB Saunders.

   Rubeiz H, Roos RP. In Johnson RT, Griffin JW, eds: *Current therapy in neurologic disease*, ed 4, St Louis, 1993, Mosby.

   Whitley RJ: Viral encephalitis, *N Engl J Med* 323:242-250, 1990.

ENCEPHALOPATHY   *(see also Coma, Dialysis, Electrolyte Disorders, Glucose, Thyroid, Uremia)*

A nonspecific term for diffuse brain dysfunction, usually the result of a systemic condition. Initially, there is impaired attention, confusion, and disorientation. Later, there may be progression to stupor and coma, or in some cases the presentation may be coma of unknown cause. Associated features may include agitation, hallucinations, myoclonus, asterixis, generalized seizures, or EEG slowing or triphasic waves.

ENCEPHALOPATHY, PERINATAL HYPOXIC-ISCHEMIC

Hypoxic-ischemic encephalopathy (HIE) is caused by both diminished oxygen delivery and diminished blood perfusion to the brain. Timing of the insult may be antepartum (20%), intrapartum (35%), both (35%), or postnatal (10%).

Infants who have sustained serious intrauterine asphyxia exhibit a "neonatal neurologic syndrome" described by Volpe. Symptoms during the first 12 hours of life include stupor or coma, respiratory irregularity, dysconjugate eye movements, hypotonia, and seizures. Between 12 to 24 hours such infants show an apparent increase in level of alertness, jitteriness, seizures, weakness, and apnea. From 24 to 72 hours consciousness again deteriorates, respiratory arrest may occur, and there are frequently other signs of brainstem dysfunction. After 72 hours, if the infant survives, consciousness improves, and there may be persistent hypotonia and weakness as well as poor feeding because of poor coordination of suck and swallow.

Management of an asphyxiated infant includes ensuring adequate ventilation, oxygenation, and perfusion, avoidance of hyperviscosity, maintenance of blood glucose level between 75 and 100 mg/dl, prevention of fluid overload, and control of seizures. A lumbar puncture should be performed to rule out meningitis. If the infant's condition is not stable enough for this procedure, a full course of empiric antibiotics is indicated. EEG usually shows voltage suppression and slowing. Ultrasound is sensitive for hemorrhagic lesions but is less sensitive for ischemic lesions, especially early in the disease. CT may show loss of gray-white differentiation (associated with neuronal loss), cerebral edema, or focal ischemic lesions.

Prognosis: A recognizable neonatal neurologic syndrome is the single most useful predictor of neurologic outcome. Infants who never develop such a syndrome will have a good outcome. Infants with a mild syndrome whose examination results and EEG normalize by 1 week of age have a good neurologic prognosis. Infants with a severe syndrome almost always have a poor neurologic outcome. Seizures, especially in the first 12 hours of life, and a burst-suppression pattern on EEG are associated with poor outcome.

Although HIE is an important cause of neurologic morbidity, the majority of infants who experience hypoxic-ischemic insults do *not* exhibit an overt neonatal neurologic syndrome or later evidence of brain injury.

REF: Volpe JJ, ed: Hypoxic-ischemic encephalopathy. In *Neurology of the newborn*, ed 2, Philadelphia, 1987, WB Saunders.

ENDOCRINE DISORDERS   *(see Electrolyte Disorders, Glucose, Muscle Disorders, Pituitary, Thyroid)*

EPIDURAL ABSCESS   *(see Abscess, Epidural)*

EPIDURAL HEMORRHAGE   *(see Hemorrhage)*

EPILEPSY
DEFINITIONS AND CLASSIFICATIONS

The epilepsies are a group of conditions marked by recurrent seizures, which are the clinical manifestations of abnormal electrical discharges in the brain. Epileptic seizures are classified as *focal* (partial and local) when they begin in a part of one hemisphere and as *generalized* when they begin bilaterally, or they are *unclassified* as to focal or generalized beginnings. Focal seizures that subsequently evolve to generalized seizures are said to exhibit secondary generalization. On clinical examination partial seizures are either *simple*, that is, without impairment of consciousness, or *complex*, that is, with impairment of consciousness. The epilepsies are classified in regard to both the seizures they produce and their origins. In *primary epilepsies*, which probably have a strong genetic predisposition, there is no underlying structural, metabolic, or pathologic process and interictal neurologic function is generally normal. *Symptomatic epilepsies* are the consequence of a known or suspected disease of the brain, and in *cryptogenic epilepsies* the cause is unknown but presumed to be symptomatic.

International Classification of Epileptic Seizures

I. Partial (focal, local) seizures.
   A. Simple partial seizures.
      1. With motor signs.
      2. With somatosensory or special sensory symptoms.
      3. With autonomic symptoms or signs.
      4. With psychic symptoms.
   B. Complex partial seizures.
      1. Simple partial onset.
      2. With impairment of consciousness at onset.
   C. Partial seizures evolving to secondarily generalized seizures.
      1. Simple partial seizures evolving to generalized seizures.
      2. Complex partial seizures evolving to generalized seizures.
      3. Simple partial seizures evolving to complex partial seizures that evolve to generalized seizures.
II. Generalized seizures (convulsive or nonconvulsive).
   A. Absence seizures.
      1. Typical absence.
      2. Atypical absence.
   B. Myoclonic seizures.
   C. Clonic seizures.
   D. Tonic seizures.
   E. Tonic-clonic seizures.
   F. Atonic seizures (astatic seizures).
III. Unclassified seizures.

REF: Commission on Classification: *Epilepsia* 22:489-501, 1981.

REVISED INTERNATIONAL CLASSIFICATION OF EPILEPSIES, EPILEPTIC SYNDROMES, AND RELATED SEIZURE DISORDERS

I. Localization-related (focal, local, partial).
   A. Idiopathic (primary).
      1. Benign childhood epilepsy with centrotemporal spikes ("benign rolandic epilepsy").
      2. Childhood epilepsy with occipital paroxysms.
      3. Primary reading epilepsy.
   B. Symptomatic (secondary).
      1. Temporal lobe epilepsies.
      2. Frontal lobe epilepsies.
      3. Parietal lobe epilepsies.
      4. Occipital lobe epilepsies.

    5. Chronic progressive epilepsia partialis continua of childhood (Koshevnikoff's disease).

    6. Syndromes characterized by seizures with specific modes of precipitation (e.g., reflex epilepsy or startle epilepsies).

  C. Cryptogenic, defined by:

    1. Seizures type.

    2. Clinical features.

    3. Causes.

    4. Anatomic localization.

II. Generalized

  A. Primary (idiopathic), in order of age of onset.

    1. Benign neonatal familial convulsions.

    2. Benign neonatal convulsions.

    3. Benign myoclonic epilepsy in infancy.

    4. Childhood absence epilepsy (pyknolepsy).

    5. Juvenile absence epilepsy.

    6. Juvenile myoclonic epilepsy (of Janz).

    7. Epilepsy with generalized tonic-clonic convulsions on awakening.

    8. Other generalized idiopathic epilepsies.

    9. Epilepsies with seizures precipitated by specific modes of activation.

  B. Cryptogenic or symptomatic, in order of age of onset.

    1. West's syndrome.

    2. Lennox-Gastaut syndrome.

    3. Epilepsy with myoclonic-astatic seizures.

    4. Epilepsy with myoclonic absences.

  C. Symptomatic (secondary).

    1. Nonspecific origin.

      a. Early myoclonic encephalopathy.

      b. Early infantile epileptic encephalopathy with suppression bursts.

      c. Other symptomatic generalized epilepsies.

    2. Specific syndromes such as neurologic diseases with seizures as a prominent feature.

III. Epilepsies not determined to be focal or generalized.

  A. With both focal and generalized seizures.

    1. Neonatal seizures.

    2. Severe myoclonic epilepsy of infancy.

    3. Epilepsy with continuous spike waves during slow-wave sleep.

      4. Acquired epileptic aphasia (Landau-Kleffner syndrome).
      5. Other undetermined epilepsies.
IV. Special syndromes.
   A. Situation-related seizures.
      1. Febrile convulsions.
      2. Isolated seizures or isolated status epilepticus.
      3. Seizures occurring only with acute metabolic or toxic events related to factors such as alcohol, drugs, eclampsia, and nonketotic hyperglycemia.

REF: Committee on Classification, *Epilepsia* 30:389-399, 1989.

DIFFERENTIAL DIAGNOSIS OF EPILEPSY

Conditions producing symptoms or signs that may be mistaken for epileptic seizures include the following:

1. Syncope.
2. Transient ischemic attacks.
3. Migraine.
4. Metabolic derangements (e.g., hypoglycemia).
5. Parasomnias.
6. Transient global amnesia.
7. Paroxysmal movement disorders (e.g., paroxysmal kinesiogenic choreoathetosis).
8. Nonepileptic seizures (pseudoseizures).

Nonepileptic seizures are common and may coexist in patients with epileptic seizures. They are associated with a variety of psychiatric syndromes, including somatoform disorders, panic disorders, dissociative disorders, psychotic disorders, factitious disorders, and malingering. They may be difficult to distinguish from epileptic seizures, especially those of mesial temporal, basal frontal, and supplementary motor area origins. Seizures originating from these areas may not be associated with scalp ictal EEG changes (see Electroencephalography).

REF: Gates JR et al. In Rowan A, Gates JR, eds: *Non-epileptic seizures*, Boston, 1993, Butterworth-Heinemann.

SELECTED EPILEPSY SYNDROMES
Idiopathic Syndromes

   Benign childhood epilepsy with centrotemporal spikes (benign rolandic epilepsy) is a common autosomal dominant syndrome producing nocturnal generalized convulsions in otherwise normal children. Focal motor or sensory seizures, often involving the face, may occur. The EEG shows characteristic interictal centrotemporal spikes. Seizures are easily controlled with phenytoin or carbamazepine and spontaneously disappear before adulthood.

Childhood absence epilepsy (pyknolepsy) occurs in genetically predisposed but otherwise normal children and is marked by typical absence seizures with a corresponding 3-Hz generalized spike-and-wave EEG discharge. Typical absences are not preceded by an aura or followed by postictal confusion. Generalized tonic-clonic seizures may also occur. Treatment consists of ethosuximide, which is effective only for absence seizures, and valproic acid, which is effective both for isolated absence seizures and for absences with or complicated by generalized tonic-clonic seizures. Absence seizures rarely persist into adulthood.

Juvenile myoclonic epilepsy (of Janz) is a genetic epilepsy syndrome whose gene has been mapped to chromosome 6. It becomes evident in normal teenagers with early morning myoclonic jerks and generalized tonic clonic seizures. Sleep deprivation and photic stimulation are often activating influences. The interictal EEG typically shows 4- to 6-Hz generalized irregular spike-wave or polyspike-wave discharges with normal background. Valproate is highly effective, but relapses are the rule when therapy is discontinued.

Symptomatic or Cryptogenic Syndromes

West's syndrome consists of the triad of infantile spasms, developmental arrest, and the interictal EEG pattern of hypsarrhythmia, which consists of multifocal spikes of very high voltage, sharp waves, and slow waves in a chaotic distribution. The syndrome may be cryptogenic or symptomatic of a variety of brain insults and is generally treated with ACTH (typically 40 units IM daily, increasing by 10 units per week as needed to maximum of 80 units daily) or other corticosteroids. Prognosis is unfavorable and is worse in the cryptogenic than in the symptomatic group. *Lennox-Gastaut syndrome* is characterized by multiple seizure types that are difficult to control, especially atonic seizures and atypical absences, in addition to generalized convulsions, mental retardation, and an abnormal interictal EEG with generalized 2- to 2.5-Hz slow spike and wave discharges. The syndrome often follows West's syndrome in an affected child and is associated with a poor prognosis. Valproate is the drug of choice because of its efficacy against the multiple seizure types, and felbamate has also recently been shown to be beneficial (Felbamate Study Group, 1993). Polytherapy may be necessary. Surgical section of the corpus callosum is sometimes effective in controlling drop attacks.

REF: Felbamate Study Group: N *Engl J Med* 428:29-33, 1993.

Symptomatic Syndromes

Temporal lobe epilepsy (TLE), the most common symptomatic, localization-related epilepsy, causes simple partial, complex partial, and secondarily generalized seizures as a result of ictal discharges typically arising from limbic structures such as the hippocampus or amygdala. The interictal EEG often shows unilateral or bilateral, usually anterior, temporal spikes. The most commonly associated lesion is hippocampal (mesial temporal) sclerosis; others include hamartomas, neoplasms (especially low-grade gliomas), cortical dysplasia, and vascular malformations. Magnetic resonance scanning by means of thin coronal sections through temporal structures is the imaging modality of choice and may show unilateral hippocampal atrophy with enlargement of the ipsilateral temporal horn and increased hippocampal signal on T2 weighted images, suggestive of hippocampal sclerosis. Phenytoin and carbamazepine are equally effective in treating symptomatic partial epilepsies such as TLE. Valproate is equally effective in treating secondarily generalized seizures but not as effective for partial seizures. Surgical resection, typically anterior temporal lobectomy, eliminates seizures in about 70% of medically refractory patients in whom the epileptogenic lesion can be accurately localized. Posttraumatic epilepsy typically begins 6 months to 2 years after head trauma. Risk factors include intracranial hemorrhage, depressed skull fracture, early seizures, or duration of posttraumatic amnesia greater than 24 hours. Phenytoin reduces the incidence of seizures within the first week after head trauma but is not effective as prophylaxis against the development of posttraumatic epilepsy.

REF: Mattson RH et al: N *Engl J Med* 327:765-771, 1992.

Temkin NR: N *Engl J Med* 323:497-502, 1990.

Other Syndromes

Febrile seizures are typically generalized convulsions that occur in children between 3 months and 5 years of age and are associated with fever but without evidence of intracranial infection or defined cause. They are common, occurring in 2% to 5% of children in the United States, and tend to run in families. Febrile seizures usually occur during the early, rising-temperature phase of an infectious illness. Most febrile seizures are *simple*, last less than 15 minutes, and are without focality; if the seizure is prolonged or focal, it is *complex* and is associated with a higher risk of subsequent afebrile epilepsy. Other risk factors include more than one seizure in 24 hours, abnormal results of neurologic examination, and afebrile seizures in a parent or sibling. Afebrile epilepsy develops in 6% to 13% of patients with two or more risk factors and in 0.9% of patients without risk factors. There is no evidence that prophylactic treatment with anticonvulsants prevents future epilepsy. Although phenobarbital, diazepam, and valproate (but not phenytoin or carbamazepine) reduce the rate of recurrent febrile seizures, in most cases they are not recommended, since two thirds of children never have another febrile seizure and there is no evidence of mental or neurologic impairment as a result of febrile seizures. Rectal benzodiazepines may be useful for prevention of recurrent complicated febrile seizures.

Neonatal seizures are nearly always symptomatic, occurring as a result of different types of brain insults; idiopathic syndromes are rare. The most common causes include hypoxic-ischemic encephalopathy, hypoglycemia, hypocalcemia, hyponatremia and hypernatremia, intraventricular or periventricular hemorrhage, central nervous system infections, cerebral malformations, inborn errors of metabolism, and drug withdrawal or intoxication. Neonatal seizures are classified as subtle, tonic, clonic, and myoclonic (Volpe, 1989); generalized tonic-clonic convulsions are rare in the neonatal period. Neonatal seizures commonly occur on EEG without clear clinical change and may become evident on clinical examination without a clear EEG ictal pattern. Jitteriness is a benign nonepileptic phenomenon that consists of rapid, stimulus-sensitive movements of all four extremities and is abolished by passive restraint of the limbs. Treatment of neonatal seizures most commonly involves phenobarbital (loading dose 20 mg/kg followed by maintenance dose of 3 to 4 mg/kg per day to achieve blood level of 16 to 40 mcg/ml) or phenytoin (loading dose 15 to 20 mg/kg followed by maintenance dose of 3 to 5 mg/kg per day to achieve blood level of 6 to 14 mcg/ml). Hypocalcemia is treated with 5% calcium gluconate, 4 ml/kg IV, and hypomagnesemia with 50% magnesium sulfate, 0.2 ml/kg IV. If seizures continue and the cause is uncertain, pyridoxine 50 to 100 mg IV should be given. Duration of treatment once seizures are controlled is controversial.

REF: Engel J Jr: *Seizures and epilepsy*, Philadelphia, 1989, FA Davis.

Volpe JL: *Pediatrics* 84:422-428, 1989.

Wyllie E, ed: *The treatment of epilepsy: principles and practice*, Philadelphia, 1993, Lea & Febiger.

STATUS EPILEPTICUS

Generalized tonic-clonic status epilepticus (GTCSE) is a medical emergency diagnosed either when repeated convulsions occur without recovery of consciousness or when a seizure is sufficiently prolonged to create a fixed and lasting condition. The likelihood of brain damage or death is directly related to the duration of GTCSE. GTCSE is more easily controlled when no new structural brain insult has occurred, as in withdrawal from anticonvulsants, other drugs, or alcohol. Refractory cases may be seen in anoxic encephalopathy, stroke, hemorrhage, neoplasm, trauma, infection, or metabolic derangement. In general the longer the duration of GTCSE, the more difficult it is to treat. A characteristic progression of EEG patterns in GTCSE has been described as follows: (1) discrete seizures, (2) waxing and waning ictal discharges, (3) continuous ictal discharges, (4) continuous ictal discharges punctuated by flat periods, and (5) bilateral periodic epileptiform discharges on a flat background. In the later stages the patient may exhibit only subtle or no motor activity. Management of GTCSE must be carried out quickly. Treatment protocols are based on the pharmacologic properties of commonly used drugs (see Tables 20 to 25).

REF: Browns TR: *Neurology*, 40(suppl 2):28-32, 1990.

Treiman DM: *Adv Neurol* 34:377-384, 1983.

Treiman DM, Walton NY, Kendrick C: *Epilepsy Res* 5:49-60, 1990.

Absence status epilepticus (spike-wave stupor) constitutes continuous generalized spike-wave discharges with alteration of consciousness. It occurs more commonly in children with secondarily generalized epilepsy such as Lennox-Gastaut syndrome rather than with pyknolepsy. It may also occur sporadically in adults with no prior history of epilepsy. Treatment of the childhood condition consists of IV diazepam (0.3 to 0.5 mg/kg no faster than 1 to 2 mg/min) followed by valproic acid. The adult form responds to the protocol listed for GTCSE (see Table 21). Because absence status epilepticus is not life-threatening and residual brain damage is unproven, use of general anesthesia is not generally recommended.

Simple partial status epilepticus (epilepsia partialis continua) most commonly involves continuous clonic focal motor seizures, but other

TABLE 20
Comparison of Medications Commonly Used to Treat Status Epilepticus

Time	Diazepam	Lorazepam	Phenytoin	Phenobarbital
To enter brain	10 sec	2-3 min	1 min	20 min
To peak brain concentration	< 5 min	30 min	15-30 min	30 min
To stop status epilepticus	1 min	< 5 min	15-30 min	20 min
Effective half-life	15 min	6 hr	> 22 hr	50-120 hr

TABLE 21

Approach To the Treatment of Generalized Tonic-Clonic Status Epilepticus

Action	Cumulative Time Frame
1. *Stabilization and diagnosis:* Secure an airway, administer oxygen, and be prepared to intubate quickly; assess vital signs, including rectal temperature, and treat hyperpyrexia appropriately; insert two large-bore IVs; obtain ECG CBC count, and levels of anticonvulsants, glucose, BUN, electrolytes, calcium, and magnesium; obtain serum and urine toxicology screens and arterial blood gas levels; administer 100 mg thiamine IV and 50 ml of 50% glucose IV; obtain history and perform neurologic examination; consider possibility of non-epileptic seizures.	0-15 min
2. *Stop seizures:* Through one IV, administer phenytoin 20 mg/kg no faster than 50 mg/min. Contraindications to phenytoin include documented allergy, significant heart block, or severe bradycardia. (If phenytoin is contraindicated, administer phenobarbital as described below). ECG should be monitored continuously, and blood pressure taken frequently. If significant rhythm disturbances or hypotension occurs during phenytoin infusion, reduce the rate to 25 mg/min.	15-60 min
If additional seizures occur while phenytoin is being infused, administer either diazepam (no faster than 2 mg/min, to maximum 20 mg) or lorazepam (no faster than 2 mg/min, to maximum 0.1 mg/kg) through the second IV, to avoid interrupting the phenytoin infusion. Benzodiazepines may cause respiratory depression.	

TABLE 21—cont'd

Approach To the Treatment of Generalized Tonic-Clonic Status Epilepticus

Action	Cumulative Time Frame
3. *If seizures persist* after infusion of phenytoin, administer an additional 7 mg/kg phenytoin IV, no faster than 50 mg/min.	
4. *If seizures persist:* Intubate the patient, if not already done. Obtain emergency EEG monitoring; administer phenobarbital IV no faster than 100 mg/min, up to 20 mg/kg or until seizures stop. Carefully monitor blood pressure and ECG.	60-120 min
5. *If seizures persist:* Induce general anesthesia with short (thiopental) or intermediate (pentobarbital) half-life barbiturates. Pentobarbital is given IV as a 5- to 10-mg/kg loading dose (no faster than 25 mg/min), followed by initial maintenance dose of 1 to 3 mg/kg per hour. Adjust dose to achieve burst-suppression pattern on EEG without depressing blood pressure. Pressor agents may be required.	120 min
6. *Other maneuvers:* Concurrently with above, treat metabolic or toxic conditions; if there is clinical suspicion for new brain insult, obtain neuroimaging once generalized tonic-clonic status epilepticus is aborted; if there is clinical suspicion for CNS infection, perform lumbar puncture after neuroimaging and treat appropriately.	

Engel J Jr: *Seizures and epilepsy*, Philadelphia, 1989, FA Davis.
Leppik IE: *Neurology* 40(suppl 2):4-9, 1990.

TABLE 22
Common Antiepileptic Drugs: Prescribing Information

Drug	Preparations	Average Plasma Concentrations*	Monotherapy Dosage	Approximate Half-Life (hr)	Protein Binding (%)
Phenytoin (Dilantin)	Caps, 30, 100 mg; tabs, 50 mg; elixir, 30, 125 mg/ml	10-20 μg/ml (6-14 μg/ml in neonates to 12 weeks of age)	*Neonates:* 15-20 mg/kg, then 3-5 mg/kg/day in divided doses *Infants:* 15 mg/kg, then 3-5 mg/kg/day in three to four doses *Children:* 15 mg/kg, then 5-15 mg/kg/day in two doses *Adults:* 15 mg/kg, then 5 mg/kg/day, once daily	Variable	90
Phenobarbital (Luminal)	Tabs, 15, 30, 60, 130 mg; elixir, 20 mg/5 ml	15-40 μg/ml	Infants, children: 6-16 mg/kg, then 3-8 mg/kg/day Adults: 4-8 mg/kg, then 2-4 mg/kg/day, single dose	40-70 50-120	50
Primidone (Mysoline)	Tabs, 50, 250 mg; elixir,	5-12 μg/ml (metabolized also	Children: 50 mg/day, increasing 50 mg q 3	10-12	~0

Drug	Preparations	Therapeutic plasma concentration	Dosage		
	250 mg/5ml	to phenobarbital)	days to 15-25 mg/kg in two to four doses; Adults: 250 mg/day in two doses; start with 100 mg at bedtime and increase by 100 mg c 3 days to 10-20 mg/kg/day in two to four doses		75
Carbamazepine (Tegretol)	Tabs, 100, 200 mg; suspension, 100 mg/5 ml	6-12 μg/ml	Children: 100 mc bid, increasing 100 mg qod to 15-20 mg/kg/day in three to four doses Adults: 200 mg bid, increasing 100 mg qod to 7-15 mg/kg/day in three to four doses	5-27	
Ethosuximide (Zarontin)	Caps, 250 mg; elixir, 250 mg/5 ml	400-100 μg/ml	Children: 250 mg/day, increasing 250 mg q 4-7 days to 15-40 mg/kg/day in three to four doses	30	0

*Many patients respond at different plasma concentrations below or above the average plasma concentrations.

TABLE 22—cont'd
Common Antiepileptic Drugs: Prescribing Information

Drug	Preparations	Average Plasma Concentrations*	Monotherapy Dosage	Approximate Half-Life (hr)	Protein Binding (%)
			Adults: 250 mg bid, increasing 250 mg q 4-7 days to 15-30 mg/kg/day in three to four doses	50-60	
Valproic acid (Depakene)	Tabs, 250 mg; elixir, 250 mg/ 5 ml	50-100 µg/ml	Children: 10-15 mg/kg/day, increasing 5-10 mg/kg/day q 1 week to 15-100 mg/kg/day in three to four doses	4-14	75-90 (inverse to concentration)
			Adults: 10-15 mg/kg/day, increasing 5-10 mg/kg/day q 1 week to 15-45mg/kg/day in three to four doses	6-16	
Divalproex Sodium (Depakote)	Tabs, 125,250, 500 mg	50-100 µg/ml	Same as for valproic acid except given in two to three doses	Same as for valproic acid	75-90 (inverse to concentration)

Drug	Preparation	Therapeutic level	Dosage	Half-life (h)	% Protein binding
Clonazepam (Klonopin)	Tabs, 0.5, 1, 2 mg	20–80 ng/ml	Children: 0.01–0.03 mg/kg/day, increasing 0.25–0.5 mg q 3 days to 0.1–0.2 mg/kg/day in three doses	18–50	85
			Adults: 1.5 mg/day, increasing 0.5–1.0 mg/day q 3 days to 20 mg/day in three doses	18–50	
Felbamate (Felbatol)	Tabs, 400, 600 mg; elixir, 600 mg/5 ml	20–80 µg/ml	Children (adjunctive): 15 mg/kg/day three or four times daily	14–20	25
			Adult: 1200 mg/day, increasing 600 mg q 2 weeks up to 3600 mg/day		
Lamotrigine (Lamictal)	Not available in United States	0.5–3.0 µg/ml	50 mg q hs, increasing 50 mg q 2 weeks, as tolerated, divided into two doses	12–50	55
Gabapentin (Neurontin)	Tabs, 100, 300, 400 mg	2–3 µg/ml	300 mg/day, increasing up to 900–1800 mg/day over 2–3 days divided into three to four doses	5–7	0

TABLE 23
Dose-Related Adverse Effects of Antiepileptic Drugs

Drug	Side Effects	
	Acute	Chronic
Phenytoin	Drowsiness, ataxia, diplopia, GI complaints, choreoathetosis, nausea, hypotension (after parenteral use), heart block	Gingival hyperplasia, hirsutism, folate deficiency, megaloblastic anemia, osteomalacia with vitamin D deficiency, peripheral neuropathy, encephalopathy, cerebellar dysfunction, pseudolymphoma, hemorrhage in the newborn
Phenobarbital	Sedation, behavior disturbance, ataxia	Attentional difficulty, hemorrhage in the newborn
Primidone	Sedation, nausea, vertigo, ataxia	Behavior disturbances (in children), loss of libido, attentional difficulties, hemorrhage in the newborn

Carbamazepine	Diplopia, vertigo, blurred vision, sedation, dry-mouth stomatitis, syndrome of inappropriate secretion of diuretic hormone, headache, diarrhea, constipation, paresthesias	Liver enzyme induction, leukopenia, nervousness, hemorrhage in the newborn
Ethosuximide	Nausea, vertigo, vomiting, hiccups, headache	Insomnia, nervousness
Valproate	Sedation, GI disturbances	Weight gain, hepatic enzyme elevation, hyperammonemia, granulopenia, thrombocytopenia, alopecia, tremor, hemorrhage in the newborn
Clonazepam	Sedation, ataxia, irritability, hypersalivation	Behavior disturbances, tolerance, withdrawal syndrome
Felbamate	GI disturbances, insomnia, headache, fatigue, nausea, vomiting	Weight loss, aplastic anemia
Lamotrigine	Diplopia, sedation, dizziness, ataxia, headache, nausea and vomiting, rash	
Gabapentin	Sedation, fatigue, dizziness nausea, weight gain, ataxia, headache	

TABLE 24
Factors Affecting Serum Concentrations of Antiepileptic Drugs (AEDs)

Drug	Change in Level	Other AEDs	Other Drugs	Disease or Condition
Phenytoin	Increased by	Phenobarbital, valproic acid, ethosuximide, felbamate, diazepam, primidone	Alcohol (acute intoxication), amphetamines, aspirin, chloramphenicol, chlordane, chlorpromazine, cimetidine, disulfiram, dicumarol, estrogens, isoniazid, methylphenidate, phenylbutazone, propoxyphene, sulfaphenazole, tolbutamide	Hepatic disease
	Decreased by	Phenobarbital, carbamazepine, clonazepam	Alcohol (chronic intoxication), theophylline, nitrofurantoin, nicotine	Pregnancy, renal disease, mononucleosis, acute hepatitis
Phenobarbital	Increased by	Valproic acid, phenytoin, felbamate		Renal disease, hepatic disease, acidic urine

	Decreased by	Clonazepam	Alkaline urine
Primidone	Increased by	Valproic acid, clonazepam	
	Decreased by	Phenytoin	
Carbamazepine	Increased by	Felbamate (↑ 10, 11 epoxide)	Hepatic disease
	Decreased by	Phenytoin, phenobarbital, primidone, felbamate, ethosuximide, valproic acid	Pregnancy
Valproic acid	Increased by	Felbamate	Hepatic disease
	Decreased by	Carbamazepine, phenytoin, phenobarbital, primidone	
Ethosuximide	Increased by	Valproic acid	

Dicumarol, chloramphenicol, phenylbutazone

Propoxyphene, erythromycin, cimetidine, isoniazid

Leppik IE, Wolff DL: *Neurol Clin* 905-921, 1993.

Continued.

TABLE 24—cont'd
Factors Affecting Serum Concentrations of Antiepileptic Drugs (AEDs)

Drug	Change in Level	Other AEDs	Other Drugs	Disease or Condition
Clonazepam	Increased by	Phenytoin		
	Decreased by	Phenobarbital		
Felbamate	Decreased by	Phenytoin, carbamazepine		
Lamotrigine	Increased by	Valproic acid		
	Decreased by	Phenytoin, carbamazepine		
Gabapentin	Minimal drug interactions			

TABLE 25

Idiosyncratic Adverse Effects of Antiepileptic Drugs*

Effect	Drug Type
Skin rash	All antiepileptic drugs
Erythema multiforme	All; more likely with ethosuximide
Stevens-Johnson syndrome	All
Exfoliative dermatitis	All
Systemic lupus erythematosus	Phenytoin, ethosuximide
Bone marrow depression	Most, including phenytoin, primidone, carbamazepine, ethosuximide, valproic acid/divalproex Na$^+$, felbamate
Thrombocytopenia	Valproic acid; rare with phenytoin, phenobarbital, clonazepam
Lymphadenopathy	Phenytoin, ethosuximide
Hepatic toxicity	Valproic acid/divalproex Na$^+$ (usually in first 6 months of therapy), phenytoin, carbamazepine
Pancreatic toxicity	Valproic acid/divalproex Na$^+$

Adapted from Dreifuss FE. In Ward AA, Penry IK, Purpura D, eds: *Epilepsy*, ed 1, New York, 1983, Raven.

manifestations such as aphasia, head and eye deviation, somatosensory changes, visual disturbances, and autonomic symptoms may occur. Ictal EEG recording may be normal. Focal motor status is often seen in the setting of metabolic derangements, particularly nonketotic hyperglycemia. Treatment in this case consists of correcting metabolic abnormalities. Slow loading with IV diazepam or lorazepam to avoid respiratory depression, followed by phenytoin, may also be used.

Complex partial status epilepticus may consist of repeated discrete complex partial seizures without full clearing of consciousness or may occur as a more continuous clouding of consciousness mimicking a confusional state. EEG is diagnostic. Treatment initially is identical to the protocol listed for GTCSE (see Table 21), although the use of general anesthesia if initial maneuvers fail is controversial.

Generalized convulsive status epilepticus in children is treated as in adults with the following modifications. Use diazepam 0.25 mg/kg IV, no faster than 1 to 2 mg/min. If there is a delay in obtaining an IV in a small child, this dose may be administered rectally via a feeding tube flushed with saline. Phenytoin 18 to 20 mg/kg is given IV over 20 minutes. If seizures persist, be prepared to intubate, and give phenobarbital 15 to 20 mg/kg IV no faster than 60 mg per min, with additional doses of 10 mg/kg as needed to control seizures.

Neonatal status epilepticus must be diagnosed using EEG monitoring because of the frequent dissociation between electrographic and clinical seizure activity. Treatment is as outlined for neonatal seizures, above. Diazepam 0.3 to 0.5 mg/kg IV or lorazepam 0.1 mg/kg IV may be given in refractory cases but is contraindicated in jaundiced neonates.

REF: Engel J Jr: *Seizures and epilepsy*, Philadelphia, 1989, FA Davis.

Leppik IE: *Neurology* 40 (suppl 2):4-9, 1990.

ANTIEPILEPTIC DRUGS

Use of antiepileptic drugs begins with the appropriate selection of a single drug based on clinical and electrographic identification of the patient's epilepsy syndrome and seizure type. The dose is increased until seizures are controlled or clinical toxicity develops. The lowest dose that will control seizures is used. If the drug is ineffective when taken in toxic doses, it is generally recommended that another monotherapy with another agent be attempted before drug combinations are used. Drug levels may provide useful adjunctive information but should be measured to answer specific questions regarding compliance, toxicity, or individual pharmacokinetics, not routinely (Dodson, 1989). Determinations of free levels of drugs that are highly protein bound, such as phenytoin, carbamezepine, or valproic acid, may be helpful during hypoalbuminemic states, renal or hepatic disease, pregnancy, malignancy, sepsis, or burns or in the presence of other drugs that displace protein binding. The use of routine serial laboratory monitoring to identify and prevent serious idiosyncratic complications of anticonvulsants is of little value, except in high-risk patients (children under age 2, especially those receiving polytherapy, are at higher risk of developing valproic acid–related hepatotoxicity, as are patients with urea cycle defects, organic acidurias, mitochondrial disorders, GM_1 gangliosidosis, and neurodegenerative diseases) and in patients with a history of adverse drug reactions. Abnormalities such as mild leukopenia or elevated hepatic enzyme levels are not predictive of severe complications. Current recommendations include the following:

1. Obtain initial baseline blood work before therapy is initiated, including complete blood cell count with differential and platelet count; evaluation of serum chemistry; determinations of levels of calcium, magnesium, phosphorus, BUN, creatinine, uric acid, iron, cholesterol, bilirubin, alkaline phosphatase, AST, ALT, total protein, and albumin; and prothrombin time and partial thromboplastin time.
2. Refrain from subsequent routine monitoring in asymptomatic patients.
3. Counsel patients and family to notify you immediately should any of the following develop: bruising, bleeding, rash, abdominal pain, vomiting, jaundice, lethargy, coma, or marked increase in seizure frequency, which may herald serious side effect and would require evaluation and laboratory monitoring.
4. For multiply handicapped, institutionalized patients who may not be able to communicate the above, annual routine blood monitoring may be of value (Pellock 1991). Several new antiepileptic medications have recently been released in the United States or are under active investigation at this time: felbamate, gabapentin, lamotrigine, vigabatrin, progabide, tiagabine, topiramate, oxcarbazepine, and phenytoin prodrug.

REF: Dodson WE: *Neurology* 39:1009-1010, 1989.

Pellock JM, Willmore LJ: *Neurology* 41:961-964, 1991.

ETHOSUXIMIDE *(see Epilepsy)*

ETHYL ALCOHOL *(see Alcohol)*

EVOKED POTENTIALS

Evoked potentials (EPs) are recordable changes in the electrical activity of the nervous system in response to an external stimulus. They are an adjunct to the history and physical exam and may provide corroborative evidence of disease of the nervous system. EPs utilize the functional integrity of the nervous system to provide information about the anatomical location of lesions. They may detect the presence of lesions that are not clinically apparent but are of little value in providing clues to the origin or cause of the lesions.

The clinically useful EPs are derived from stimulation of one of the modalities of the sensory system—visual (VEP), brain stem auditory (BAEP), and somatosensory (SEP)—and are recorded from electrodes on the scalp. Because of the low voltage of EPs (100 times smaller than the scalp EEG), multiple stimulations with averaging and filtering are necessary to separate the signal from background noise. The actual signal recorded may be either "near-field" (the electrode is placed *near* the generator of the signal in the cortex, for example, P100 wave of the VEP generated by the occipital cortex) or "far-field" (the electrode is placed *far* from the generator of the signal, which is volume conducted through the tissues of the body to the recording electrodes on the scalp, for example, P11 wave of the SEP generated by the dorsal root entry zone). In general, the latency from stimulus to recorded potential is more important than signal amplitude. The potentials are usually designated by the letter "P" or "N" followed by a number. "P100" is a wave of *positive* deflection occurring at a latency of 100 ms. "N20" is a wave of *negative* deflection occurring at a latency of 20 ms. By convention, "positive" is a downward and "negative" an upward needle deflection. It should be remembered that *absolute latencies and standard deviations are quite laboratory specific* (Figure 15).

Electroretinograms (ERGs) are derived from stimulation of the retina with light while recording electrical activity directly from the cornea. When combined with VEPs, ERGs can be useful in prognosis for recovery of visual function and differentiation of retinal from optic nerve disease.

Motor-evoked potentials (MEP) are derived from stimulating the CNS motor system with magnetically induced or directly applied electrical current. Recordings are made from electrodes placed over muscles. MEPs have yet to gain significant clinical use and will not be discussed further.

Visual-evoked potentials are primarily used to detect *anterochiasmatic* lesions of the visual system. Their usefulness in retrochiasmatic lesions is minimal. The most useful VEPs are generated by checkerboard pattern-reversal stimuli that evoke large, reproducible potentials. Check sizes subtending greater than 40 degrees of arc preferentially stimulate retinal luminance channels. Those less than 30 degrees stimulate contrast and spacial frequency detectors, and those less than 15 degrees mainly stimulate the fovea. *P100* is the most useful and re-

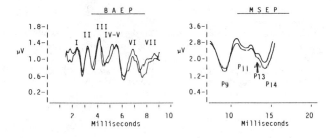

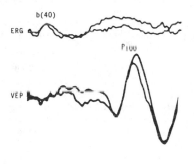

FIGURE 15
Normal evoked potentials.

producible wave. It is generated by the striate cortex as a near-field potential and recorded from electrodes placed over the occipital cortex. A significant prolongation of latency between eyes with alternate *full-field monocular* stimulation is evidence for anterochiasmatic disease on the side with prolonged latency. P100 may be bilaterally absent or prolonged with chiasmatic lesions. Refractive errors and macular disease can affect both the latency and amplitude of VEPs (see also "Electroretinograms" below).

Brainstem auditory-evoked potentials detect lesions of the auditory system and mid-upper brainstem. Click stimuli of 50 to 100 μs square-wave pulses to headphones or ear-insert transducers are used to elicit seven recordable potentials at the scalp. Waves I through VII occur within 10 ms after stimulation and are generated by propogating action potentials within the eighth cranial nerve (CN) and central auditory pathways. They are volume conducted to the scalp and recorded there as far-field potentials. The specific generators of the waves are controversial, but most authorities agree with the following schema: I—distal CN VIII; II—proximal CN VIII; III—bilateral superior olivary complex; IV—ascending auditory fibers in the rostral pons; V—inferior colliculus; VI—medial geniculate nucleus; VII—distal auditory radiations. Waves VI and VII are often unobtainable or inconsistent and are clinically useless. Waves II and IV may be buried in, or fused to other waves, and are not as important as waves I, III, and V. Absolute latencies are not as important as the I-III-V interpeak latencies (IPLs).

Commonly recognized abnormal BAEP patterns include the following:

1. *Absence of all waves:* Peripheral hearing loss, excessive background noise, technical error (rarely in Friedreich's ataxia, distal CN-VIII lesions, or system atrophies).
2. *Wave I only (or increased I-III IPL):* Lesions of the proximal acoustic nerve or pontomedullary junction near the root entry zone (peripheral demyelination or inflammation, Cerebellopontine (CP) angle tumors, pontine glioma, MS, leukodystrophies, neonatal anoxia, or brainstem infarct).
3. *Waves I-III only (or increased III-V IPL):* Lesions sparing the pontomedullary junction but affecting the pons to low midbrain (most commonly seen with MS, any disorder of pontine tegmentum, or large extrinsic masses compressing the brainstem—especially CP angle tumors opposite the stimulated ear).
4. *Increased I-III, III-V, and I-V IPL:* Diffuse or multifocal disease such as demyelination, brainstem glioma, and especially hypothermia. (NOTE: BAEPs are extremely stable over wide ranges of metabolic derangement. Diffuse prolongation of IPLs should not be explained by metabolic abnormality.)

Somatosensory-evoked potentials are obtained from electrical stimulation of the median nerve at the wrist (MSEP) or the posterior tibial nerve at the ankle (PTSEP). Analysis of SEPs can give information about the integrity of the sensory component of peripheral nerves, spinal cord, brainstem, and to a lesser extent, the cortex. Recordings of far-field potentials are made over the scalp, and both near- and far-field potentials may be obtained at other points along the proximally propogating action potential.

MSEP: Four clinically useful "early" components of MSEPs and their presumed generators have been identified and are consistent and reproducible regardless of position of scalp electrodes. *P9* originates from the distal brachial plexus, *P11* from the dorsal root entry zone, *P13* from the dorsal columns of the cervical cord, and *P14* from the medial lemniscus of the brainstem. It can be seen that absence of a component or increased IPL provides evidence of a lesion along the course of propogation. Other "late" components (approximately N19, P23, N32, P40, and N60) have been identified and probably correspond to thalamic or suprathalamic generators. They are prolonged with decreasing levels of arousal and are not reproducible from person to person, or from the same person at different times or with changes of state. They also vary with different recording montages. Their usefulness is seen only when simultaneous bilateral stimulation produces assymetries.

PTSEP: This is the most "laboratory specific" EP, with widely differing waveform designations and terminology. PV (propogated volley) is the designation given to the near-field potential recorded over the lower spine, which roughly corresponds to the cauda equina and lower gracile tract. It increases in latency with more proximal recording sites. N22 is probably generated by axon collaterals in the dorsal columns near the thoracolumbar junction. Later components can be recorded from the scalp and represent more rostral brainstem, thalamic, and cortical generators. Their usefulness is proportional to the technique and reliability of the given laboratory. As with MSEPs, PTSEPs can give localizing information pertaining to lesions along the course of propogation.

Electroretinograms: Two types of ERGs are in common use. Flash ERGs are useful for detecting retinal lesions and will not be discussed. Pattern ERGs (P-ERGs) utilize a checkerboard pattern-reversal stimulus. When a small enough check size is used (less than 2.4 degrees of arc), the major positive wave recorded from the cornea (b-wave) represents retinal ganglion cell function. The latency of "b" is about 40 ms and is prolonged or abolished by disease processes in or distal to the ganglia. When "b" is subtracted from the simultaneously recorded P100 of the VEP, retinocortical time (RCT) can be determined

(RCT = P100 − b). RCT is a more accurate reflection of optic nerve integrity proximal to the retinal ganglia and is independent of macular disease.

Three abnormal patterns of P-ERG/VEP have been identified:

1. *Normal P-ERG, delayed VEP and RCT*: Demyelination of the optic nerve.
2. *Normal P-ERG, absent VEP*: Acute total block of optic nerve fibers.
3. *Absent P-ERG, absent VEP*: Severe macular disease or long-standing severe optic nerve disease with retrograde degeneration of retinal ganglion cells.

There is also evidence that decreased amplitude of P-ERGs in recent optic neuritis has a poor prognosis for visual recovery, and progressive loss of P-ERG amplitude correlates with the development of optic nerve atrophy.

Evoked potentials and multiple sclerosis: EPs are most useful in the evaluation of MS (1) to demonstrate sensory abnormalities when the history or exam is equivocal and (2) to demonstrate clinically inapparent lesions when demyelination is suspected in other areas of the nervous system. Less important uses are (3) to define the distribution of the disease process and (4) to monitor changes in a patient's status. *When the diagnosis of MS is clinically definite, EPs will add little additional information.*

Abnormal VEPs are present in about 95% of cases of optic neuritis, regardless of how remote and regardless of whether vision has returned. About 50% of MS patients have abnormal VEPs even without clinical evidence of optic nerve involvement. Whereas about 35% of patients with progressive myelopathy have abnormal VEPs, only about 10% show abnormality after a single episode of transverse myelitis.

Forty-six percent of patients with MS have abnormal BAEPs, regardless of clinical classification. Thirty-eight percent of patients without clinical findings of brainstem involvement show abnormalities. The most common abnormalities are decreased or absent wave V or increased III-V IPL.

Of 1000 MS patients with varying classifications, 58% had abnormal MSEPs and 76% had abnormal PTSEPs.

The differential sensitivity of EPs in detecting white matter lesions in MS is related to the length of fiber tract being tested (i.e., the order of sensitivity is SEP greater than VEP and BAEP). *As the degree of clinical certainty of the diagnosis increases from possible to probable to definite, the detection rate of lesions will be greater but the usefulness of the information obtained will be less.*

Evoked potentials and other neurologic diseases: Many attempts have been made to use EPs as prognostic indicators of disease and trauma. In general, results are conflicting and no better than following clinical signs and symptoms. There is currently no definite role for EPs in the evaluation of brain death or recovery from coma. Intraoperatively, SEPs (during spinal cord surgery) and BAEPs (during posterior fossa surgery) may provide an early indication of compromise of neural tissue. In cervical spondylosis, PTSEPs may eventually help predict which patients are more likely to develop a significant cord deficit so that early surgical intervention can be considered. Flash VEPs have been used by some centers to monitor changes in intracranial pressure, but this is controversial.

REF: Gilmore R (ed): *Neurologic clinics*, Philadelphia, 1988, WB Saunders.

EYE MOVEMENTS   *(see Calorics, Eye Muscles, Gaze Palsy, Graves' Ophthalmopathy, Nystagmus, Ocular Oscillations, Ophthalmoplegia, Optokinetic Nystagmus, Vertigo, Vestibulo-ocular Reflex)*

EYE MUSCLES

Because of their insertional properties the six extraocular muscles affect eye movements in three planes in primary position (see Table 26). In testing muscle strength, the optical axis is aligned with a muscle's main vector. The superior and inferior rectus muscles insert on the anterior globe at 23 degrees temporal to the primary position. Therefore these muscles function solely in the vertical plane only when the eye is abducted 23 degrees. The oblique muscles insert on the posterior globe at 51 degrees nasal to primary position. Thus adduction maximizes the depressor effect of the superior oblique, whereas abduction maximizes intorsion (Figure 16).

Diplopia testing in paralytic strabismus begins with measurement of visual acuity, confrontation visual fields, and observation of any abnormal head posture. Head tilt occurs in the direction of action of the weak muscle. Range of motion in each eye is tested in the nine cardinal positions of gaze with the opposite eye covered (ductions) and

TABLE 26
Actions of Eye Muscles in Primary Position

Muscle	Primary Action	Secondary Action	Tertiary Action
Lateral rectus	Abduction		
Medial rectus	Adduction		
Superior rectus	Elevation	Intorsion	Adduction
Inferior rectus	Depression	Extorsion	Adduction
Superior oblique	Intorsion	Depression	Abduction
Inferior oblique	Extorsion	Elevation	Abduction

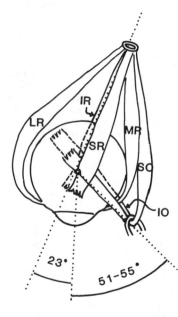

FIGURE 16
Insertion of ocular muscles on the globe. *LR* = lateral rectus; *MR* = medial rectus; *SR* = superior rectus; *IR* = inferior rectus; *SO* = superior oblique; *IO* = inferior oblique.

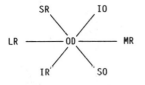 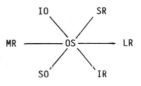

FIGURE 17
Main field of action of individual eye muscles.

with both eyes viewing (versions). Misalignment can be seen in the corneal reflection of a penlight and is tested in directions of gaze (Hirschberg's test).

Subjective diplopia testing relies on the principles that the disparate images are maximally separated in the main field of action of the paretic muscle and that the more peripheral image belongs to the paretic eye (Figure 17). The Maddox rod tests primarily for phoria because it disrupts fusion; therefore only noncomitant deviations (unequal in different fields of gaze) should be considered abnormal. If the paretic eye and the position of gaze producing the maximum separation of the images can be determined, the paretic muscle can be identified.

Objective tests include the cover-uncover test for tropia and the alternate cover test for phoria, which are performed in primary position and in each cardinal position. Deviation of the nonparetic eye when covered (secondary deviation) is always greater than the deviation of the paretic eye when covered (primary deviation).

REF: Leigh RJ, Zee DS: *The neurology of eye movements*, ed 2, Philadelphia, 1991, FA Davis.

FACIAL NERVE

The *course of the facial nerve* (cranial nerve (CN) VII) is depicted in Figure 18. The numbers in the figure refer to the following *locations of the lesions:*

1. Peripheral to chorda tympani in facial canal or outside stylomastoid foramen. Peripheral upper and lower facial weakness (motor aspects of CN VII) only. Usually related to trauma.
2. Facial canal (mastoid), involving chorda tympani. In addition

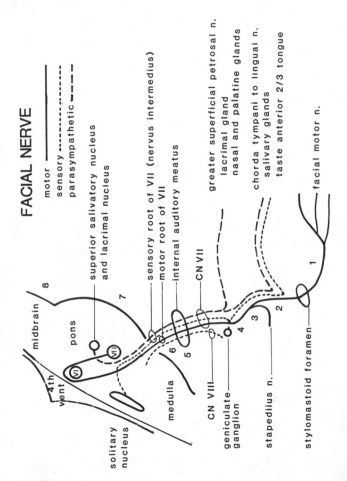

FIGURE 18
Facial nerve.

to upper and lower facial weakness, patients have loss of taste over the anterior two thirds of tongue and decreased salivation.

3. Facial canal, involving the stapedius nerve. As in 1 and 2, plus hyperacusis.

4. Geniculate ganglion. Usually associated with pain in the ear. May have decreased lacrimation.

5. Internal auditory meatus. Complete CN VII (facial weakness; decreased taste, salivation, and lacrimation) plus CN VIII dysfunction (deafness and, perhaps, vestibular symptoms).

6. Extrapontine, subarachnoid. May have other cranial nerve involvement. Hemifacial spasm is more commonly associated with more proximal lesions of CN VII.

7. Pontine (nuclear or infranuclear). Millard-Gubler, Foville's and Brissaud's syndromes (see Ischemia).

8. Supranuclear. Lesions may occur anywhere from mid-pons to motor cortex and are usually associated with other findings such as hemiparesis, hemisensory deficit, language disturbance, and homonymous hemianopia, depending on location. Taste, salivation, and lacrimation are not involved. Lower facial weakness is much more prominent than upper because of bilateral input to the portions of the facial nucleus controlling the upper face; input for the lower face is from contralateral cortex. Mild weakness may appear only as slight drooping of the angle of the mouth, slight widening of the palpebral fissure, or flattening of the nasolabial fold.

Causes of facial nerve palsies are many, although "idiopathic" Bell's palsy (occasionally related to herpes simplex) is most common. Other treatable and potentially serious causes should be excluded by careful history, examination, and where indicated, neuroradiologic and electrodiagnostic studies.

Bell's palsy is attributed to swelling of the nerve or nerve sheath in the facial canal. Seventh-nerve findings are variable, depending on the site and extent of lesion. Recovery is spontaneous and complete in up to 90% of cases. Electromyographic evidence of denervation indicates a worse prognosis for complete recovery. Partial or incomplete recovery may be associated with contractures, synkinetic motor movements (e.g., angle of mouth and lids), excessive tearing with salivary gland stimulation (crocodile tears), or gustatory sweating. Ramsay-Hunt syndrome refers to herpes zoster of the geniculate ganglion; herpetic lesions are often visible on the tympanic membrane, external auditory canal, and pinna.

Other causes of peripheral facial weakness include trauma (facial, skull fracture), surgery (middle ear, mastoids, cranial nerve V), neoplasms (schwannoma, neurofibroma, nasopharyngeal carcinoma, leukemia, lymphoma, hemangioma, glomus tumors, cholesteatoma, parotid tumors), and infections involving the subarachnoid space, petrous portion of the temporal bone, middle ear, mastoid, parotid, or the facial nerve itself. Involvement may result from granulomatous infiltration of the meninges or, as in the case of sarcoid, with parotid gland swelling. Facial weakness may be congenital, as in the Möbius' syndrome, with greater upper than lower facial diplegia, paralysis of abduction of the eye, ptosis, and, occasionally, abnormal musculature of the tongue, sternocleidomastoid, and muscles of mastication. Recurrent facial paralysis and facial swelling (Melkersson's syndrome) occurs rarely and may be associated with a furrowed tongue (Melkersson-Rosenthal syndrome). The nerve itself may be involved in Guillain-Barré syndrome, acute intermittent porphyria, and lead poisoning. Facial weakness may also be seen in myasthenia gravis and various myopathies. Rarer causes include osteopetrosis, thiamine deficiency, and hemorrhage into the facial canal. Bilateral facial paralysis can be seen with brainstem diseases, meningitis, sarcoidosis, myasthenia, facioscapulohumeral muscular dystrophy, Guillain-Barré syndrome, porphyria, and heavy-metal intoxications.

Pontine involvement is most commonly vascular but may result from infection, hemorrhage, trauma, neoplasm (most commonly pontine glioma), or demyelinating disease. Facial myokymia may occur with pontine lesions. *Supranuclear* causes are many and include vascular, neoplastic, traumatic, and infectious causes.

Blepharospasm is bilateral, episodic, involuntary contractions of orbicularis oculi muscles of undetermined origin. When lower facial muscles are involved, blepharospasm may be part of Meige's disease (see Dystonia).

Hemifacial spasm is painless unilateral facial spasms, either repetitive or lasting up to several minutes. It is frequently exacerbated by alkalosis. Differential diagnosis includes focal seizures. Aberrant vascular loop compressing the facial nerve as it exits the pons is often the cause. Treatment is carbamazepine, botulinum toxin, or surgical decompression.

Facial myokymia is often benign and self-limited. Persistent myokymia may be seen in multiple sclerosis or brainstem neoplasm or after stroke.

Treatment of facial nerve disorders is aimed at the primary cause. Corneal exposure should be prevented with lubricating ointment but may also require tarsorrhaphy. Electrical physiotherapy may be detrimental and should not be used. Corticosteroid treatment within the first 2 days of "idiopathic" Bell's palsy may prevent the progression to complete denervation. The contraindications and side effects of corticosteroid therapy should be reviewed in each case. Prednisone, 1 mg/kg, is given in divided doses for 5 to 6 days and tapered over 5 days if paralysis is incomplete, but continued for another 10 days and tapered over the subsequent 5 days if paralysis is complete.

FAINTING *(see Syncope)*

FASCICULATION *(see Electromyography, Motor Neuron Disease)*

FEBRILE SEIZURE *(see Epilepsy)*

FEMORAL NERVE *(see Peripheral Nerve, Pregnancy)*

FLOPPY INFANT *(see Hypotonic Infant)*

FOLIC ACID DEFICIENCY *(see Nutritional Deficiency Syndromes)*

FONTANEL *(see also Macrocephaly)*

The anterior fontanel is an interosseous space located at the juncture of the sagittal and coronal sutures; the posterior fontanel is located at the juncture of the sagittal and lambdoidal sutures. At birth both fontanels are open. The posterior fontanel becomes fused in the first few months of life. By age 7 months, the anterior fontanel is fibrous; by age 2 years, it is palpable as a midsagittal depression. The anterior fontanel may be quite large at birth; this has little significance unless associated with palpably split sutures. If the infant has been delivered vaginally, the cranial bones may override each other and the fontanel may be difficult to palpate. When the infant cries, the fontanel may be tense and bulging. At other times it should be soft and flat and may pulsate. A "full" or "tense" fontanel when the infant is quiet is a sign of increased intracranial pressure. Causes of delayed closure of the anterior fontanel (persistently large) include prematurity, malnutrition, increased intracranial pressure, chromosomal abnormalities (trisomies 13, 18, and 21), metabolic disorders (hypothyroidism, rickets, and hypophosphatasia), and primary bone disorders (achondroplasia, cleidocranial dysostosis, and osteogenesis imperfecta).

FRIEDREICH'S ATAXIA *(see Spinocerebellar Degeneration)*

FRONTAL LOBE

The frontal lobe consists of the motor, premotor, and prefrontal areas. Three behavioral syndromes with lesions affecting the prefrontal regions have been described:

1. The *orbitofrontal syndrome* is characterized by disinhibition, impulsive behavior, emotional lability, euphoria, poor judgment, and easy distractibility.
2. The *frontal convexity syndrome* is characterized by apathy, psychomotor retardation, poor word-list generation, motor perseveration and impersistence, and inability to execute multistepped behaviors.
3. The *medial frontal syndrome* is characterized by paucity of spontaneous movement, sparse verbal output, lower extremity weakness, and incontinence.

These syndromes may exist in pure or mixed forms.

FUNGAL INFECTION *(see Abscess, Cerebrospinal Fluid, Encephalitis, Meningitis)*

GAIT DISORDERS

Gait depends both on maintenance of equilibrium and on mechanisms of locomotion. Classification of gait disorders has traditionally been based on visual recognition of typical gaits such as those seen in spasticity, parkinsonism, chorea, ataxia, and hysteria. A better classification is based on the level of dysfunction. Lowest-level gait disorders arise because of musculoskeletal, peripheral nervous system, vestibular, or sensory dysfunction. Middle-level gait disorders encompass hemiplegic, paraparetic, cerebellar ataxic, parkinsonian, choreic, and dystonic gaits. Highest-level gait disorders are due to difficulties in frontal planning and execution and include cautious gait, frontal and subcortical dysequilibrium, gait ignition failure (gait apraxia) and frontal gait disorders. Diagnosis of gait disorders is based on history and associated neurologic findings. Isolated gait disorders in the elderly are frequently due to treatable disorders such as Parkinson's disease, cervical myelopathy, or normal-pressure hydrocephalus.

REF: Nutt JG, Marsden CD, Thompson PD: *Neurology* 43:268–279, 1993.

GANGLIOSIDOSES *(see Degenerative Diseases of Childhood, Chorea)*

GAUCHER'S DISEASE *(see Degenerative Diseases of Childhood)*

GAZE PALSY *(see also Ophthalmoplegia, Progressive Supranuclear Palsy)*

Horizontal gaze palsies: A unilateral gaze (saccadic and pursuit) palsy may indicate a contralateral cerebral hemispheric (frontoparietal), contralateral midbrain or ipsilateral pontine lesion. Except when the pontine lesion is at the level of the abducens nucleus, either involving the nucleus itself or the paramedian pontine reticular formation, the eyes can be driven toward the side of the palsy with cold caloric stimulation of the ipsilateral ear. Hemispheric lesions characteristically produce transient defects; brainstem lesions may be associated with enduring defects. An acute cerebellar hemispheric lesion can result in an ipsilateral gaze palsy that can be overcome with calorics. Unilateral saccadic palsy with intact pursuit is unusual and indicates an acute frontal lesion. Unilateral impaired pursuit with normal saccades is usually due to an ipsilateral deep posterior hemispheric lesion with a contralateral hemianopia.

Vertical gaze palsies: The rostral interstitial nucleus of the medial longitudinal fasciculus (riMLF) in the upper midbrain contains the cells that generate vertical eye movements. A medially placed lesion will result in both an up-gaze and a down-gaze palsy. An isolated down-gaze palsy is due to bilateral or lateral midbrain lesion. Isolated up-gaze palsies occur with lesions of the posterior commissure, bilateral pretectal regions, and large unilateral midbrain tegmental lesions. In the dorsal midbrain (Parinaud's) syndrome the paralysis of upward gaze is usually associated with convergence-retraction nystagmus, lid retraction, and light-near dissociation of the pupils. An acute bilateral pontine lesion at the level of the abducens nucleus may result in a transient up-gaze paralysis in addition to an enduring bilateral horizontal gaze palsy.

Conjugate eye deviations: Horizontal deviations are associated with acute gaze palsies as described above and with irritative cerebral foci (seizure or intracerebral hemorrhage), which usually drive the eyes to the side opposite the lesion. Ipsiversive eye and head movements, however, are reported with focal seizures. Upward deviations occur in the oculogyric crisis of postencephalitic parkinsonism and, more commonly, as an idiosyncratic reaction to phenothiazines. They may also occur in coma, usually as a result of anoxic encephalopathy. Downward deviations may occur transiently in normal neonates but also in infantile hydrocephalus and in adults with metabolic encephalopathy, bilateral thalamic infarction, or hemorrhage.

REF: Daroff RB et al. In Duane TD, ed: *Clinical ophthalmology*, Philadelphia, 1988, Lippincott.

   Leigh RJ, Zee DS: *The neurology of eye movements*, ed 2, Philadelphia, 1991, FA Davis.

GEGENHALTEN   *(see Rigidity)*

GERMINOMA   *(see Tumor)*

GERSTMANN'S SYNDROME

A clinical tetrad of agraphia, acalculia, right-left disorientation, and "finger agnosia." Finger agnosia may be manifest by bilateral difficulties in finger naming (finger anomia), movement of fingers to command, matching of fingers to demonstration ("show me this finger"), and recognition of stimuli ("wiggle the finger that I touch"). When all features are present, a dominant parietal or posterior perisylvian lesion is highly likely. The syndrome is almost always accompanied by aphasia, alexia, or constructional apraxia.

REF: Benton AL: *Arch Neurol* 49:445-447, 1992.

GIANT CELL ARTERITIS   *(see Vasculitis)*

GILLES DE LA TOURETTE'S SYNDROME   *(see Tourette's Syndrome)*

GLASGOW COMA SCALE   *(see Coma)*

GLOMUS JUGULARE TUMOR   *(see Tumor)*

GLOSSOPHARYNGEAL NERVE   *(see Cranial Nerves, Neuralgia)*

GLUCOSE

Hypoglycemia: Symptoms arise from neuroglucopenia and endogenous release of catecholamines. Mild hypoglycemia produces hunger, weakness, dizziness, blurred vision, anxiety, tremor, tachycardia, pallor, diaphoresis, headache, and mild confusion. With severe hypoglycemia the preceding symptoms are followed by seizures (blood glucose levels of less than 30 mg/100 ml) and (at glucose levels of less than 10 mg/100 ml) progression to coma, pupillary dilation, hypotonia, and extensor posturing. The presence of paresthesias may be related to hyperventilation. Focal findings may mimic cerebrovascular disease. Symptoms, signs, and residual neurologic deficit depend on the rate of onset, duration, and severity of hypoglycemia. Patients with chronic hypoglycemia may have no sympathetic symptoms but may have cognitive or behavioral disturbances. Repeated severe attacks of hypoglycemia may result in dementia.

Hyperglycemia: Diabetic ketoacidosis is the most common cerebral complication of diabetes and is frequently accompanied by decreased levels of consciousness and, occasionally, coma. Muscle cramps, hyperesthesias, dysesthesias, and diffuse abdominal pain may occur. The neurologic changes correlate best with serum osmolarity, although dehydration, acidosis, and associated electrolyte disorders contribute. *The treatment of diabetic ketoacidosis may lead to fatal cerebral edema if blood osmolarity is rapidly lowered relative to brain osmolarity.* Treatment may also cause hypophosphatemia, hypokalemia, and hypoglycemia.

Hyperglycemia nonketotic states result in CNS complications that are due to extracellular hyperosmolarity. Neurologic manifestations can be seen with blood glucose levels of more than 425 mg/dl. These include hallucinations, depression, apathy, irritability, seizures (typically focal and resistant to anticonvulsant medication), other focal signs (either postictal or in isolation), flaccidity, diminished deep tendon reflexes, tonic spasms, myoclonus, meningeal signs, nystagmus, tonic eye deviations, and reversible loss of vestibular caloric responses. As the blood glucose level rises above 600 mg/dl, coma may develop. Thrombosis of cerebral vessels and sinuses may occur. Seizures generally improve within 24 hours of rehydration and correction of hyperglycemia.

Persistent hypoglycorrhachia with normal serum glucose levels has been attributed to a defective glucose transport across the blood-brain barrier, resulting in seizures and developmental delay. These long-term neurologic sequelae may be prevented by a ketogenic diet.

REF: De Vivo et al: *N Engl J Med* 325:703–709, 1991.

GLYCOGEN STORAGE DISEASE   *(see Degenerative Diseases of Childhood, Myopathy)*

GRAVES' OPTHALMOPATHY   *(see also Thyroid)*

Graves' ophthalmopathy refers to any thyroid-associated ophthalmopathy. Graves' hyperthyroidism occurs in about 90% of these patients. There is an association with autoimmune hypothyroidism in half of the remaining patients; the others have no overt thyroid abnormalities on biochemical study.

Patients with Graves' ophthalmopathy frequently complain of dryness, "gritty" sensation, lacrimation, photophobia, blurring of vision, deep orbital pressure, or diplopia. Diplopia is due to fibrosis of ocular muscles that do not extend fully when their antagonist contracts. Fibrosis of the inferior rectus, the most frequently affected muscle, causes diplopia on upward gaze. Other findings on examination are periorbital and lid edema, lid retraction, lid lag, conjunctival chemosis and injection, and exposure keratitis. Some patients have compressive optic neuropathy with decreased visual acuity, optic disc changes, dulling of color perception, and visual field defects.

Diagnostic evaluation of thyroid eye disease includes thyroid function tests of free thyroxine, triiodothyronine, TSH, serum thyrotropin receptor antibody, and serum antimicrosomal and antithyroglobulin antibodies. Enlarged extraocular muscles can be demonstrated by ultrasonography, CT, or MRI.

The rapidity, type, and degree of intervention for management depend on visual status, rapidity and severity of ocular symptoms, systemic thyroid status, and the stage of extraocular muscle involvement, that is, fibrotic versus inflammatory involvement. Treatments include artificial tears, corticosteroids, orbital radiation, and surgical decompression. Generally, ocular findings, except proptosis, are ameliorated with control of hyperthyroidism, although they progress in a minority of patients despite thyroid ablation.

REF: Char DH: *Med Clin North Am* 75(1):97–118, 1991.

Fells P: *Lancet* 338:29 32, 1991.

Weetman AP: *Lancet* 338:25–28, 1991.

GUILLAIN-BARRÉ SYNDROME *(see Neuropathy, Cerebrospinal Fluid)*

GUSTATORY SENSE *(see Taste)*

H REFLEX *(see Electromyography)*

HALLERVORDEN-SPATZ DISEASE *(see Chorea, Degenerative Diseases of Childhood, Dystonia)*

HALLUCINATIONS

The DSM IV R defines hallucinations as a "sensory precept without external stimulation of the relevant sensory organ." Some distinguish true hallucinations (experiences perceived as real and outside the body) from pseudohallucinations (perceived as occurring within the body or known to be unreal). Phenomona include lilliputian (small animals or people), brobdingnagian (giants), and autoscopic (seeing one's self from outside) characteristics, as well as palinopsia, voices, palinacusis, crawling sensations, shooting pains, smells, and other features.

I. Differential diagnosis of visual hallucinations.
   A. Ocular disorders: Associated with reduced vision. These are usually formed, bright, colored images. Charles Bonnet syndrome is isolated visual hallucinations, usually of ocular cause. Ocular causes of visual hallucinations include enucleation; cataracts; macular, choroidal, and retinal disease; and vitreous traction.
   B. CNS disorders: May be due to lesions anywhere along the optic pathways and visual association cortices. Also seen with midbrain disease ("peduncular hallucinosis"; complex forms, usually with other brainstem signs), dementias, epilepsy, migraine, and narcolepsy. Hypnagogic hallucinations occur just before falling asleep, and hypnopompic hallucinations occur on awakening.

    C. Medical disorders: Seen in 40% to 75% of delirious patients; usually brief, nocturnal, and emotionally charged. Causes include alcohol and drug withdrawal, hallucinogens, sympathomimetics, and metabolic encephalopathies.

    D. Psychiatric disorders: Schizophrenia, mania or depression, and hysteria.

    E. Normal Individuals: Dreams, hypnagogic hallucinations, hypnosis, childhood (imaginary companion), sensory deprivation, sleep deprivation, intense emotional experiences.

II. Differential diagnosis of auditory hallucinations.

    A. Diseases of the ears or peripheral auditory nerves.

    B. CNS diseases: Epilepsy, neoplasms, and occasionally, vascular lesions.

    C. Toxic or metabolic: Alcoholic hallucinosis, encephalopathies.

    D. Psychiatric: Schizophrenia (60% to 90% of patients), affective disorders, conversion reactions, multiple personality disorder.

III. Tactile, somatic, and phantom limb hallucinations. Phantom limb is the sensation of persistent presence of an amputated extremity and is found in almost all amputees; usually described as the phantom limb being numb or tingling, of normal size, correctly aligned, with peripheral areas more prominent, and recedes gradually. This may occur after acute hemiplegia or loss of any body part. Tactile hallucinations occur commonly in patients with schizophrenia (15% to 50%) and affective disorder (25%). Formication (the sensation of insects crawling) is found in alcohol and drug withdrawal (especially sympathomimetics) and dementias.

IV. Olfactory and gustatory hallucinations. Medial temporal lobe lesions and complex partial seizures ("uncinate fits") may produce olfactory hallucinations. They may also occur in migraine, dementias, toxic and metabolic conditions, depression and Briquet's syndrome (20% to 25% of patients). Gustatory hallucinations may be seen in manic-depressive illness, schizophrenia, Briquet's syndrome, and partial seizures.

REF: Cummings JL: *Clinical neuropsychiatry*, New York, 1985, Grune & Stratton.

HEADACHE

Headache disorders are extremely common. The lifetime prevalence of headache (any kind), migraine, and tension-type headache have been estimated as 93%, 8%, and 69% for men and as 99%, 25%, and 88% for women. The prevalence for tension-type headache decreases with increasing age, whereas migraine shows no correlation to age.

CLASSIFICATION

The full classification by the International Headache Society can be found in *Cephalalgia*, 1988.

1. *Migraine*. Migraine is characterized by unilateral, pulsating, moderate to severe headache, often increasing with physical activity and helped by sleep. It is often accompanied by nausea or vomiting, photophobia, and phonophobia. Migraine may be preceded or accompanied by auras, most commonly visual fortification spectra, scintillating scotomas, or flashes of light (photopsias). Migraine subtypes include those with aura (classic, complicated, ophthalmic, hemiparesthetic, hemiplegic, or aphasic) and without aura (common migraine), ophthalmoplegic migraine (most commonly complete oculomotor palsy), retinal migraine, basilar migraine, and childhood periodic syndromes (migraine equivalents), including acute confusional states, benign positional vertigo, cyclic vomiting, "Alice in Wonderland" syndrome, paroxysmal leg pains, and alternating hemiplegia of childhood. Occasional migraines may be pure "acephalgic" auras without headache, but these may require investigation to rule out other intracranial processes. Complications of migraine include status migranosus and migraine stroke.

2. *Cluster headache*. Predominantly affect men in a ratio of 4.5 to 6.7:1; may occur at any age, but most often occur in the late twenties. Periodicity is the main feature of cluster headaches; the average cluster period lasts 2 to 3 months and recurs every year or two. Cluster headaches are nocturnal in more than 50% of patients and in many patients are characterized by a circadian regularity. They are often precipitated by alcohol use (during the cluster). Cluster headaches can be episodic or chronic.

   There is no associated aura. The pain reaches it peak 10 to 15 minutes after onset and generally lasts for 45 to 60 minutes, occurring at a frequency of 1 to 3 per day. The pain is usually felt in the trigeminal nerve distribution and is excruciating, penetrating, and nonthrobbing. Signs associated with cluster headache are conjunctival injection, lacrimation, nasal congestion, rhinorrhea, forehead and facial sweating, miosis, ptosis, and eyelid swelling.

Symptomatic cluster headache treatment includes 100% O_2 and ergotamine, which are very effective. Prophylactic treatment consists of lithium, the effectiveness of which is known within a week, calcium channel blockers, methysergide, corticosteroids, and ergotamine. For episodic cluster headache the preferred abortive treatment is O_2; the prophylactic treatment of choice is a combination of ergotamine and verapamil. The most effective treatment for chronic cluster headache is a combination of lithium and verapamil, to which ergotamine can be added for resistant headaches. If these fail, a 2-week tapering course of corticosteroids may break the cycle.

3. *Chronic paroxysmal hemicrania.* A type of cluster headache in which there is severe unilateral orbital or supraorbital pain, or both, always on the same side. Headaches last from 2 to 10 minutes and occur daily up to 15 times a day. This type of headache also has the same associated signs as cluster headache. A diagnostic-therapeutic test for chronic paroxysmal hemicrania is that attacks show an absolute, specific responsiveness to indomethacin (150 mg or less).

4. *Tension-type headaches.* These headaches are episodic but may transform into the chronic variety. The headaches are diffuse, bilateral, pressing or "tightening" in quality, and mild to moderate in severity. Pain often involves the posterior aspects of the head and neck. Photophobia, phonophobia, or mild nausea may occur rarely. Vomiting is not a feature of chronic tension-type headache.

5. *Drug-induced headache.* When used frequently and in excessive quantities, symptomatic medications used for acute relief of headaches may perpetuate headaches. Two main forms of drug-induced headache occur: analgesic-rebound headache and ergotamine-rebound headache. The features of a drug-induced headache are a self-sustaining, rhythmic, headache-medication cycle characterized by daily or near-daily headache and a predictable use of pain medication as the only means of relief. Distinguishing drug-induced headache from a primary headache disorder such as tension or migraine is difficult, since

migraine patients may manifest some features of migraine without the typical pattern of the attacks. Other accompanying symptoms include asthenia, nausea, restlessness, irritability, memory problems, difficulty with concentration, behavior problems, sleep abnormalities, and tolerance to symptomatic medications. After the initial withdrawal period, there is improvement in the previously mentioned symptoms, as well as a reduction in the frequency and severity of headache. The use of excessive amounts of daily symptomatic medications nullifies the beneficial effects of concomitant prophylactic medications

6. *Headache associated with other medical conditions.* Headache may be a symptom of local cranial disease (sinusitis, otitis, dental conditions), upper cervical spine conditions (see Craniocervical Junction), or systemic diseases. Acute severe headache raises the possibility of life-threatening conditions such as subarachnoid hemorrhage or meningitis. Headache is a cardinal feature of pseudotumor cerebri and temporal arteritis. Brain tumor headache is not always localized and often simulates tension or migraine. The classic pattern of headaches that are worse on awakening is often not present. Headache is present in 25% of strokes but is not a reliable localizing finding. Headache is common after head trauma and may be indistinguishable from migraine or tension headache.

7. *Medication-related headaches.* Nitrates, caffeine, alcohol, ergotamine, analgesic abuse.

HEADACHE THERAPY

Three components of a systematic approach to treating headache are psychologic, physical, and pharmacologic. Psychologic therapy involves reassurance and counseling, as well as stress management, relaxation therapy, and biofeedback as appropriate. Physical therapy involves identifying headache triggers, such as diet, hormone variations, and stress, whose alteration may be helpful in treating selected cases. A headache calendar documenting the occurrence, severity, and duration of headaches; the type and efficacy of medication taken; and any triggering factors should be recorded by the patient. Pharmacotherapy can be divided into two approaches, symptomatic and prophylactic.

I. *Symptomatic or abortive therapy.*
   A. Routine analgesics (aspirin, acetaminophen, and nonsteroidals, including ibuprofen, naproxen, naproxen sodium, indomethacin, ketorolac, and others).

B. Narcotic analgesics should be avoided but are useful for occasional, severe headaches.

C. Ergotamine preparations are available for oral, sublingual, and rectal administration and by inhalation.

1. Sumatriptin 6 mg IM provides relief in up to 80% of patients with acute migraine. Failure to respond to the initial dose makes it unlikely that response will be observed after subsequent doses. Response is often seen within 1 hour and may be repeated once every 24 hours.

2. Ergotamine 1 mg PO q½h up to 5 mg per attack.

3. Ergotamine 1 mg and caffeine 100 mg (Cafergot), 1 or 2 tabs PO q½h up to 5 tabs per attack.

4. Ergotamine 2 mg sublingually q½h up to 3 per day.

5. Ergotamine and caffeine (Cafergot) suppository, 1 pr; may repeat in 1 hr prn.

6. Dihydroergotamine (D.H.E. 45) (see Table 27).

D. Isometheptene two capsules at onset and 1 q1h prn up to 5 capsules per headache.

E. Ibuprofen 400 to 800 mg PO at onset and repeat q4h prn.

F. Metoclopramide 10 mg IM, IV, or PO 15 minutes before other analgesic agents has proven useful.

G. Prednisone 40 to 60 mg PO qd over a short course may break "status migranosus."

H. Biofeedback and behavior therapy.

II. *Prophylactic treatment of migraine.*

A. Avoid any precipitants.

B. Avoid inciting dietary factors such as red wine, aged cheese, chicken liver, pickled herring, chocolate, tuna, sour cream and yogurt, ripe avocado and banana, smoked meats, and foods with monosodium glutamate or nitrates.

C. Conduct trial when patient is not using oral contraceptives and nitrates, if possible.

D. Prophylactic medication for those with frequent or disabling attacks includes the following.

1. Beta blockers.

a. Propranolol, starting at 20 mg PO bid and gradually increasing prn to 80 mg tid. Has been used in children.

b. Others: Nadolol (80 to 240 mg); atenolol (Tenormin) (50 to 100 mg); timolol, (20 to 100 mg).

2. Methysergide 2 mg PO tid or qid. Need drug holiday every 6 months for 1 month to prevent fibrotic retroperitoneal or mediastinal changes.

TABLE 27
Protocol for Severe, Persistent Headaches

I. Dihydroergotamine (D.H.E. 45) and metoclopramide protocol is tried initially. It is contraindicated in pregnancy and in Prinzmetal's angina. For patients over 60 years of age, monitor cardiac status during first two doses of D.H.E. 45. Side effects include diarrhea, leg pains, vasospasm, chest pain, and supraventricular arrhythmia.

  A. Metoclopramide 10 mg IV plus D.H.E. 45, 0.5 mg IV over 2 to 3 min.

  B. If nausea and headache are absent, continue D.H.E. 45, 0.5 mg IV q8h for 3 days with metoclopramide 10 IV. Stop metoclopramide after sixth dose.

  C. If no nausea is present and headache is persistent, repeat D.H.E. 45, 0.5 mg IV in 1 hour without metoclopramide; if nausea does not recur, give D.H.E. 45 1 mg q8h for 3 days with six doses of metoclopramide. If nausea recurs with the second dose of D.H.E. 45, reduce D.H.E. 45 dose to 0.75 mg.

  D. If nausea and headache persist, hold D.H.E. 45 for 8 hours, then give D.H.E. 45, 0.3 to 0.4 mg q8h for 3 days, with metoclopramide for six doses.

II. Protocol for those unable to tolerate D.H.E. 45.

  A. Prednisone 80 mg per day (short, rapidly tapering dosage).

  B. Neuroleptics: Haloperidol 5 mg PO or IM, thiothixene 5 mg PO or IM, or chlorpromazine 10 to 50 mg PO or 25-mg suppository.

  C. Opiate analgesics: Meperidine 75 to 100 mg, hydromorphone 4 mg, or morphine 10 mg.

Raskin NH: *Neurol Clin* 8:857-865, 1990.

---

   3. Naproxen sodium (550 bid).

   4. Calcium channel blockers: Nifedipine 10 mg PO tid or verapamil 80 mg PO tid, starting dose.

   5. Amitriptyline starting at 25 mg PO qhs and increasing to 50 to 100 mg qhs.

   6. Other tricyclics.

   7. Phenelzine sulfate 15 mg PO qd, qod, or bid.

   9. Ergonovine 0.2 mg PO tid up to 2 mg qd.

  10. Combination Ergotamine, belladonna, and phenobarbital (Bellergal) 2 to 4 tabs PO qd.

      11. Cyproheptadine 2 to 4 mg PO qid.
      12. Vascular-headache diet combined with any of the above.
      13. Depakote 250 tid to therapeutic doses.
      14. Phenytoin 200 to 400 mg per day; especially useful in children.

III. *Treatment of cluster headache.*
    A. Treat as for migraine (ergotamine, methysergide, sumatriptin).
    B. 100% O_2 by mask at 6 l per min up to 15 minutes per attack.
    C. Lidocaine 4% intranasal; 15 drops ipsilateral to headache with head extended and rotated away from side of headache.
    D. Prednisone 40 to 60 mg PO qd over short course; rebound headaches can occur after discontinuation.
    E. Lithium carbonate 300 mg PO bid-qid titrated to lithium levels (0.6 to 1.2 mEq/l) is especially useful for chronic cluster headaches.
    F. Indomethacin 25 to 50 mg PO tid for cluster headache variants and atypical migraines (exertional migraine, benign orgasmic cephalgia, chronic paroxysmal hemicrania, cough headache, and ice-pick headache).

IV. *Chronic daily headache.*
    A. Discontinuation of the offending medications, especially analgesics used to excess.
    B. Use of pharmacotherapeutic agents in attempt to break the cycle of continuous headache.
    C. Initiation of prophylactic pharmacotherapy (often tricyclic or beta blocker).
    D. Concomitant behavioral intervention, including biofeedback therapy, individual behavioral counseling, family therapy, physical exercise, and dietary instruction.
    E. Adequate instruction on ill effects of medications with special focus on analgesics.
    F. Continuity of care.

REF: *Cephalagia*, ed 1, vol 8, suppl 7, Norwegian University Press.

Mathew NT: *Neurology* 42(suppl 2):22–31, 1992.

Mathew NT: *Neurology* 43(suppl 3):26–33, 1993.

Sculman EA, Silberstein SD: *Neurology* 42(suppl 2):16–21, 1992.

Welch KMA: *N Engl J Med* 329:1476–1483, 1993.

HEAD CIRCUMFERENCE   *(see Child Neurology)*

HEARING

Bedside testing of hearing should include examination of the external ear and the tympanic membranes. Auditory acuity can be grossly assessed by whispering into each ear while closing the other and by comparing the distance from the ear at which the patient and the examiner can hear a ticking watch or fingers rubbing together. *Tuning fork tests* are commonly used. In Weber's test a 256-Hz tuning fork is placed at the midline vertex of the skull; sound referred to an ear with decreased acuity indicates conductive hearing loss. In Rinne's test a tuning fork placed on the mastoid and one held in front of the ear are compared; if bone conduction is greater, conductive loss is implied.

Audiologic tests are used to quantitate and localize (conductive, sensorineural, cochlear, and retrocochlear) hearing loss. *Pure-tone threshold* determines auditory threshold for tones over various frequencies and intensities for both air and bone conduction. Impairment of both air and bone conduction, especially at high frequencies, indicates sensorineural hearing loss. When bone conduction is greater than air conduction, conductive hearing loss is present. Other tests of loudness function are the alternate binaural loudness balance and the short-increment sensitivity index. Bekesy audiometry, tone decay tests, speech discrimination tests, the stapedius reflex (pathway from cochlea to eighth cranial nerve to facial nerve to stapedius muscle), and brain stem auditory evoked potentials (BAEP) help distinguish retrocochlear from cochlear lesions. Rarely, cortical deafness or auditory agnosia occurs with bitemporal lesions and BAEPs are normal.

Causes of nonretrocochlear hearing loss include bacterial, viral, or fungal infections of the external, middle, or inner ear; presbycusis; otosclerosis; cholesteatoma and glomus tumor; ototoxic drugs such as aminoglycosides, aspirin, and diuretics; Meniere's disease; and trauma.

Causes of retrocochlear (eighth cranial nerve and CNS) hearing loss include the following:

1. Tumors: Acoustic neuroma, cholesteatoma, meningioma, pontine glioma.
2. Vascular: Vertebrobasilar ischemia and inferior lateral pontine infarction or basilar occlusion.
3. Demyelinating diseases.
4. Congenital malformations: Arnold-Chiari, Klippel-Feil syndromes.

5. Degenerative diseases: Hereditary ataxias, hereditary neuropathies; Refsum disease, xeroderma pigmentosum, Cockayne's syndrome, Usher's syndrome (retinitis pigmentosa and deafness), and other rare hereditary degenerative disorders.
6. Infectious: meningitis, encephalitis, syphilis.
7. Inflammatory: Vogt-Koyanagi-Harada syndrome, Behçet's syndromes; sarcoidosis.
8. Mitochondrial diseases: Kearns-Sayre syndrome.

REF: Rudge P: *Clinical neuro-otology*, New York, 1983, Churchill Livingstone.

HEMANGIOBLASTOMA   *(see Tumor)*

HEMANGIOMA   *(see Angioma)*

HEMATOMA   *(see Hemorrhage)*

HEMIANOPIA   *(see Visual Fields)*

HEMORRHAGE   *(see also Aneurysm, Angioma)*

Primary intraparenchymal hemorrhage (intracerebral hemorrhage) accounts for 10% of all strokes. Hypertension is the predominant risk factor. Chronic hypertension causes lipohyalinosis of the small, intraparenchymal arteries, resulting in arteriolar wall weakness and subsequent rupture. Location of hemorrhage in decreasing order of frequency is as follows: putamenal (35% to 50%), subcortical white matter (30%), cerebellar (15%), thalamic (10% to 15%) and pontine (5% to 12%). Active bleeding usually lasts only a short time; later clinical deterioration is most often ascribed to surrounding edema and ischemia than to continued hemorrhage.

The signs and symptoms of cerebral hemorrhage correlate with anatomic location, size, and degree of associated mass effect. Headache is a frequent accompanying symptom.

Putamenal hemorrhage is associated with contralateral hemiparesis, hemianesthesia, and homonymous hemianopsia with aphasia or neglect (depending on which hemisphere is involved). There is also decreased level of consciousness, ipsilateral eye deviation, and normal pupils.

Thalamic hemorrhage produces contralateral hemisensory loss with variable hemiparesis, contralateral homonymous hemianopsia, vertical or lateral-gaze palsies (including "wrong way" deviation), and occasionally, nystagmus.

Cerebellar hemorrhage is associated with severe occipital headache, sudden nausea and vomiting, and truncal ataxia. It is a potential neurosurgical emergency when brainstem compression is imminent.

Pontine hemorrhage causes coma, pinpoint pupils (reactive to light), bilateral extensor posturing, impaired ocular motility, and caloric testing.

Acute mortality in intracerebral hemorrhage is usually due to mass effect with herniation or brainstem compression. Mortality may be high, especially in posterior fossa hemorrhage. The long-term prognosis for recovery of function may be better than in infarction, since there is usually displacement of tissue instead of primary tissue damage and necrosis.

Diagnosis is made by CT; acutely blood appears hyperdense. Angiography may be necessary to exclude underlying vascular malformation or tumor.

Management may require an intensive care setting with frequent neurologic evaluation. Maintain adequate ventilation, pulmonary and pharyngeal toilet, and adequate fluid and electrolyte balance. Antiedema agents (corticosteroids, osmotic diuretics) may be used but their efficacy is uncertain. Hyperventilation with induction of hypercapnia can also be used to decrease intracranial pressure.

Blood pressure management is controversial; injudicious lowering of the pressure is contraindicated. Neurosurgical evaluation should be obtained for superficially located cerebral hemorrhages and all cerebellar hemorrhages.

Other causes of intraparenchymal hemorrhage account for 25% to 50% of nonhypertensive cerebral hemorrhage and include the following:

1. Trauma.
2. Ruptured arteriovenous malformation (see also Angiomas).
3. Ruptured aneurysm with parenchymal extension.
4. Metastatic carcinoma, especially of the lung, choriocarcinoma, melanoma, and renal adenocarcinoma.
5. Primary neoplasms (glioblastoma multiforme, pituitary adenoma).
6. Embolic infarction with secondary hemorrhage (up to one third of embolic infarcts).
7. Hematologic disorders, including leukemia, lymphoma, thrombocytopenic purpura, aplastic anemia, sickle cell ane-

mia, hemophilia, hypoprothrombinemia, afibrinogenemia, Waldenström's macroglobulinemia.

8. Anticoagulant therapy.
9. Cerebral amyloid angiopathy. Usually becomes evident as multiple, recurrent hemorrhages in the white matter or cortex, sparing deep gray (as opposed to hypertensive hemorrhages). Amyloid angiopathy may be the cause in 5% to 10% of sporadic intracerebral hemorrhages. It is associated with dementia in about 30% of cases; familial cases are associated with mutations in the amyloid precursor protein on chromosome 21 (Dutch and Icelandic forms). Attempts at surgical evacuation are usually futile, since the vessels are fragile, bleeding is difficult to control, and the incidence of recurrent hemorrhages is high.
10. Vasculopathies such as lupus, polyarteritis nodosa, and granulomatous arteritis.
11. Cortical vein thrombosis with secondary hemorrhage.
12. Drugs, including methamphetamine, amphetamine, pseudoephedrine, phenylpropanolamine, and cocaine.

Subarachnoid hemorrhage occurs with an incidence of 15 per 100,000; peak incidence is at 55 to 60 years of age. Most cases are due to rupture of cerebral aneurysm or trauma (see Aneurysm).

Subdural hemorrhage (SDH) may be acute or chronic. Acute SDH is usually due to trauma with tearing of bridging veins. There may be an initial loss of consciousness with regaining of consciousness (lucid interval), followed in several hours by progressive deterioration of mental status and headache. Lateralizing signs may be present. Diagnosis is based on clinical course, emergency CT (appears as hyperdensity over cortex), and if necessary, angiography. Treatment consists of neurosurgical evacuation. Dialysis patients and alcoholics are particularly prone to SDH.

Chronic SDH is less clearly related to trauma and may follow minor head trauma in elderly patients and patients receiving anticoagulants. Symptoms and signs resemble those in acute SDH but develop gradually over several days to months. Lateralizing signs are common. Mental status changes may suggest dementia. Diagnosis is as for acute SDH, although the lesion on CT is usually hypodense or isodense. Treatment is neurosurgical evacuation.

The prognosis for survival and recovery in surgically treated patients is generally good.

Acute epidural hemorrhage results from skull fracture with laceration of the middle meningeal artery and vein. The clinical course is similar to that for acute SDH but is more rapidly progressive. Rapid herniation, respiratory depression, and death may ensue. The CT appearance is a lens-shaped hyperdensity. Treatment is a neurosurgical emergency.

REF: Powers WJ: *Neurology* 43:461–467, 1993.

Selman WR, Ratcheson RA. In Bradley WG et al, eds: *Neurology in clinical practice*, Boston, 1991, Butterworth-Heinemann.

HEPARIN THERAPY   *(see Ischemia)*

HEPATOLENTICULAR DEGENERATION   *(see Wilson's Disease)*

HERNIATION   *(see also Intracranial Pressure)*

Herniation is displacement of the cerebral or cerebellar structures from their normal compartments to another, which results from pressure differences between compartments. Most commonly, increased pressure is due to a focal lesion (e g , tumor with edema, hemorrhage, infarct, or abscess). Diffuse elevations of intracranial pressure, as in pseudotumor cerebri, rarely produce herniation. There are four common herniation syndromes: cingulate, central transtentorial, uncal or lateral transtentorial, and cerebellar. The latter may be either upward through the transtentorial notch or downward, causing the cerebellar tonsils to herniate through the foramen magnum. These syndromes are accompanied by characteristic clinical signs that correspond to the anatomic structures involved (see Table 28).

A rostral-caudal progression of clinical signs is seen with both central and lateral transtentorial herniation, indicating worsening herniation (see Table 29). The progression begins with diencephalic involvement, and mesencephalic, pontine, and finally medullary involvement follow. In two infrequent exceptions to this orderly progression, signs skip from the hemispheres or diencephalon to the medulla, bypassing the rostral brain stem. (1) Acute cerebral hemorrhage with extravasation into the ventricles produces a pressure wave that compresses the medullary respiratory center in the floor of the fourth ventricle and (2) when lumbar puncture is performed on patients with incipient transtentorial herniation, the procedure may induce enough of a pressure change to produce tonsillar herniation.

For treatment of herniation, see Intracranial Pressure.

TABLE 28
Herniation Syndromes

Syndromes	Anatomy	Signs
Central transtentorial herniation: Caudal displacement of diencephalon through tentorial notch	Reticular formation or diencephalon initially, then rostral-caudal progression	Altered consciousness
Lateral transtentorial herniation (uncal)	Ipsilateral CN III	Ipsilateral pupil dilation, then external ophthalmoplegia
	Ipsilateral posterior cerebral artery	Contralateral homonymous hemianopsia
	Contralateral cerebral peduncle (false localizing); then follows rostral-caudal progression but may skip diencephalic stage	Ipsilateral hemiparesis
Cerebellar tonsillar herniation	Medullary respiratory center	Respiratory arrest
Cingulate herniation under falx cerebri	Anterior cerebral artery	Leg weakness

TABLE 29
Rostral-Caudal Progression of Transtentorial Herniation

	Diencephalon	Midbrain-Upper Pons	Low Pons-Upper Medulla	Medulla
Consciousness, systemic	Agitated or drowsy to coma, diabetes insipidis	Hypothermia or hyperthermia, comatose	Comatose	Fluctuating pulse, blood pressure falls Coma
Breathing	Yawns, pauses, Cheyne-Stokes respirations	Central hyperventilation	Tachypnea (20-40 breaths per min) shallow	Slow and irregular or hyperapnea alternating with apnea, then breathing stops
Pupils	Small (1-3 mm) reaction, small but brisk	Irregular, midposition (3-5 mm), fixed	Small, midposition, fixed	Dilated, fixed
Eye movements	Roving, VOR* weak or brisk, fast-phase caloric response lost, loss of vertical movement	Intact VOR,† may be dysconjugate response	No VOR,* no caloric response	No VOR, no caloric response

*See Oculovestibular Reflex (VOR).
†See Calorics.

TABLE 29—cont'd
Rostral-Caudal Progression of Transtentorial Herniation

| Motor | Preexisting hemiplegia worsens, decorticate posturing to noxious stimuli, plantars extensor | Bilateral decerebrate posturing to noxious stimuli | Flaccid flexor response in LEs to noxious stimuli | Flaccid, no deep tendon reflexes |

REF: Plum F, Posner JB: *The diagnosis of stupor and coma*, ed 3, Philadelphia, 1982, FA Davis.

HERPES SIMPLEX *(see Encephalitis)*

HERPES ZOSTER *(see Zoster)*

HEUBNER'S ARTERITIS *(see Syphilis)*

HEXOSAMINIDASE DEFICIENCY *(see Degenerative Diseases of Childhood)*

HICCUPS *(Singultus, Hiccoughs)*

A recurrent reflex myoclonic contraction of the diaphragm with a forceful inspiration, associated with laryngeal spasm and closure of glottis, producing a characteristic sound. It is mediated by the phrenic nerve (afferent) and vagus and thoracic nerves (efferent). Gastrointestinal, pulmonary, and cardiovascular symptoms and signs may be present. Carcinoma, achalasia, and hiatal hernia are common pathologic causes, as well as intrathoracic distention, pulmonary or pleural irritation, pericarditis, mediastinitis or mediastinal mass, intrathoracic abscesses or tumors, and aortic aneurysms. CNS causes are many, including metabolic (acetonemia, uremia), drugs (sulfonamides), infection (encephalitis), hypothalamic disease (also associated with yawning), tumors of the fourth ventricle, and cerebrovascular disease (vertebrobasilar insufficiency). Idiopathic and psychogenic hiccups are common.

Treatment is usually not required; the hiccups tend to be self-limited. They may be intractable, especially if there is a primary cause, in which case the underlying cause is treated. Drug therapies for intractable hiccups include phenothiazines (prochlorperazine, chlorpromazine), valproic acid, phenytoin, carbamazepine, benzodiazepines (clonazepam, diazepam), and baclofen. Surgical sectioning of the phrenic nerve or selective vagotomy is occasionally required.

HIV *(see AIDS)*

HORNER'S SYNDROME *(see also Ptosis, Pupil)*

Horner's syndrome (oculosympathetic paresis) is due to disruption at any point along the course of the sympathetic pathway from the hypothalamus to the orbit (Figure 19). Signs are miosis (resulting from iris dilator weakness) most evident in dim illumination, ptosis (weakness of Müller's muscle), and anhidrosis. Heterochromia of the iris occurs in congenital Horner's syndrome.

The cause of Horner's syndrome can be determined in about 60% of cases. Lesions of the first-order neuron (central) are myriad and include stroke, tumor, hemorrhage, and demyelinating disease. Second-order neuron (preganglionic) causes include apical lung tumor, tuberculosis, radical neck dissection, trauma, and neck masses. Third-order neuron (postganglionic) lesions include internal carotid aneurysms, carotid dissection, cluster headaches, and migraine and do not have anhidrosis.

Cocaine eyedrops (4% to 10%) are used to differentiate Horner's syndrome from simple anisocoria on a pharmacologic basis. By preventing norepinephrine reuptake at sympathetic nerve endings, the eyedrops cause normal pupils to dilate. Lesions of any part of the sympathetic pathway cause failure of pupillary dilation because of lack of norepinephrine at the nerve terminal.

Evaluation for central and preganglionic lesions should include careful neck palpation, apical lordotic chest x-ray views, and possibly CT of the neck and chest. New-onset postganglionic Horner's syndrome suggests carotid artery disease. Isolated postganglionic Horner's syndrome is generally benign.

REF: Loewenfield IE: *The pupil: anatomy, physiology and clinical applications*, vol 1, Ames, IA, 1993, Iowa State University Press.

HUNTINGTON'S DISEASE

Huntington's disease (HD) is an autosomal-dominant neurodegenerative disease characterized by progressive choreoathetosis, psychological or behavioral changes, and dementia. Although chorea is generally thought to be the first sign of HD, behavioral changes may occur a decade or more before the movement disorder, with depression the most common symptom. Patients may become erratic, irritable, impulsive, and emotionally labile.

The reported mean age of onset ranges from 35 to 42 years, with an average duration from onset to death of 17 years. Three percent of patients develop signs and symptoms before the age of 15, with rigidity, myoclonus, dystonia, and seizures more evident than chorea; in these cases, the course is rapid and there is often paternal transmission.

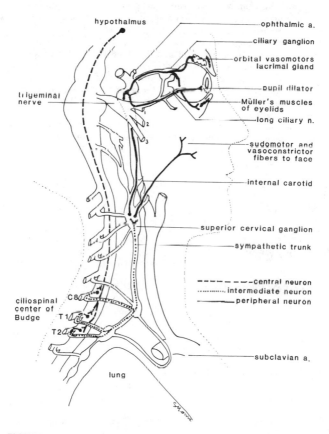

hypothalmus

ophthalmic a.

ciliary ganglion

orbital vasomotors
lacrimal gland

pupil dilator

Müller's muscles
of eyelids

long ciliary n.

trigeminal
nerve

sudomotor and
vasoconstrictor
fibers to face

internal carotid

superior cervical ganglion

sympathetic trunk

— — — — — central neuron
.... intermediate neuron
————— peripheral neuron

ciliospinal
center of
Budge

C8

T1

T2

subclavian a.

lung

FIGURE 19
Oculosympathetic pathways.

Neuropathology reveals neuronal loss that is most severe in the caudate and putamen, along with a glial response. Several neurotransmitter systems are altered, with abnormally increased or decreased levels of neurotransmitters, biosynthetic enzymes, and receptor-binding sites.

Genetic testing has been based on linkage analysis of affected families. The gene has now been identified and the disease state correlated with excess copies of a trinucleotide CAG repeat. The development of genetic tests based on this information is now underway.

CT and MRI reveal atrophy of the caudate nucleus and cortex. PET studies have revealed relative hypometabolism in the striatum of some patients at risk for the disease.

Treatment is aimed at reducing the movement disorder when it is disabling or embarrassing. Haldol has proved to be quite effective at doses of 1 to 40 mg per day but may cause adventitious movements if usage is prolonged.

REF: Huntington Disease Collaborative Research Group: *Cell* 72:971, 1993.

Martin JB, Gusella JF: *N Engl J Med* 315:267, 1986.

Meissen GJ, et al: *N Engl J Med* 318:535, 1988.

HYDRANENCEPHALY *(see Developmental Malformations)*

HYDROCEPHALUS

Hydrocephalus is characterized by an increase in volume of cerebrospinal fluid (CSF) associated with dilation of the cerebral ventricles. Three mechanisms cause hydrocephalus: (1) obstruction of CSF pathways, (2) defective absorption of CSF, and (3) oversecretion of CSF (rare but seen with choroid plexus papilloma). Hydrocephalus is classified as either communicating or noncommunicating, as normal-pressure or high-pressure, and as *ex vacuo* (Figure 20).

Noncommunicating hydrocephalus is due to intraventricular obstruction of the foramen of Monro, the third ventricle, the aqueduct of Sylvius, or the foramen of Luschka or of Magendie. Lesions causing obstruction include aqueductal stenosis, cysts, intraventricular and extraventricular tumors, inflammation, and congenital malformations.

Communicating hydrocephalus is most often due to obstruction of CSF pathways in the subarachnoid space, arachnoid villi, or draining veins. Causes include inflammation of the leptomeninges as a result

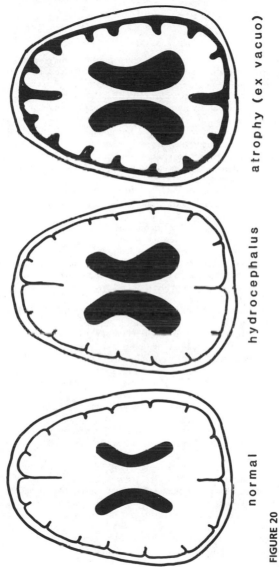

normal   hydrocephalus   atrophy (ex vacuo)

FIGURE 20
MR or CT appearance of normal and enlarged ventricles

of prior infection or hemorrhage, tumors, posttraumatic obstruction, and congenital malformations (most commonly Arnold-Chiari malformation).

Normal-pressure hydrocephalus (NPH) is a syndrome of communicating hydrocephalus without clinical evidence of intracranial hypertension. It is characterized by the triad of (1) gait disturbance characterized by low-velocity short steps with reduction of step height, (2) dementia, and (3) urinary incontinence. Diagnosis is based on history and supported by imaging and lumbar puncture with normal opening pressure. Treatment is surgical shunting. The most favorable responses occur in nondemented patients.

Hydrocephalus ex vacuo describes the phenomenon of an increase in volume of CSF under normal pressure in compensation for loss of brain mass.

Clinical presentation varies depending on age and whether the hydrocephalus is acute or chronic. In an infant the most common symptoms are irritability, poor feeding, and lethargy. On examination a bulging, tense fontanel, separation of sutures, increased head circumference, frontal bossing, globular but symmetric head shape, "setting sun" sign resulting from paralysis of upward gaze, and loss of developmental milestones may be evident. In older children (over 6 years of age) and adults the most common symptoms are headache and emesis that are worse in the morning, diplopia, loss of gross and fine motor coordination usually manifested as a gait abnormality, cranial nerve VI palsies, absent retinal pulsations, and papilledema.

Diagnosis is made by CT or MRI. A small or normal fourth ventricle usually implies obstruction proximal to it. A dilated fourth ventricle implies obstruction distally, either at the outflow of the foramina of the fourth ventricle or in the subarachnoid space. In the infant with an open anterior fontanel, ultrasonography is useful for assessing ventricular size and presence of blood.

Examination of CSF may be helpful in determining the origin of the hydrocephalus, but lumbar puncture is contraindicated when imaging studies show evidence of mass effect, such as midline shift, effacement of cortical sulci, or effacement of the suprachiasmatic, basilar, quadrigeminal, or cerebellar cisterns.

The major therapy is extraventricular shunting. Pharmacologic treatment of CSF overproduction includes carbonic anhydrase inhibitors such as acetazolamide and furosemide.

REF: Fishman RA: *Cerebrospinal fluid in diseases of the nervous system*, Philadelphia, 1992, WB Saunders.

HYPERACTIVITY *(see Attention Deficit–
                    Hyperactivity Syndrome)*

HYPERACUSIS *(see Facial Nerve)*

HYPERGLYCEMIA *(see Glucose)*

HYPERREFLEXIA *(see Reflexes)*

HYPERTENSION *(see Hemorrhage, Ischemia)*

HYPERTENSION, INTRACRANIAL *(see Herniation,
                                 Intracranial
                                 Pressure,
                                 Pseudotumor
                                 Cerebri)*

HYPERTHYROIDISM *(see Graves' Ophthalmopathy,
                      Myopathy, Thyroid)*

HYPERVENTILATION *(see also Coma, Sleep
                       Disorders)*

Inspiratory patterns reflect many factors and may provide localizing information.

Involuntary hyperventilation resulting from autonomic hyperactivity of brainstem respiratory centers is rare; hypoxemia, acid-base disorders, CSF acidosis, pulmonary disease, drug effects, and voluntary hyperventilation are more common.

Voluntary hyperventilation is usually related to anxiety. Symptoms include chest pain, palpitations, dyspnea, lightheadedness, perioral and fingertip numbness or parathesias, cramps, GI distress, insomnia, a feeling of fright, and occasionally syncope. Arterial blood gas levels should show a respiratory alkalosis during an attack. Reproduction of symptoms by hyperventilation is diagnostic.

Posthyperventilation apnea is characterized by an exaggerated apneic response to lowered $PaCO_2$ seen with bilateral hemispheric dysfunction. When more than 12 seconds of apnea follows 20 to 30 seconds of voluntary hyperventilation, the diagnosis is made (normal response, less than 10 seconds of apnea).

Cheyne-Stokes breathing, central neurogenic hyperventilation, and *apneustic* and *ataxic respirations* may occur during coma (see Coma for a discussion of these entities).

REF: Colice GL: *Neurologic disorders and respiration, Clin Chest Med* 10(4):521–543, 1989.

HYPOGLOSSAL NERVE   *(see Cranial Nerves)*

HYPOGLYCEMIA   *(see Glucose, Syncope)*

HYPOREFLEXIA   *(see Reflexes)*

HYPOTENSION   *(see Syncope)*

HYPOTENSION, INTRACRANIAL   *(see Intracranial Pressure)*

HYPOTHALAMUS   *(see Limbic System)*

HYPOTHYROIDISM   *(see Myopathy, Neuropathy, Thyroid)*

HYPOTONIC INFANT   *(see also Child Neurology, Chromosomal Disorders)*

Hypotonia in infancy can be caused by lesions at any level of the nervous system. The history and examination determine the site of dysfunction and help identify the cause of the hypotonia. Family history of disease is present in some cases (see Table 30).

In a classic case a hypotonic (floppy) infant assumes a frog-leg posture (hips abducted and externally rotated and the entire length of the limbs in contact with the flat surface). There is decreased resistance to passive movement and marked head lag with hand traction in the supine position. In ventral suspension an inverted-U shape of the back is evident, neck extension is absent, and elbow and knee flexion is minimal.

Increased reflexes indicate a CNS lesion. If they are normal, a myopathy has to be ruled out. Neuropathy causes decreased reflexes. Decreased alertness, poor response to external stimuli, and poor suck or grasp reflex suggest CNS disease. Muscle fasciculations occur with neuropathy and anterior horn cell disease. Hypotonia with weakness suggests anterior horn cell or peripheral nervous system disease.

Beyond the neonatal period hypotonic infants frequently come to medical attention with delay in achieving motor milestones. Assessment of nonmotor-dependent activity such as social response, smiling,

TABLE 30

Differential Diagnosis of the Hypotonic Infant

I. CNS disease.
  A. Perinatal hypoxia-ischemia.
  B. Congenital infection.
  C. Encephalitis, meningitis.
  D. Trauma.
  E. Hydrocephalus.
  F. Tumors.
  G. Trisomies 21 and 13.
  H. Aminoacidopathy.
  I. Storage diseases.
  J. Werdnig-Hoffmann syndrome.
  K. Poliomyelitis.
  L. Leigh syndrome disease.
  M. Prader-Willi syndrome.
II. Neuropathy.
  A. Guillain-Barré syndrome.
  B. Infantile neuropathy.
III. Neuromuscular junction.
  A. Myasthenia gravis.
  B. Infantile botulism.
IV. Muscle disease.
  A. Congenital myopathies.
  B. Myotonic dystrophy.
  C. Carnitine deficiency.
V. Nonneurologic.
  A. Ehlers-Danlos syndrome.
  B. Sepsis.
  C. Dehydration.
  D. Hypothyroidism.
  E. Hypothermia.
  F. Rickets.

and vocalization is important in determining associated intellectual delay. Mental retardation in association with hypotonia obviously suggests a CNS origin.

Once all other causes are excluded, the term "benign congenital hypotonia" may be applied to a hypotonic infant who is otherwise physically and developmentally normal.

HYPOXIA   *(see Cardiopulmonary Arrest)*

HYPSARRHYTHMIA   *(see Electroencephalography, Epilepsy)*

IMMUNIZATION

When neurologic complications are identical to naturally occurring disease, it is impossible to determine in a specific case whether the disorder and the immunization are related or coincidental. Therefore analytic population-based studies of adverse reactions are required to analyze immunization-related syndromes.

The following types of vaccines are available:

I. Killed organisms: Influenza, pertussis, and rabies vaccines are associated with toxic or allergic reactions involving the nervous system: *Haemophilus influenzae* type b and hepatitis B vaccines have no neurologic complications.

A. Influenza: Neurologic complications were rarely noted before 1976, when an increase was found in the incidence of Guillain Barré syndrome in the adult population during the 6 weeks following immunization against swine flu, but such an increase has not occurred with subsequent vaccine programs. Patients with a history of Guillain Barré syndrome should not receive influenza vaccination.

B. Pertussis: Simple febrile seizures may be a consequence of pertussis immunization if the fever has no other cause and both fever and seizures occur within 24 hours of administration. There is also a causal relationship between diptheria-pertussis-tetanus (DPT) vaccine and shocklike states or acute encephalopathy (defined in controlled studies as encephalopathy, encephalitis, or encephalomyelitis). The risk of acute encephalopathy is 0.0 to 10.5 per million immunizations. There is insufficient evidence to indicate a causal relationship between DPT vaccine and permanent neurologic damage, aseptic meningitis, learning disabilities, and attention-deficit disorder. There is evidence, however, that DPT vaccine has no causal relationship to infantile spasms, hypsarrythmia, Reye's syndrome, or sudden infant death syndrome.

C. Rabies: Some underdeveloped countries prepare whole-virus vaccines that contain myelin basic protein and are associated with encephalomyelitis and polyneuritis within 2 weeks after immunization.

II. Live-attenuated viruses: Measles, mumps, rubella, poliomyelitis, and varicella vaccines produce their natural diseases and expected complications of the natural disease.

    A. Measles: Ordinarily combined with mumps and rubella (measles, mumps, and rubella [MMR] vaccine). Except for febrile seizures in children who are genetically predisposed, neurologic complications are uncommon. The risk of encephalopathy is small compared to the 1-per-1000 risk of encephalopathy from natural measles

    B. Rubella: Transient arthralgias may develop in up to 40% of patients. No causal evidence exists for association with polyneuritis or other neuropathies.

    C. Poliomyelitis: Paralytic poliomyelitis is the only known complication of oral polio vaccine (OPV) and almost always occurs after initial immunization. Approximately one third of cases have occurred in OPV recipients, one half in contacts of recipients, and the remainder in immunodeficient recipients or contacts.

    D. Varicella: No neurologic complications have been reported.

III. Toxoids: May produce rare allergic reactions. The only contraindication is a history of neurologic or severe hypersensitivity reaction following a previous dose. Tetanus and diphtheria are often given together, making it difficult to attribute adverse reactions to one without the other. Demyelinating neuropathy with complete recovery occurs in rare instances.

REF: Aminoff MJ: *Neurology and general medicine*, New York, 1989, Churchill Livingstone.

    Howson CP, Howe CJ, Fineberg HV, eds: *Adverse effects of pertussis and rubella vaccines*, Institute of Medicine, Washington, DC, 1991, National Academy.

IMMUNOSUPPRESSION   *(see AIDS, Transplantation— Complications of)*

IMMUNOSUPPRESSIVE DRUGS   *(see Chemotherapy, Lambert-Eaton Myasthenic Syndrome, Multiple Sclerosis, Myasthenia Gravis, Vasculitis)*

IMPOTENCE

Male sexual dysfunction results from a complex interaction of psychologic, neurologic, vascular, endocrine, and physical factors. Reflex erection is mediated by the sacral plexus, pudendal nerve, and nerve erigentes. Psychogenic erection is mediated by cerebral cortex and sympathetic thoracolumbar and parasympathetic sacral plexus. Many authors believe that the limbic system also plays an important role in erection, with neurotransmitters modulating this higher cortical response.

Causes of impotence are approximately equally divided between functional and organic. Endocrine causes include diabetes (peripheral diabetic neuropathy, abnormal cystograms) and pituitary axis dysfunction (prolactin-secreting pituitary adenoma, hypogonadism). Vascular origins include atherosclerosis, arteritis, priapism, and thromboembolism. Impotence may follow cystectomy, radical prostatectomy, abdominal perineal resection of the rectum, abdominal aortic aneurysm repair, or external sphincterotomy. Spinal cord dysfunction (tumor, trauma) has been implicated; however, studies of these patients show a much higher incidence of sexual function than would be expected based on the anatomic involvement. Nondiabetic autonomic dysfunction (Shy-Drager and Riley-Day syndromes) as well as multiple sclerosis, Parkinson's disease, and syphilis may be associated with impotence. Inflammation (urethritis, prostatitis, cystitis) and mechanical factors (congenital malformation, Peyronie's disease, morbid obesity, malignancy, phimosis, hydrocele, ruptured urethra) may result in impotence. Sedating drugs may impair libido. Alcohol may cause malnutrition and peripheral neuropathy as well as sedation. Anticholinergic drug side effects may impair erection. Drugs that interfere with sympathetic neurotransmission may impair ejaculation.

History is aimed at distinguishing between functional and organic factors (adequacy of neurologic and vascular pathways) and identification of specific causes. Inquire about the following:

1. Onset and progression of sexual dysfunction.
2. Ejaculation and orgasm.
3. Morning and nocturnal erection pattern.
4. Relation to masturbation.
5. Response to different sexual partners.
6. Endocrine, vascular, or neurologic disease.
7. Previous surgery.
8. Medication, alcohol use.

Examination is aimed at identifying evidence of systemic or endocrine illness and peripheral vascular disease. Neurologic examination should seek evidence of peripheral neuropathy, autonomic neuropathy, myelopathy, or sacral radiculopathy. Urologic or gynecologic consultation should be obtained. Laboratory studies should include fasting blood glucose, prolactin, and testosterone levels. Additional urologic or neurologic studies may be necessary.

Conjoint sex therapy is the mainstay of treatment for functional impotence. After remediable organic causes have been treated, penile prosthesis implantation can be done by a urologist in refractory cases. Pelvic revascularization is largely experimental.

REF: de Groat WC, Booth AM: *Ann Intern Med* 92:329, 1980.

       Gautier-Smith PC. In Aminoff MJ, ed: *Neurology and general medicine*, New York, 1989, Churchill Livingstone.

INFARCTION—CEREBRAL   *(see Ischemia)*

INFARCTION—MUSCLE   *(see Muscle Disorders, Myoglobinuria)*

INFARCTION—SPINAL CORD   *(see Spinal Cord)*

INFECTION   *(see Abscess, Encephalitis, Meningitis)*

INSOMNIA   *(see Sleep Disorders)*

INTRACRANIAL PRESSURE   *(see also Herniation, Pseudotumor Cerebri)*

Management of intracranial pressure (ICP) requires balancing several important physiologic variables. Normal ICP is 5 to 15 mm Hg (torr), which equals 65 to 195 mm CSF or H_2O. Factors that determine the level of ICP are pressures exerted by cranial contents, arterial pressure, and intracranial venous pressure. After the cranial sutures fuse the intracranial cavity has a fixed total volume comprising three components—brain, CSF, and blood. Brain volume is 1400 ml; CSF volume is 150 ml—75 ml intracranial and the remainder spinal; and intracranial vascular volume is about 75 ml. Cerebral perfusion pressure is the difference between arterial pressure and ICP. Perfusion pressures lower than 40 to 60 mm Hg are considered detrimental to nerve cell survival. After any major cerebral injury ICP should be maintained at a level as close to normal as possible, to provide a margin of safety. Plateau waves, which consist of episodic surges in ICP sometimes exceeding 450 mm H_2O, can occur several times an hour, especially with iatrogenic maneuvers such as suctioning or pain, and are associated with increased risk of herniation. In general, slow increases in the volume of one compartment can be compensated by decreases in the volumes of others, but a rapid rise in ICP increases risk of herniation or the occurrence of global ischemia and is a neurologic emergency. For example, outcome after head trauma is inversely related to the level of ICP after acute injury.

Increased ICP occurs with space-occupying lesions, cerebral edema, trauma, hemorrhages, infections, and pseudotumor cerebri. An acute increase in blood pressure causes an elevated ICP, as seen in hypertensive encephalopathy; chronic hypertension does not cause a change in ICP. Processes that increase venous pressures cause increases in ICP, such as jugular compression, superior vena cava obstruction, congestive heart failure, or Valsalva's maneuvers. Postural effects alter the pressures in the intracranial venous sinuses, which in turn alter the CSF pressure.

The clinical presentation of increased ICP depends on the underlying process and whether it is acute or chronic. Manifestations of headache, papilledema, diplopia, or focal signs may occur. Cushing's triad of bradycardia, hypertension, and slowing of respiration may occur, as may cardiac arrhythmias such as atrial fibrillation, nodal and ventricular bradycardia, large T waves, prolonged QT intervals, and changes in ST segments.

Treatment of increased ICP may involve medical and surgical components. General measures include keeping the head elevated 30 degrees above horizontal, restricting fluid intake, and avoiding hypotonic IV solutions. Anticonvulsants are sometimes given on a prophylactic basis to prevent seizures, with subsequent rises in ICP. Hyperventilation results in cerebral vasoconstriction and rapidly decreases ICP. The pCO_2 value should be maintained between 25 and 30 mm Hg. Mannitol is given as a 20% solution, 1 gm/kg over 15 minutes, and in repeated doses at 3- to 4-hour intervals. Mannitol is best used when ICP can be directly monitored; otherwise, mannitol should be titrated to produce a serum osmolality of 315 to 320 mOsm/L. After 3 to 4 hours brain and plasma osmolalities equilibrate, requiring increasingly higher plasma osmolalities for the same effect. Urine output should be monitored. Side effects include renal failure, hyperosmolarity, and factitious hyponatremia. Hypothermia (27° to 36° C) decreases ICP by 50%, but peak effect takes several hours; hypothermia may also decrease cerebral perfusion. Glucocorticoids are useful in controlling brain edema associated with brain tumors and meningitis but are of uncertain value in other forms of cerebral edema. Barbiturate coma can decrease ICP, and is a last-resort medical therapy; complications include further sedation of comatose patients and hypotension, often requiring vasopressors to maintain blood pressure. Surgical monitoring by subdural, subarachnoid, or ventricular pressure transducers provides accurate information regarding efficacy of intervention. Surgical therapy by ventricular shunting offers immediate reduction in ICP, especially in patients with hydrocephalus.

Decreased ICP may occur in the setting of CSF leakage, either spontaneously, through openings in the dura to sinuses or mastoid or after lumbar puncture or neurosurgery, or through overshunting. Postural headache similar to that observed after lumbar puncture is a frequent symptom. Diagnosis is confirmed by demonstration of CSF leakage on cisternogram or by other evidence of CSF leakage (positive results for glucose in tests of pharyngeal secretions). MRI may show meningeal enhancement. Spontaneous remission may occur, and treatment depends on cause or origin.

REF: Fishman RA: *Cerebrospinal fluid in diseases of the nervous system*, ed 2, Philadelphia, 1992, WB Saunders.

ISCHEMIA (see also Amaurosis Fugax, Aneurysms, Angiography, Hemorrhage, Lacunar Syndromes)

A thorough medical evaluation is required for the diagnosis and management of cerebral ischemia. The history (including age, race, family history, handedness, previous medical illness, medications, activity at the time of onset of the deficit, and prior pattern of neurologic deficits), physical examination, and imaging tests determine anatomic localization, help determine the underlying pathophysiologic condition, and guide treatment.

DURATION

Cerebral ischemic events are classified by duration and the presence of residual deficit. *Stroke* is a nonspecific term that refers to the acute onset of neurologic dysfunction resulting from cerebrovascular disease (hemorrhagic or ischemic infarction) and lasting longer than 24 hours. *Transient ischemic attack* (TIA) refers to a vascular neurologic deficit (clinically defined) lasting up to 24 hours, but typical TIAs often last less than 30 minutes. *Progressing stroke* refers to a deficit with symptoms and signs that worsen, usually over a course of up to 18 hours in the carotid distribution and up to 2 to 3 days in the vertebrobasilar distribution. The term *completed stroke* indicates that a patient has a stable neurologic deficit without evidence of progression. It should be emphasized that classification by duration alone is of limited value and not an end in itself, since it does not provide detailed insight into pathophysiologic characteristics.

Central nervous system ischemia or infarction should be described in terms of its vascular anatomy (Tables 31 and 32). The cerebral vasculature is divided into anterior (carotid) and posterior (vertebrobasilar) distributions. In about 5% of patients the circle of Willis is congenitally absent. In addition, there are many variants of the classic cerebrovascular anatomy.

Figures 21, 22, and 23 show brainstem cross-sectional anatomy that correlates with brainstem syndromes described in Table 32.

REF: Wolf JK: *The classic brainstem syndromes*, Springfield, Ill, 1971, Charles C Thomas.

MECHANISM AND DIFFERENTIAL DIAGNOSIS

The identification of the ischemic mechanism is critical in determining therapy. Relatively benign conditions may mimic cerebral infarction, but these should be considered in the diagnosis only after treatable or serious conditions have been excluded.

The characteristic clinical profile of embolic infarction is sudden onset of maximal neurologic deficit that may rapidly improve. Thrombotic infarction (including "lacunar infarction") is often preceded by TIAs and may progress over hours or days in a stuttering fashion. Intraparenchymal and subarachnoid hemorrhages are typically of sudden onset with severe headache and often occur with changes in mental status. Imaging modalities have revealed many exceptions to these profiles. Serial arteriography in embolic infarction has revealed vascular occlusion that may later vanish, despite persistence of neurologic deficit, and there may be little atherosclerotic change.

Transient ischemic attacks were originally thought to result from emboli of ulcerated carotid plaques, but imaging and pathologic studies have revealed many patients with asymptomatic ulceration. Recent evidence shows that recurrent TIAs correlate more with the presence of carotid stenosis and probably represent border zone ("watershed") ischemic phenomena occurring distal to areas of critical stenosis whenever the blood pressure drops sufficiently.

Patients with a history of migraine may have transient neurologic deficits with or without headache in later life, so-called "late-life mi-

Text continued on p. 211.

TABLE 31
Signs and Symptoms of Ischemic Vascular Occlusion

Artery	Signs and Symptoms
Common carotid artery (CCA)	Ipsilateral eye, distal vessels; may be asymptomatic
Middle cerebral artery (MCA)	Contralateral hemiparesis (face and arm greater than leg); horizontal gaze palsy; hemisensory deficits; homonymous hemianopsia; language and cognitive deficits (aphasia, apraxia, agnosia, neglect)
Anterior cerebral artery (ACA)	Contralateral hemiparesis (leg greater than arm and face); contralateral grasp reflex and degeneralten; abulia; gait disorders; perseveration; urinary incontinence; may produce bilateral signs caused by involvement of a single vessel of common origin
Posterior cerebral artery (PCA)	Contralateral homonymous hemianopsia (or quadrantanopsia); may produce memory loss, dyslexia without dysgraphia, color anomia, hemisensory deficits, and mild hemiparesis; may be supplied by the anterior circulation
Cerebellar infarction:	Dizziness, nausea, vomiting, nystagmus, ataxia *Recognition is important to detect brainstem compression caused by swelling; neurosurgical decompression may be lifesaving.*

TABLE 32
Brainstem Syndromes

Syndrome	Localization	Clinical Features		
		Ipsilateral	Contralateral	
Benedikt's	Midbrain tegmentum, red nucleus, cranial nerve (CN) III, cerebral peduncle	CN III palsy	Hemiataxia, tremor, hemiparesis, hyperkinesia	
Claude's	Paramedian midbrain tegmentum, red nucleus, ND III, superior cerebellar peduncle	CN III palsy	Hemiataxia, tremor, hemiparesis	
Weber's syndrome	Ventral midbrain, CN III, cerebral peduncle	CN III palsy	Hemiparesis	
Parinaud's	Dorso rostral midbrain, posterior commissure and its interstitial nucleus	Paralysis of upward gaze and accommodation, light-near dissociation of pupil, lid retraction, convergence-retraction nystagmus		
Nothnagel's	Dorsal midbrain, brachium conjunctivum, CN III nucleus, medial longitudinal fasciculus	Ataxia, CN III palsy, vertical gaze palsy		
Raymond-Cestan	Medial mid-pons (paramedian branch, mid-basilar artery), middle cerebellar peduncle, corticobulbar tract, corticospinal tract, variable medial lemniscus	Ataxia	Hemiparesis (face, arm, and leg), variable sensory, variable oculomotor	

Syndrome	Location/structures	Clinical findings	
	Lateral mid-pons (short circumferential artery, middle cerebellar peduncle, CN V)		Ataxia, paralysis of muscles of mastication, facial hemihypesthesia
One and a half	Paramedian pontine reticular formation or CN VI nucleus, medial longitudinal fasciculus	Horizontal gaze palsy	Internuclear ophthalmoplegia
Foville's	Paramedian pontine reticular formation, CN VI, and VII corticospinal tract	Horizontal gaze palsy, CN VII palsy	Hemiparesis, hemisensory loss, internuclear ophthalmoplegia
Millard-Gubler	Ventral paramedian pons, CN VI and VII fascicles, corticospinal tract	CN VI palsy, facial palsy	Hemiparesis
Raymond's	Ventral pons, CN VI fascicles and corticospinal tract	CN VI palsy	Hemiparesis
Babinski-Nageotte	Dorsolateral pontomedullary junction	Ataxia, hemihypesthesia in face, Horner's	Hemiparesis, hemihypesthesia in body, vertigo, vomiting, nystagmus
Wallenberg's	Dorsolateral medulla, vestibular nucleus, restiform body, CN V nucleus and spinal tract, CN IX and X, lateral spincthalamics, descending sympathetics	Lateropulsion; ataxia; loss of pain and temperature in face; paralysis of soft palate, poster or pharynx, and vocal cord; Horner's	Loss of pain and temperature in body

Continued.

TABLE 32—cont'd
Brainstem Syndromes

Syndrome	Localization	Clinical Features		
		Ipsilateral	Contralateral	
Cestan-Chenais	Lateral medulla	Ataxia; paralysis of soft palate, posterior pharynx, and vocal cord; Horner's, hemiphypesthesia in face	Hemiparesis, hemiphypesthesia in body	
Avellis'	Lateral medulla, CN IX and X, lateral spinothalamics	Paralysis of soft palate, posterior pharynx, and vocal cord	Hemiparesis, hemihypesthesia	
Vernet's	Lateral medulla, CN IX, X, and XI	Paralysis of soft palate; paralysis of vocal cord, posterior pharynx, and sternocleidomastoid; decreased taste over posterior third of tongue; hemihypesthesia of pharynx	Hemiparesis	
Jackson's	Lateral medulla, CN IX, X, XI, and XII	Paralysis of soft palate, posterior pharynx, vocal cords, sternocleidomastoid, upper trapezius, and tongue	Hemiparesis, hemihypesthesia	

Tapia's	Lateral medulla, CN IX, X, XII (more commonly, there is extra-cranial involvement)	As in Schmidt's syndrome, except that sternocleido-mastoid and trapezius are not involved.
Preolivary	Anterior medulla, CN XII, pyramid	Tongue atrophy or weakness Hemiparesis

Vertebrobasilar arteries (VBA) brainstem syndromes are best described in terms of neuroanatomic localization. Eponymic descriptions in the literature vary.

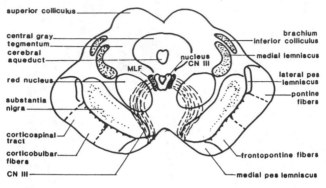

FIGURE 21
Midbrain cross-section. *MLF*, Medial longitudinal fasciculus.

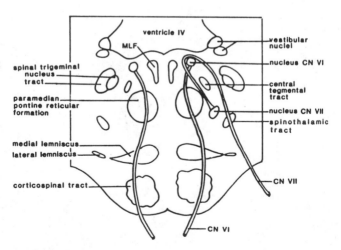

FIGURE 22
Pons cross-section. *MLF*, Medial longitudinal fasciculus.

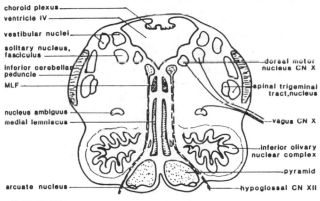

FIGURE 23
Medulla cross-section.

graine accompaniments." Careful workup is necessary to exclude vascular causes. Isolated vertigo or the feeling of lightheadedness in the absence of brainstem signs may indicate labyrinthine disease (see Vertigo) or orthostatic hypotension. Transient deficits may be a manifestation of seizures, although seizures with only "negative" manifestations are rarely diagnosed in the absence of other seizure-like features. Syncope, hyperventilation, and hypoglycemia can also mimic TIAs.

NATURAL HISTORY AND RISK FACTORS

The recognition and reduction of risk factors is the most effective way to prevent stroke. Risk factors for stroke vary with age and race. In young adults trauma, migraine, and, occasionally, spontaneous arterial dissection are the most common causes of stroke. In patients 50 years of age and older, hypertension, TIAs, coronary heart disease, congestive heart failure, and diabetes mellitus are important time-dependent risk factors. Smoking, obesity, increased fibrinogen level, maternal history of death from stroke, and excessive alcohol use are also recognized as risk factors. Other studies have shown that established chronic atrial fibrillation (AF) carries a lower risk than paroxysmal and new-onset AF. The asymptomatic carotid bruit (ACB) is more an indicator of systemic atherosclerosis than of a localized anatomic problem. Patients with ACB are at four times greater risk of dying as a result of cardiac causes than as a result of stroke-related causes; stroke is nearly as likely to occur in the distribution of the opposite carotid artery.

The prognosis in individuals with TIA varies considerably. Some patients may have dozens of TIAs without sequelae, whereas others may have only one or a brief flurry that presages a major ischemic event. Overall the incidence of stroke after a TIA is 20% in the first year and 5% per year (five times the normal age-adjusted risk) thereafter. The major risk period is the first 2 months. The frequency with which TIAs precede thrombotic stroke is unclear.

The overall mortality rate in patients with TIA is about 6% per year; death resulting from myocardial infarction (MI) occurs at a rate of 5% per year. Thus patients with TIA have a much higher chance of dying of MI than of stroke, even in the absence of angina or ECG abnormalities.

Fifty percent of TIAs resolve within an hour, and 90%, within 4 hours. Neurologic deficits that resolve completely after 4 hours are frequently associated with small strokes on pathologic examination or imaging, although they are classified as TIAs. An interval greater than 2 weeks between TIAs of the same vascular distribution reduces the probability that a severe arterial lesion exists.

CLINICAL AND LABORATORY EVALUATION

In addition to the history and neurologic examination attention should be given to blood pressure (in both upper extremities and with postural changes), cardiac examination, carotid and cranial bruits, facial pulses, fundoscopy, and evidence of peripheral emboli.

A CT scan is performed on all patients to exclude the presence of hemorrhage. Unless a subarachnoid hemorrhage is suspected (10% have negative results on CT; see Aneurysm), CSF examination is usually not necessary nor, if there is a large mass effect, desirable. Magnetic resonance imaging (MRI) is more sensitive for the detection of small strokes, particularly in the brainstem and posterior fossa. Additional studies should include complete blood cell and platelet counts; determinations of erythrocyte sedimentation rate, blood chemistry values, prothrombin time (PT), and partial thromboplastin time (PTT); Venereal Disease Research Laboratory (VDRL) test for syphilis; urinalysis; chest x-ray; EEG; and in selected patients, sickle cell testing. Duplex carotid ultrasonography is useful as an initial screening examination, especially for patients with carotid-distribution ischemic events, but it is operator dependent (see Ultrasonography). History of heart disease or abnormality on cardiac examination suggests the need for echocardiography.

Additional evaluation, such as determinations of antinuclear antibodies, anticardiolipin antibody levels, serum viscosity, protein electrophoresis, and serum amino acid levels as well as hematology consultation, may prove useful, especially in younger patients who have ischemia without an obvious cause. An EEG may help exclude a focal seizure disorder with Todd's paralysis. Serial blood cultures should be obtained if there is suspicion of endocarditis, such as cardiac embolism in patients at risk for endocarditis (those with artificial valves, intravenous drug abusers, and those with congenital heart disease). Holter monitoring is used when arrythmia is suspected in the cause of ischemia.

Angiography is still considered by most to be the "gold standard" in studying the cranial vasculature. It is indicated in the acute phase of an infarct when there is either an unclear or a potentially treatable condition. Angiography is not justified if an established maximal deficit is present or if no therapy is contemplated. As a general guideline, patients with TIA in the carotid distribution should have angiography if they are considered candidates for surgery after evaluation of their general medical status and severe carotid stenosis is established by examination and noninvasive carotid ultrasound examination. MRI angiography is a noninvasive technique for imaging the large extracranial and intracranial vessels that is undergoing intensive clinical investigation.

Transcranial Doppler is useful for noninvasive evaluation of the large cerebral arteries. It can demonstrate large vessel occlusion and helps assess collateral flow in ischemic territories (see Ultrasonography).

THERAPY

The treatment of acute and chronic ischemia is controversial. Decisions must take into consideration the patient's medical condition and life expectancy and the risk of therapy versus long-term benefits.

A number of common complications in stroke patients may be minimized with attentive care. Venous stasis in paralyzed limbs should be prevented by the use of elastic hose and low-dose heparin (with the precautions as noted later for large or embolic strokes). Decubiti and stasis may be prevented by means of mobilization of the extremities and trunk. Aspiration pneumonia occurs frequently in patients with stroke, and any patient with depressed gag reflexes or dysphagia should be carefully evaluated to determine whether he or she can tolerate oral feeding. Alterations in bladder function are common after stroke; urine output should be monitored for signs of retention; intermittent catheterization is preferable to indwelling catheters.

Once ischemia occurs, little can be done to reverse neuronal loss after perfusion has been halted for more than a few minutes. The area surrounding an infarct, however, is thought to be at continued risk because of impaired autoregulation. Rapid lowering of blood pressure should be avoided. Although considerable controversy exists regarding optimal blood pressure control in the period immediately after a stroke, there is probably greater risk in lowering blood pressure than in allowing it to remain at high levels. Indications for pressure reduction include systemic reasons for antihypertensive therapy, such as acute renal failure or myocardial infarction. Bed rest is recommended during and immediately after a stroke to prevent postural changes in blood pressure, which, when coupled with impaired autoregulation, may exacerbate ischemia. Unlike the situation with blood pressure, most authorities advocate tight control of glucose level, since lactic acidosis may compromise ischemic, noninfarcted tissue surrounding the infarct. Other underlying medical conditions such as polycythemia and endocarditis must be treated.

ANTICOAGULATION THERAPY AND THE MANAGEMENT OF ACUTE STROKE AND TIA

There are a number of relative *indications* for anticoagulation (AC) therapy in the presence of acute ischemia. Despite anecdotal evidence, no well-controlled studies have demonstrated a clear benefit, and the issue remains controversial. Heparin may be useful in preventing further thrombosis and total occlusion of a major cerebral vessel in TIA or progressing stroke or during a period of fluctuating deficit. Contraindications include the presence of a large, acute infarct or hemorrhage and those mentioned later. Large (particularly embolic) strokes have an increased risk for hemorrhagic transformation during the first few days. As a result, heparin AC therapy is often delayed. If AC therapy is indicated, one approach is beginning warfarin therapy immediately because of the delay in the onset of effective therapy. Indications for long-term AC therapy may be found on arteriography: severe stenosis of a major vessel in an inoperable location, distal stump thrombus, or, possibly, ulceration of an atheromatous plaque.

ANTICOAGULATION THERAPY IN CEREBRAL EMBOLISM OF CARDIAC ORIGIN

Long-term AC therapy with warfarin (prothrombin time [PT], international normalized ratio [INR] 1.2 to 1.5 times the control value) is indicated (in the absence of the usual contraindications) in patients with symptomatic atrial fibrillation, atrial fibrillation with coexisting cardiomyopathy, mechanical prosthetic cardiac valves, and symptom-

atic mitral valve prolapse and in the presence of intracardiac mural
thrombus. Some of these are high-risk conditions that require anticoagulation therapy, even without a history of TIA or stroke. Short-term
AC therapy is recommended in patients with newly installed bio-
prosthetic valves and in the case of atrial fibrillation when cardioversion
is being performed. In rheumatic heart disease with atrial fibrillation,
there is good evidence that AC therapy reduces the risk of future
embolization. Since the risk of stroke in atrial fibrillation and sinus
node disease is five times greater than normal, many argue that all
patients with atrial fibrillation should receive AC therapy.

When embolic stroke is associated with a prosthetic valve, AC
therapy should be withheld while arteriography and contrasted CT
scans are performed to exclude the presence of ruptured mycotic aneurysm. When a large embolic stroke occurs in association with a
known cardiac source (such as mural thrombus), there may be no
entirely satisfactory course of action, since AC therapy may worsen the
neurologic deficit through hemorrhagic transformation, whereas with-
holding AC therapy may lead to repeated embolization. Management
of such cases must be highly individualized. AC therapy provides no
benefit in patients with embolism resulting from marantic endocarditis,
calcific valves, or atrial myxoma.

USE OF ANTICOAGULANTS

Anticoagulation therapy is usually achieved rapidly with IV heparin
administration and then maintained with oral administration of warfarin. AC therapy is contraindicated in patients with bleeding diatheses,
predispositions to hemorrhage (peptic ulcer disease or neoplasm), severe
liver disease, endocarditis, or uremia, and in those at risk for frequent
falling. Anticoagulation therapy is appropriate only in compliant patients whose condition can be followed up closely, and generally only
after exclusion of hemorrhage by CT.

Heparin is administered IV. A bolus of 5,000 to 10,000 units
followed by continuous infusion of 15 units/kg per hour or 600 to
1000 units per hour may be used. Some prefer to avoid all bolus
administrations and use only continuous infusion because of the risk
of hemorrhagic complications. The heparin infusion rate is adjusted
to maintain the activated partial thromboplastin time at 1.5 times the
control value. Patients should be monitored for evidence of excessive
anticoagulation (petechiae, microscopic hematuria, or occult blood in
stool), and clinical status. Heparin AC therapy can be reversed in
minutes with protamine sulfate.

Warfarin loading is unnecessary. Warfarin is initiated with a maintenance of 10 to 15 mg per day. Prothrombin time is determined daily,

and the dosage adjusted to maintain the PT at an INR 1.2 to 1.5 times the control value. Greater degrees of anticoagulation are associated with a greater incidence of hemorrhagic complications. Because numerous factors, including many drugs and liver disease, influence the response to warfarin, great care is required in using this drug. Heparin may also affect the PT. After satisfactory anticoagulation is attained with warfarin, the PT should be determined at least every 2 weeks. Excessive prolongation of the PT can be corrected with vitamin K; however, vitamin K reversal significantly prolongs the time required to re-initiate AC therapy with warfarin.

ANTIPLATELET AGENTS

The rate of infarction and death is reduced after treatment with 1200 mg per day of aspirin for TIAs in the carotid and vertebrobasilar distributions. Many different doses of aspirin, however, as low as 80 mg per day, can be used effectively. Lower doses are associated with lowered risk of bleeding complications. Ticlopidine, a new antiplatelet agent, is slightly more efficacious than aspirin. The use of ticlopidine necessitates initial monitoring of complete blood cell counts every other week for the first 3 months of therapy because of the risk of neutropenia.

SURGICAL TREATMENT OF STROKE

Carotid endarterectomy (CEA) is the most common vascular surgical procedure; approximately 100,000 CEAs per year are performed in the United States. The North American Symptomatic Carotid Endarterectomy Trial (NASCET) has shown that patients with artery narrowing of 70% to 99% benefit from CEA. Thus the current standard of practice is to perform CEA in patients with severe (>70%) carotid stenosis and a history of symptoms or clinical events. There are neither well-controlled studies nor significant clinical experiences to support CEA after "completed" carotid occlusion or asymptomatic carotid stenosis. Some authorities claim emergent thrombolysis, CEA, or embolectomy may have benefit in acute cases of stroke. Although controversial, surgery is usually deferred for 4 weeks after an ischemic insult.

REHABILITATION

Although it has been traditional to begin the various forms of therapy early in the course after stroke, large prospective studies have not indicated a specific beneficial effect and many patients improve spontaneously. Nonetheless, the use of physical and other modalities of therapy provides a means of early mobilization and motivation for the patient. Speech therapy may benefit patients with aphasia whose language deficits persist more than several weeks.

PROGNOSIS

Factors that favor a poor prognosis include hemorrhagic stroke, impaired consciousness, heavy alcohol use, older age, male sex, hypertension, heart disease, and leg weakness. The mortality rates at 1 month are 17% for patients with carotid distribution and 18% for patients with vertebrobasilar territory infarction.

DIFFERENTIAL DIAGNOSIS OF CEREBRAL INFARCTION

I. Cerebrovascular thrombosis associated with vascular disease.
   A. Atherosclerosis.
   B. Lipohyalinosis.
   C. Dissection.
   D. Chronic progressive subcortical encephalopathy (Binswanger's disease).
II. Cerebral embolism.
   A. Cardiac source.
      1. Valvular (mitral stenosis, prosthetic valve, infective endocarditis, marantic endocarditis, Libman-Sacks endocarditis, mitral annulus calcification, mitral valve prolapse, calcific aortic stenosis).
      2. Atrial fibrillation, sick sinus syndrome.
      3. Acute myocardial infarction, left ventricular aneurysm, or both.
      4. Left atrial myxoma.
      5. Cardiomyopathy.
      6. Acute and subacute bacterial endocarditis.
      7. Prosthetic valve dysfunction.
      8. Chagas' disease, trichinosis.
   B. Paradoxic embolism and pulmonary source.
      1. Pulmonary arteriovenous malformations (including Osler-Weber-Rendu syndrome).
      2. Atrial and ventricular septal defects with right-to-left shunts.
      3. Patent foramen ovale with right-to-left shunt.
      4. Pulmonary vein thrombosis.
      5. Pulmonary and mediastinal tumors.
   C. Artery-to-artery embolism.
      1. Cholesterol emboli.
      2. Atheroma thrombus.
      3. Complications of vascular and neck surgery.
      4. Idiopathic carotid mural thrombus, embologenic aortitis.
      5. Emboli distal to unruptured aneurysm.
      6. Arterial dissection.

D. Other.
  1. Fat embolism syndrome.
  2. Air embolism.
III. Arteriopathies.
  A. Inflammatory
    1. Takayasu's disease.
    2. Allergic granulomatosis (Churg-Strauss syndrome).
    3. Granulomatous angiitis (isolated CNS vasculitis).
    4. Infectious: Syphilis, mucormycosis, ophthalmic zoster, tuberculosis, malaria, severe tonsillitis, lymphadenitis.
    5. Associated with amphetamine, cocaine abuse.
    6. Associated with systemic disease (lupus erythematosus, Wegener's granulomatosis, polyarteritis nodosa, rheumatoid arthritis, Sjögren's syndrome, scleroderma, Degos' Behçet's syndromes, acute rheumatic fever, inflammatory bowel disease).
  B. Noninflammatory.
    1. Spontaneous dissections.
    2. After radiation therapy. (See Radiation Injury)
    3. Fibromuscular dysplasia.

REF: Gasecki AP et al: *Nebr Med J* 77:121-123, 1992.

Liu GT et al: *Neurology* 42:1820-1822, 1992.

Marshall RS, Mohr JP: *J Neurol Neurosurg Psychiatry* 56:6-16, 1993.

Miller VT, Hart RG: *Stroke* 19:403-406, 1988.

Phillips SJ: *Stroke* 20:295-298, 1989.

van Gijn J: *Neurol Clin* 10:193-208, 1992.

KAYSER-FLEISCHER RINGS   *(see Wilson's Disease)*

KEARN-SAYRE SYNDROME   *(see Myopathy, Ophthalmoplegia)*

KORSAKOFF'S SYNDROME   *(see Alcohol, Memory, Nutritional Deficiency Syndromes)*

KRABBE'S DISEASE   *(see Degenerative Diseases of Childhood)*

KUGELBERG-WELANDER DISEASE   *(see Motor Neuron Disease)*

KUSSMAUL'S RESPIRATION   *(see Electrolytes, Metabolic Acidosis)*

LABYRINTHINE DYSFUNCTION   *(see Calorics, Dizziness, Nystagmus, Vertigo, Vestibulo-Ocular Reflex)*

LACUNAR SYNDROMES   *(see also Ischemia)*

Lacunar syndromes are clinical manifestations of infarcts up to 20 mm (most <10 mm) in diameter that are located in the subcortical cerebrum and brainstem and result from occlusion (lipohyalinosis) of small arteries (40 to 200 μm). A small cavity or lacune forms after healing. Lacunes are frequently associated with hypertension (60% to 90%) and atherosclerosis of large and middle-sized intracranial arteries. Although the true incidence is unknown, lacunes are infrequently associated with embolism and extracranial carotid occlusive disease. Lacunes occur in the lenticular nuclei (37%), caudate nucleus (10%), thalamus (14%), internal capsule (10%), pons (16%), corona radiata, external capsule, pyramids, and other brainstem structures.

Clinical presentations of lacunar infarction (see Table 33) are probably related to the size of the lesion and range from asymptomatic through the classic lacunar syndromes to more complex syndromes. Onset is often gradual or stepwise. Approximately 30% are preceded by transient ischemic attacks.

Head CT demonstrates up to 70% of lesions within 7 days. Multiple lacunes are present in 30% of patients. MRI is more sensitive. Thirty percent of lesions on imaging studies are asymptomatic. Autopsy studies have shown that lacunar infarcts are often unrecognized during life.

Treatment consists of low-dose aspirin and control of hypertension and other vascular risk factors. Cerebral angiography is not recommended in pure lacunar syndromes. However, in the absence of history or signs of hypertension (such as retinopathy and left ventricular hypertrophy) some authors recommend aggressive workup for sources of embolus, large vessel disease, or unusual causes of stroke. Prognosis is usually favorable, but probability of recurrence is high.

TABLE 33
Most Common Lacunar Syndromes

Syndrome	Localization	Clinical Features
Pure sensory stroke	Ventricular posterior thalamus	Sensory loss face, arm, leg—same side; no weakness; no visual field deficits; no "cortical" signs
Pure motor hemiparesis	Posterior limb interior capsule, basis pontis, cerebral peduncle	Weakness face, arm, leg—same side; no sensory loss; no visual field deficits; no "cortical" signs
Ataxic hemiparesis	Basis pontis, Ventricular anterior thalamus and adjacent interior capsule	Cerebellar ataxia and weakness—same side; often leg > face
Dysarthria—clumsy hand syndrome	Basis pontis, genu interior capsule	Facial weakness, dysarthria, dysphagia, slight weakness and clumsiness of hand—same side

Of more than 20 different lacunar syndromes that have been described, four classic syndromes are presented in Table 33.

REF: Caplan LR: *Neurology* 39:1246–1250, 1989.

LAMBERT-EATON MYASTHENIC SYNDROME

The Lambert-Eaton myasthenic syndrome (LEMS) is an autoimmune disorder of neuromuscular transmission. IgG antibodies directed at the voltage-gated calcium channels (VGCCs) on presynaptic cholinergic nerve terminals are responsible for the disease. Decreased numbers of VGCCs lead to a decreased probability of nerve impulse-induced release of acetylcholine (ACh) vesicles from presynaptic nerve terminals. Presynaptic ACh stores and the postsynaptic response to individual quanta are normal.

The most frequent presenting symptom is proximal leg or arm weakness. Muscle aching and stiffness worsened by prolonged exercise are common. There may be difficulty combing the hair or rising from a chair. Unlike myasthenia gravis, initial symptoms resulting from cranial nerve dysfunction are rare. However, transient diplopia, ptosis, dysphagia, dysarthria, and neck flexion weakness can develop in later stages. Eighty percent of patients have autonomic involvement, usually dry mouth and impotence and occasionally, constipation, blurred vision, and impaired sweating. Sensory complaints are rare.

On examination proximal weakness of the lower limbs greater than in the upper limbs is the most consistent finding. A progressive increase in strength after a few seconds of sustained contraction is usual, with fatigue after continued contraction. Muscle wasting is rare and when present, mild. Limb reflexes are decreased or absent in more than 90% of cases. However, a potentiation of reflexes after maximal contraction of the involved muscle for 10 to 15 seconds is usually present.

Lambert-Eaton myasthenic syndrome is associated with small cell lung carcinoma in approximately two thirds of cases; the bulk of the remaining third of cases are of idiopathic origin. Other neoplasms associated with LEMS include carcinomas of the rectum, kidney, stomach, and breast and leukemia. Autoimmune diseases such as systemic lupus erythematosus, rheumatoid arthritis, and Sjögren's syndrome are occasionally related to LEMS. Lambert-Eaton myasthenic syndrome usually precedes the diagnosis of cancer by an average of 10 months. Onset after a diagnosis of small cell lung cancer is unusual. The survival rate of tumor-associated LEMS is poor (8.5 months), usually because of progression of the underlying malignancy. In patients without serious underlying disease the prognosis is good. The ratio of men to women affected by LEMS is 1.8:1.

Definitive diagnosis rests on electrophysiologic studies. The amplitude of the compound muscle action potential is low, and additional decrement is observed with repetitive stimulation at low frequency (2 Hz). At high frequencies (>10 Hz) of stimulation a profound incremental response (post-tetanic potentiation) occurs. A similar phenomenon is present after sustained voluntary exercise (postexercise facilitation). Nerve conduction velocities and latencies are normal. Patients with LEMS sometimes respond to edrophonium testing.

Treatment is directed at the responsible tumor or underlying autoimmune disorder. Guanidine 10 mg/kg per day may improve strength but is not well tolerated. Response to cholinesterase inhibitors is variable. Plasmapheresis, immunosuppressive agents (such as azathioprine), and prednisone (100 mg/day for 1 week, followed by a gradual taper to 60 mg every other day) may help, particularly if the LEMS is due to autoimmunity. A drug that facilitates synaptic transmission, 3,4-diaminopyridine (DAP), may improve strength in patients with LEMS in doses of 15 mg four times a day (1 mg/kg per day). Anticholinesterases may facilitate the effect of DAP.

REF: Rosenfeld MR, Dalmau J: *Semin Neurol* 13:291–298, 1993.

LANDRY-GUILLAIN-BARRÉ SYNDROME   *(see Neuropathy, Cerebrospinal Fluid)*

LANGUAGE DISORDERS   *(see Aphasia)*

LEARNING DISABILITIES   *(see also Attention Deficit Hyperactivity Disorder)*

Learning disability (LD) is defined as difficulty in the acquisition and use of language, reasoning, mathematical abilities, or social skills. It may coexist with but should not be the direct result of other handicapping conditions.

In preschoolers LD usually becomes evident as language delay. A child who has no meaningful words by age 18 months, no meaningful phrases by age 24 months, or speech unintelligible to strangers by age 3 years should be evaluated for hearing loss and referred for speech therapy.

In school-aged children LD usually becomes evident as unexpected school failure in a child of at least average intelligence. Selective reading disability is a common form of LD that can lead to general failure in school if not recognized early. There is often a family history of learning problems. Standard intelligence and achievement tests should be administered to verify normal intelligence and failure to achieve the expected level of school performance.

The medical history should search for evidence of perinatal insult, cerebral infarction, head injury, lead poisoning, or seizures. The general examination should encompass vision, hearing, head circumference, skin lesions, and dysmorphic features. The results of neurologic examination, like those of the general examination, are usually normal but may reveal "soft" signs (especially clumsiness). Manifestations of attention deficit hyperactivity disorder should be sought (see Attention Deficit Hyperactivity Disorder). EEG is useful only when seizures (especially absence seizures) are suspected. Other diagnostic tests are usually not helpful in the absence of abnormal results of neurologic examination. Treatment of LD involves special class placement for specialized instruction and reliance on the assistance of allied health personnel.

REF: Ehrenberg G: Learning disabilities: an overview, *Semin Neurol* 11(1):1, 1991.

Rapin I: Disorders of higher cerebral function in preschool children, *Am J Dis Child* 142:1119–1124, 1988.

LEIGH'S DISEASE   *(see Degenerative Diseases of Childhood)*

LENNOX-GASTAUT SYNDROME   *(see Degenerative Diseases of Childhood, Electroencephalography, Epilepsy)*

LEUKODYSTROPHY   *(see Degenerative Diseases of Childhood)*

LEWY BODIES   *(see Parkinson's Disease)*

LHERMITTE'S SIGN   *(see Multiple Sclerosis, Radiation)*

LIMBIC SYSTEM

An area of the brain consisting of the cingulate, parahippocampal and subcallosal gyri, hippocampal formation, dentate gyrus, hypothalamus, mammillary bodies, amygdaloid complex, epithalamus, medial tegmental region of the midbrain, septal nuclei, anterior and dorsomedial thalamic nuclei, and fibrous pathways (fornix, mamillothalamic tract, medial forebrain bundle, and stria terminalis). Lesions and disease in the limbic system lead to abnormalities of memory, emotion, motivation, behavior, and autonomic and endocrine control.

REF: Carpenter MB: *Core text of neuroanatomy*, ed 4, Baltimore, 1991, Williams & Wilkins.

Strub RL, Black FW: *Neurobehavioral disorders: a clinical approach*, Philadelphia, 1988, FA Davis.

LIPID STORAGE DISEASES OF MUSCLE   *(see Myopathy)*

LOCKED-IN SYNDROME   *(see Coma)*

LUMBAR PUNCTURE   *(see Cerebrospinal Fluid)*

LUMBOSACRAL PLEXUS

The lumbosacral plexus comprises the anastomoses derived from the ventral primary rami of T12-S4 (Figure 24). Causes and origins of lumbosacral dysfunction include neoplasm, retroperitoneal hemorrhage, psoas abscess (resulting from osteomyelitis), diabetes, injections, herpes zoster infections, pyelonephritis, appendicitis, retroperitoneal masses, aortic aneurysms, and trauma. Pain, weakness, loss of deep tendon reflexes, and sensory changes may occur in the appropriate distribution (see also Dermatomes and Myotomes).

Idiopathic lumbosacral plexus neuropathy (less common than idiopathic brachial plexopathy) is characterized by a sudden onset of severe pain in the thigh or buttock (followed 5 to 10 days later by weakness in the distribution of the involved plexus).

Radiation plexopathy usually occurs 1 to many years after radiation therapy. Findings include unilateral or bilateral distal leg weakness, mild pain, and EMG showing myokymic discharges (50%). In contrast, plexopathy resulting from tumor is associated with severe pain at onset and weakness involving proximal and unilateral leg muscles.

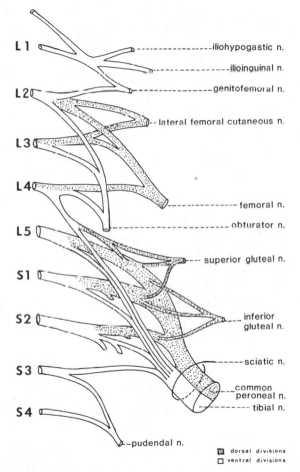

FIGURE 24
Lumbosacral plexus.

CT scan is the imaging procedure of choice for visualizing the retroperitoneal space and lumbosacral plexus.

REF: Brazis PW, Masdeu JC, Biller J: *Localization in clinical neurology*, ed 2, Boston, 1990, Little, Brown.

Dyck PJ, Thomas PK: *Peripheral neuropathy*, ed 3, Philadelphia, 1993, WB Saunders.

LUPUS *(see Vasculitis)*

LYME DISEASE

Lyme disease, also called Lyme borreliosis, is a widely distributed multisystem disease caused by a tick-transmitted spirochete, *Borrelia burgdorferi.*

Stage 1: Localized infection. Usually begins 3 days to 1 month after a tick bite. Manifests as a red macule or papule and expands centrifugally to form an annular red lesion with central clearing. Regional adenopathy and mild systemic symptoms of headache, neck stiffness, lethargy, or mild encephalopathy are also present. The CSF is usually normal. Treatment of this stage includes giving doxycycline 100 mg PO bid for 10 to 30 days or amoxicillin (with probenecid) 500 mg PO qid for 10 to 30 days.

Stage 2: Disseminated infection. Within days or weeks the spirochete may spread hematogenously, become evident on clinical examination as erythema migrans, lymphocytoma, migratory musculoskeletal pain, acute arteritis, generalized adenopathy, splenomegaly, carditis, severe malaise, and fatigue.

Weeks to months after illness the most common neurologic abnormality is lymphocytic meningitis with or without accompanying CNS parenchymal involvement. Radiculoneuritis, when present, may be asymmetric, painful, and be associated with dermatomal sensory and myotomal motor abnormalities. Variations include mononeuritis, mononeuritis multiplex, brachial or lumbosacral plexopathy, and Guillain-Barré–like syndrome. Electrophysiologic testing usually points to axonal degeneration in distal nerves and roots.

Cranial neuropathies develop in about 60% of patients. Facial palsy is most common, occurring in 70% to 80% of patients in stage 2 and in 10% of all patients. Cranial nerves III, IV, VI (13%), V (6%), VIII (5%), and II (3%) may also be involved.

CSF findings in stage 2 include increased blood cell count (100 to 200 white blood cells (WBC)/mm^3 with >90% lymphocytes), decreased glucose level (<⅔ serum glucose) and increased protein concentrations (35% of patients; usually 100 to 300 mg/dl). Treatment in stage 2 with Bell's palsy is the same as for stage 1. Other neurologic involvement requires giving penicillin G, 20 to 24 million units per day IV for 10 to 14 days, ceftriaxone 2 g/day IV for 2 to 4 weeks, cefotaxime 2 g IV tid for 2 to 4 weeks, or doxycycline 100 to 200 mg PO bid for 10 to 30 days. Parenteral antibiotics are preferred for neurologic lyme disease associated with CSF abnormalities and CNS lyme syndromes, regardless of CSF findings.

Stage 3: Late or persistent infection. Occurs months to years after initial infection. Stage 3 becomes evident as attacks of arthritis, persistent skin infection, and persistent, often progressive neurologic abnormalities, sometimes with a long latency. These neurologic manifestations include chronic progressive encephalomyelitis (meningitis, encephalitis, myelitis, cranial neuritis, and radiculoneuritis), focal encephalitis, mild encephalopathy, distal axonopathy, and asymmetric polyneuropathy. CSF findings are similar to those in stage 2. Treatment is the same as for stage 2, except that doxycycline is given for 30 days. Nonspecific problems (fatigue, joint pain, and muscle ache) may persist several months after treatment.

Features that support a diagnosis of Lyme disease include erythema migrans, tick bite or exposure to travel in an endemic area, extraneural involvement, and suggestive neurologic syndromes (that is, unilateral or bilateral Bell's palsy, aseptic meningitis, atypical Guillain-Barré syndrome, and mild polyneuropathy).

Today antibody is measured by enzyme-linked immunosorbent assay (ELISA); assays utilizing western blots are not currently standardized. CSF Lyme antibody index confirms neurologic Lyme disease but is not invariably elevated. Currently used experimental CSF studies have limited availability.

B. burgdorferi is virtually impossible to culture, and routine biopsy is not helpful.

REF: Coyle PK: *Semin Neurol* 12:200–208, 1992.

         Finkel MF: *Semin Neurol* 13:299–304, 1993.

MACROCEPHALY   *(see Child Neurology for head circumference norms)*

Head circumference greater than 2 SDs above the mean for age, sex, and gestation. Differential diagnosis includes hydrocephalus (as a result of neoplasm, arteriovenous malformation, infection, or trauma), subdural fluid collections, CNS structural malformation (hydranencephaly), megalencephaly (increased brain substance with abnormal cytoarchitecture; may be associated with neurocutaneous syndromes or CNS metabolic diseases), benign familial megalencephaly (may be autosomal dominant; may be clumsy but otherwise neurologically and developmentally normal; cytoarchitecture is normal).

Evaluation includes review of prior head circumference measurements to assess rate of head growth (a rapidly growing head that is crossing percentile lines suggests hydrocephalus), assessment of head shape (frontal bossing is associated with hydrocephalus, lateral bulging with infantile subdural hematoma), measurement of head circumferences of parents and siblings (benign familial megalencephaly), and CT, MRI, or ultrasound. If the infant is neurologically and developmentally normal and there are no risk factors for hydrocephalus, close observation may be all that is necessary.

A useful rule of thumb for normal rate of head growth follows:

Prematures	1 cm/wk
1 to 3 mo	2 cm/mo
3 to 6 mo	1 cm/mo
6 to 12 mo	½ cm/mo

MACULA   (see Retina and Uveal Tract)

MAGNESIUM   (see Electrolyte Disorders)

MAGNETIC RESONANCE IMAGING (MRI)

Magnetic resonance imaging (MRI) is a form of computed tomography that creates images based on the behavior of various tissues exposed to strong magnetic fields, controlled magnetic field gradients, and radiofrequency (RF) pulses. Image intensity and contrast depend on the concentration of unpaired protons, typically from hydrogen nuclei; the motion of these nuclei; nuclear magnetic relaxation parameters; and the type of sequence or acquisition that the MRI device is performing.

When tissue protons are placed in a magnetic field, they tend to align themselves either longitudinally (parallel) in a low-energy state or transversely (antiparallel) in a high-energy state to the vector of the imposed magnetic field, although they flip periodically between the two states. Since low-energy states are preferred, more protons align longitudinally than transversely at any given moment. The net magnetization vector, therefore, is longitudinal to the imposed magnetic field (the equilibrium state). A 90-degree RF pulse can be applied, exciting the protons and changing them from longitudinal to transverse alignment. As these protons return to equilibrium within the magnetic field (that is, longitudinal alignment), they emit energy (as RF signal), which can be detected and converted into meaningful data—the image—by means of certain manipulations discussed in the following sections.

TECHNICAL PARAMETERS IN MRI

1. *Repetition time* (TR) defines a duration of a cycle, that is, the time between successive 90-degree RF pulses. It also sets the "starting intensity" from which the signal decay (T2) is measured.

2. *Echo time* (TE) defines a sampling interval during the cycle, that is, the time between giving the RF pulse and measuring the amount of RF signal being emitted by the tissue, or "the echo." Single or multiple echoes may be sampled during a given cycle.

3. *Relaxation time* is the time it takes the protons to return to equilibrium within the magnetic field after an RF pulse has been given. MRI signal is based mainly on the relaxation times of the protons within lipids and water. Protons within protein, DNA, and solid structures such as bone have relaxation properties that are undetectable by typical MRI imaging. Relaxation time is determined by two processes called $T1$ and $T2$.

T1 relaxation is based on how fast the protons return to equilibrium (longitudinal alignment) after being energized. At any given time after the RF pulse is given (TE), those elements whose protons re-equilibrate fastest, (for example, lipids, with the highest percentage of protons in the longitudinal position) appear brightest on images where the T1 characteristics are selected for (T1-weighted images [T1-Wi]). Elements whose protons re-equilibrate slower, for example, water, appear darker (see Table 34). The shorter the TE, the greater the difference between the elements. At short TE a large percentage of the lipid protons have reattained their longitudinal position, whereas few water protons have done so. At longer TE a large percentage of both lipid and water protons are realigned. The greater the difference between the two elements (the shorter the TE), the greater the contrast on T1-Wi (T1-weighted images have short TR and short TE).

T2 relaxation is determined by how fast an element "decays" from the transverse alignment to the longitudinal alignment. In this situation the longer an element maintains its transverse alignment (slower decay), the stronger the signal it emits (that is, the brighter, on T2-weighted images (T2-Wi) (see Table 35). At shorter TE, high percentages of

TABLE 34
T1-Weighted Image

Dark (Low Signal, Long T1)	Bright (High Signal, Short T1)
CSF	Lipid
Deoxyhemoglobin (in intact red blood cells)	Gadolinium
Calcium	Methemoglobin (free or in red blood cells)
Air	Proteinaceous substances
Edema	Hepatic failure (globus pallidus)
Most pathologic lesions	Hypoxia (caudate, putamen)
	Melanotic tumors

TABLE 35
T2-Weighted Image

Dark (Low Signal, Short T2)	Bright (High Signal, Long T2)
Solids	CSF
Cortical bone	Liquids
Calcium	Edema
Hemosiderin	Most pathologic lesions
Deoxyhemoglobin (in intact red blood cells)	
Methemoglobin (in intact red blood cells)	
Ferritin	
Mucinous metastatic lesions	
Air	

both lipid and water protons are made in transverse alignment. At a longer TE most of the lipid protons have returned to longitudinal alignment (fast decay), whereas most of the water protons remain in transverse alignment, (slow decay). Therefore, for greatest contrast of T2-Wi images, choose longer TE (T2-Wi, long TE and long TR).

The degree of brightness or darkness on T1-Wi and T2-Wi can thus be determined by tissue fat and water content. In general, pathologic conditions are dark on T1-Wi, bright on T2-Wi, and bright on spin density images (see Tables 36 and 37).

TABLE 36
Gradient Echo T2 Weighted Image

Dark (Low Signal)	Bright (High Signal)
Hemosiderin	Flow-related enhancement
Deoxyhemoglobin	
Calcium	
Ferritin	

TABLE 37
Hematoma

	T1-WI	T2-WI
Acute	—	Bright rim (intact red blood cells)
	—	Dark core (deoxyhemoglobin)
	—	Edema
Subacute	Bright rim (methe-moglobin)	—
	Dark to bright core (methemoglobin)	—
	Less edema	—
Chronic	—	Dark rim (hemosiderin)
	—	No edema

The acquisition of data may be performed in a variety of patterns or *sequences*, which emphasizes these differences in tissue properties.

A typical example is the spin echo (SE) sequence, in which an initial 90-degree pulse is given and the echo is recalled at a predetermined point with an additional 180-degree pulse. The 180-degree pulse is necessary because of "dephasing" or spreading of the magnetic vectors of individual protons as they decay; they would eventually cancel each other out until the net vector became so weak that the signal emitted would be undetectable. The 180-degree pulse "rephases" or brings back together the individual proton vectors so that the echo emitted can be detected. T1-Wi, T2-Wi, and intermediate (also called spin density [SD]) images may be obtained with this sequence. SD images utilize tissue characteristics between T1-Wi and T2-Wi, i.e., long TR and short TE.

Another frequently used acquisition sequence is the gradient echo (GE), a "fast scanning" technique that replaces the protons for sampling by means of reversing the magnetic field gradient. The sequence takes less scanning time and is useful for imaging flowing blood (flow-related enhancement) and detecting calcification or hemorrhage and for mild myelogram effect (white CSF) in the spinal canal. GE images, like the SE, may be T1- or T2-weighted; usually only T2-W1 or SD images are employed.

CLINICAL USES OF MRI

1. Vascular: Strokes appear earlier and in better detail on MRI than on CT. However, this sensitivity has not proven clinically useful except in the posterior fossa, where CT images are poor. For arterio-venous malformations, MRI and magnetic resonance angiogram (MRA) are the noninvasive examinations of choice. For aneurysms, MRI and MRA are excellent for screening, bur conventional angiography can exclude smaller aneurysms.

MRI with magnetic resonance venography (MRV) is superior for venous sinus thrombosis. MRI can visualize (early) all types of hemorrhage, including hypertensive, tumoral, and other intraparenchymal, subdural, and epidural bleeds. CT, however, can image blood at least as well and less expensively. MRI is poor for detecting subarachnoid blood. MRI should be chosen when a subtle hemorrhage (such as a small contusion) is suspected.

2. Tumors: MRI is the examination of choice in ruling out small tumors or for tumor delineation. The ability to map the extent of a tumor (especially with the use of gadolinium) and the multiplanar capability of MRI make it useful in surgical planning.

3. Infections: With MRI, cerebritis is well visualized and abscess is well delineated.

4. Meningeal process: MRI is more sensitive than CT for visualizing both infected and neoplasm-infiltrated meninges.

5. Trauma: In acute cases MRI is not the examination of choice because of the lack of bony detail and the length of time needed to obtain images. CT should be used.

6. Demyelinating disease: MRI is the examination of choice because of the excellent delineation of white matter pathology. Active lesions of multiple sclerosis are enhanced with gadolinium.

7. Congenital and structural abnormalities: MRI is excellent for showing heterotopias and other anatomic abnormalities.

8. Spine imaging: Because the spinal cord is a thin, inherently low-contrast structure, MRI is the noninvasive examination of choice

for all spine disease. Vertebral bone is well imaged on spinal MRI because it contains fatty marrow. However, small spinal column fractures are better seen on CT.

9. Pregnancy: The safety of MRI in pregnancy has yet to be determined; therefore risk versus benefit must be considered.

ADVANTAGES OF MRI

1. Multiple planar capability: the magnetic field can be adjusted to image in any plane without moving the patient.

2. No ionizing radiation.

3. Superficial soft tissue contrast. Subtle differences in soft tissue proton relaxation characteristics enable visual distinction between soft tissues. This distinction is considered an "inherent" contrast of the soft tissue that can be significantly more appreciated with MRI than with any other modality.

4. Vascular anatomy. Characteristics of flowing blood are different from those of stationary soft tissue. Vessels can be imaged in more detail with MRI than with other noninvasive modalities, and MRAs and MRVs reconstructed by subtracting out the background stationary tissue signal (via longer relaxation times) from the signal obtained from moving protons. Unidirectional flow can be enhanced by computer to select for the arterial or venous systems.

5. MRI can easily image areas that are poorly visualized by CT, for example, areas surrounded by thick bones, such as the posterior fossa and temporal lobes.

6. Gadolinium is a paramagnetic IV contrast agent analogous to iodinated contrast of x-ray CT, which enhances tissues that are highly vascular or have a damaged blood-brain barrier. Unlike traditional contrast agents, gadolinium has few contraindications, and adverse reactions are rare. Contrast-enhanced MRI is generally obtained with T1-Wi, in which gadolinium enhancement appears bright.

DISADVANTAGES AND LIMITATIONS OF MRI

1. Longer imaging time. MRI can take between 1½ and 3 hours, depending on the anatomic area being studied and the complexity of the image acquisition.

2. Sensitivity to motion is high, resulting in poor image quality with slight patient movement. Movement is a particular problem when the patient is delirious or does not fully understand the procedure. Chloral hydrate, benzodiazepines, barbiturates, or other medications can be used as a sedative, but timing and dosage are important considerations to be monitored.

3. Claustrophobia often occurs because of tighter confinement and longer imaging times than with CT. Sedation may be necessary.

4. Metal and electronic devices such as pacemakers, cochlear implants, and foreign bodies often contraindicate MRI. A list may be obtained from a neuroradiologist.

5. Calcium is not well visualized. Therefore, bone signal is restricted to that given off by marrow fat and is usually black on MRI.

6. Artifacts are common on MRI because of the complex interactions of several types of information, any of which can distort the final image.

REF: Atlas SW, ed: *Magnetic resonance imaging of the brain and spine*, New York, 1991, Raven.

MALABSORPTION *(see Nutritional Deficiency Syndromes)*

MALIGNANT NEUROLEPTIC SYNDROME *(see Neuroleptics)*

MARCHIAFAVA-BIGNAMI SYNDROME *(see Alcohol, Demyelinating Diseases, Nutritional Deficiency Syndromes)*

MARCUS GUNN PUPIL *(see Pupil)*

McARDLE'S DISEASE *(see Muscle Disorders, Myoglobinuria, Myopathy)*

MEASLES *(see Electroencephalography, Encephalitis, Immunization)*

MEDIAN NERVE *(see Carpal Tunnel Syndrome, Neuropathy, Peripheral Nerve)*

MEDULLARY SYNDROMES *(see Ischemia)*

MEDULLOBLASTOMA *(see Cerebrospinal Fluid, Computed Tomography, Tumor)*

MEIGE'S SYNDROME   *(see Dystonia)*

MEMORY   *(see also Mental Status Testing)*

Memory comprises the mental processes of encoding, storage, and recall of experiences and information. Memory can be divided into immediate recall and long-term memory or subtypes such as declarative (episodic and semantic) and nondeclarative (including classic conditioning, priming, and procedural) memory. The anatomy of memory involves many widely distributed neural structures. The medial temporal lobe memory system is involved in the processing and storage of long-term memory and involves the hippocampus, amygdala, and adjacent related entorhinal, perirhinal, and parahippocampal cortices and their connections to neocortex. Damage to basal forebrain structures (septum, nucleus basalis of Meynert, and orbitofrontal regions), as occurs in Alzheimer's disease, is associated with a memory disorder often accompanied by other frontal lobe abnormalities. Damage to diencephalic structures, particularly dorsomedial and other thalamic nuclei, as in Korsakoff's syndrome, leads to amnesia, possibly by disconnection of cortical areas involved in memory processing.

Amnestic syndromes include retrograde or anterograde amnesia. Retrograde amnesia commonly follows head injury and involves loss of memory for a variable time before the event. Anterograde amnesia, the inability to incorporate ongoing experience into memory stores, is seen in Wernicke-Korsakoff's psychosis or bilateral limbic lesions (hippocampal-amygdala complex). The latter is usually due to occlusive vascular disease or encephalitis. Total global retrograde amnesia, in which an individual loses all prior memory, is never due to organic dysfunction.

In the syndrome of "transient global amnesia" an individual behaves in an apparently automatic fashion for minutes to hours without recollection of those events and has a retrograde amnesia that may be spotty. The syndrome occurs in middle-aged or elderly individuals and rarely recurs. Its pathogenesis is unknown but may be a manifestation of migraine, transient vascular insufficiency, or partial complex seizure.

REF: Bauer RM, Tobias B, Valenstein E. In Heilman KH, Valenstein E, eds: *Clinical neuropsychology*, ed 3, New York, 1993, Oxford University.

Squire LR, Zola-Morgan S: *Science* 253:1380–1386, 1991.

MENIERE'S DISEASE   *(see Vertigo)*

MENINGEAL CARCINOMATOSIS   *(see Cerebrospinal Fluid, Meningitis, Tumors)*

MENINGIOMA   *(see Computed Tomography, Tumor)*

MENINGITIS

Meningitis is an infectious or inflammatory process involving the subarachnoid space. Bacterial meningitis (invariably associated with a cortical encephalitis and often with a ventriculitis) is a medical emergency and should be suspected in any patient with an acute onset of nuchal rigidity, headache, altered mental status, fever, emesis, and photophobia. Meningeal signs are often absent in infants younger than 6 months of age and in elderly individuals. If the diagnosis of acute bacterial meningitis is suspected, blood cultures and head CT are obtained immediately. Antibiotic therapy should be begun before the patient leaves the emergency room for the CT. Antibiotics are chosen based on patient age, severity of clinical situation, and possible organisms (see Table 38). If the CT result is normal, a CSF examination must be performed and sent for appropriate studies, including blood cell and differential cell counts, glucose and protein levels, and cultures (bacterial, viral, fungal, and mycobacterial, as appropriate). Organism-specific studies, including cryptococcal antigen studies and counterimmunoelectrophoresis specific for some strains of *Haemophilus influenzae*, *Neisseria meningitides*, *Streptococcus pneumoniae*, β-hemolytic streptococci, and *Escherichia coli* are often useful, especially if results of initial CSF cultures are negative (see Table 39).

Laboratory evaluation of CSF begins with a Gram stain and india ink examination of centrifuged CSF sediment. Cell counts > 1000/mm^3, protein levels > 50 mg/dl, and glucose levels < 30 mg/dl suggest bacterial infection. There is overlap with ranges more typical of fungal, tuberculous, and viral meningitis (see Cerebrospinal Fluid). A polymorphonuclear (PMN) predominance is more common with bacterial meningitis, and a lymphocytosis with aseptic meningitis. Approximately 10% of bacterial meningitides show a lymphocytosis. Early viral meningitis, especially as a result of mumps, may show a PMN predominance. Hypoglycorrhachia (low CSF glucose level) occurs in bacterial, tuberculous, fungal, carcinomatous, or chemical meningitis.

In the subacute presentation (more than 24 hours of symptoms), unless mental status is impaired, a more detailed workup may be done before starting antibiotic therapy. Signs and symptoms of meningoencephalitis lasting for at least 4 weeks with persistently abnormal results

TABLE 38

Wide-Coverage Antibiotics Used in Initial Treatment of Acute Meningitis Before Return of Cultures

Patients	Antibiotic Therapy
Neonates	Ampicillin or penicillin G IV IM; aminoglycoside or ampicillin and cefotaxime; appropriate dosages depend on age and weight
Children 1–3 mo	Ampicillin 200 mg/kg per day IV divided q6h and cefotaxime 200 mg/kg per day IV divided q6h
Children >3 mo	Cefotaxime 200 mg/kg per day IV divided q6h or ceftriaxone 100 mg/kg per day divided q12h
Adults	Cefotaxime 1 g IV q8h to 2 g IV q4h or ceftriaxone 1 to 2 g IV q12h

For severe penicillin allergy consider giving chloramphenicol and trimethoprim–sulfamethoxazole. If methicillin-resistant *Staphylococcus* organisms are a consideration, vancomycin 1 g IV q12h is recommended.

of CSF study are consistent with chronic meningitis. Recurrent meningitis is defined as repetitive episodes of meningitis associated with an abnormal result of CSF study followed by symptom-free periods during which the CSF is normal (see Table 40). *Mollaret's meningitis*, also called benign recurrent aseptic meningitis, has recently been associated with herpes simplex virus, type 2, and may improve on administration of prophylactic acyclovir.

Mortality rates for the different forms of meningitis are variable. The three most common bacterial meningitides (pneumococcal, meningococcal, and those caused by *H. influenzae*) have an average mortality rate of 10%; neurologic deficits occur in about 20% of survivors. The less common bacterial meningitides can have much higher mortality rates. The frequency of complications correlates with increased duration of symptoms before treatment. Mental status changes, in particular, agitation and confusion, are poor prognostic signs, as is an underlying malignancy, alcoholism, diabetes, or pneumonia. Com-

TABLE 39

Causative Organisms in Meningitis According to Patient Age and Clinical Setting*

Infants < 6 wk old: Group B streptococci, *E. coli*, *S. pneumoniae*, *L. monocytogenes*, *Salmonella* organisms, *P. aeruginosa*, *S. aureus*, *H. influenzae*, *Citrobacter* organisms, herpes simplex II

Children 6 wk to 15 yr old: *H. influenzae*, *S. pneumoniae*, *N. meningitidis*, *S. aureus*, viruses

Older children and young adults: *N. meningitidis*, *S. pneumoniae*, *H. influenzae*, *S. aureus*, viruses

Adults > 40 yr old: *S. pneumoniae*, *N. meningitidis*, *S. aureus*, *L. monocytogenes*, gram-negative bacilli

Diabetes mellitus: *S. pneumoniae*, gram-negative bacilli, staphylococci, *Cryptococcus* organisms, Mucorales

Alcoholism: *S. pneumoniae*

Sickle cell anemia: *S. pneumoniae*

Pneumonia or upper respiratory infection: *S. pneumoniae*, *N. meningitidis*, viruses, *H. influenzae*

AIDS or other abnormal cellular immunity: *Toxoplasma*, *Cryptococcus*, *Coccidiodes*, and *Candida* organisms; *L. monocytogenes*, *M. tuberculosis* and *avium-intracellulare*, *T. pallidum*, *Histoplasma* organisms, *Nocardia*, *S. pneumoniae*, gram-negative bacilli

Abnormal neutrophils: *P. aeruginosa*, *S. aureus*, Candida and Aspergillus organisms, Mucorales

Immunoglobulin deficiency: *S. pneunomiae*, *N. meningitidis*, *H. influenzae*

Ventricular shunt infections: *S. epidermidis*, *S. aureus*, gram-negative bacilli

Penetrating head trauma, skin lesions, bacterial endocarditis or other heart disease, severe burns, IV drug abuse: *S. aureus*, streptococci, gram-negative bacilli

Closed head trauma, CSF leak, pericranial infections: *S. pneumoniae*, gram-negative bacilli

Following neurosurgical procedures: *S. aureus*, *S. epidermidis*, gram-negative bacilli

Tick bites: *B. burgdorferi*

Swimming in fresh water ponds: *Naegleria* organisms

Contact with water frequented by rodents or domestic animals: *Leptospira* organisms

Contact with hamsters or mice: Lymphocytic choriomeningitis virus

Exposure to pigeons: *Cryptococcus* organisms

Travel in southwestern United States: *Coccidioides* organisms

*Adapted from Mandell GL et al: *Principles and practice of infectious diseases*, ed 2, New York, 1985, John Wiley & Sons.

TABLE 40

Causes of Aseptic, Chronic (C), and Recurrent (R) Meningitis

Infectious
Actinomyces sp. (C)*
Amebas
Blastomyces sp. (C)*
Brucella sp. (C)
Borrelia sp. (C,R)
Candida sp. (C)
Coccidioides sp. (C)
Cryptococcus sp. (C)
Cysticercosis (C)*
Fungi (C,R)
Herpes simplex I and II
Histoplasma sp. (C)
Human immunodeficiency virus (C)
Leptospira sp. (C,R)
Listeria sp.
M. tuberculosis (C,R)
Mycoplasma sp.
Nocardia sp.*
Parameningeal suppurative foci (R)
Partially treated meningitis (R)
Rickettsia sp.
T. pallidum (C)
Toxoplasma sp. (C)*

Noninfectious
Behcet's syndrome (C,R)
Chemical
Drugs (ibuprofen, isoniazide, sulindac, sulfamethoxazole)
Granulomatous angiitis (C)
Lupus erythematosus (R)
Meningitis-migraine syndrome (R)
Mollaret's meningitis (R)
Neoplasm (C,R)
Rupture of cyst (R)
Sarcoid (C,R)
Uremia
Uveomeningoecephalitis (C,R)
Viruses (R)

*More commonly cause brain abscess or focal lesion.

mon sequelae include hearing loss, vestibular dysfunction, cognitive and behavioral changes, and seizures.

Glucocorticoid administration suppresses the inflammatory response, with resultant decreased brain edema and lowered intracranial pressure. Children with meningitis who receive treatment with dexamethasone 0.6 mg/kg per day in four divided doses for the initial 4 days of antibiotic therapy have lower rates of sensorineural hearing loss and neurologic sequelae. The advantages of corticosteroids in the treatment of adults with meningitis are unclear, although such treatment may benefit those with increased intracranial pressure.

REF: Durand ML et al: N Engl J Med 328:21–28, 1993.

Quagliarello V, Scheld WM: N Engl J Med 327:864–872, 1992.

MENINGOCELE   *(see Developmental Malformations)*

MENTAL RETARDATION   *(see Chromosomal Defects, Microcephaly)*

MENTAL STATUS TESTING

Bedside mental status examination should allow for quick screening of focal and global abnormalities. Elements of the mental status examination include state of awareness, attention, mood and affect, speech and language, memory, visual spatial function, praxis, and other aspects of cognition such as calculations, thought content, and judgment. Patients who appear to have difficulties on screening examinations should have a more detailed survey of their cognitive abilities, ranging from short, standardized tests such as the Mini mental state examination or short Blessed test to more detailed neuropsychologic evaluation (Figure 2).

Interpretation of mental status testing cannot be performed in isolation. An inattentive patient may not perform well on memory tasks or language comprehension, but this is not indicative of primary language or memory disturbance. Visual impairment may complicate constructional testing and naming. General information and proverb testing, although useful as a screening test, is highly dependent on educational level, socioeconomic status, and cultural background.

REF: Crum R et al: JAMA 269(18):2386–2391, 1993.

Katzman R et al: Am J Psychiatry 140:734–739, 1983.

Actual	Possible	
		Orientation
_____	5	What is the date, year, month, day, season?
_____	5	Where are we: state, county, town, hospital, floor?
		Registration
_____	3	Name three objects: 1 second to say each. Then ask the patient to name all three after you have said them. Give one point for each correct answer. Then repeat them until patient learns all three. Count trials and record. Trials _____
		Attention and calculation
_____	5	Serial 7's. One point for each correct. Stop after five answers. As an alternative, spell "world" backwards.
		Recall
_____	3	Ask for the names of the three objects repeated above. Give 1 point for each correct name.
		Language
_____	2	Name a pencil and a watch.
_____	1	Repeat the phrase "No ifs, ands, or buts."
_____	3	Follow a three-stage command. "Take the paper in your right hand, fold it in half, and put it on the floor."
_____	1	Read and obey the following: "Close your eyes."
_____	1	Write a sentence.
_____	1	Copy the design shown here.

_____ **Total** (maximum score, 30)

Assess level of consciousness along the following continuum:

Alert Drowsy Stupor Coma

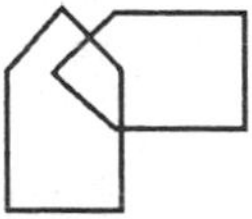

FIGURE 25
Mini mental state examination. (From Folstein MF, Folstein SE, McHugh PR: *Psychiatr Res* 12:189-98, 1975.

Strub RL, Black FW: *The mental status examination in neurology*, Philadelphia, 1993, FA Davis.

MERALGIA PARESTHETICA *(see Neuropathy, Peripheral Nerve)*

METABOLIC ACIDOSIS *(see Electrolyte Disorders)*

METABOLIC ALKALOSIS   *(see Electrolyte Disorders)*

METABOLIC DISEASES OF CHILDHOOD)   *(see also Degenerative Diseases of Childhood)*

Congenital metabolic diseases include disorders of amino acid metabolism and transport; carbohydrate, glycoprotein, lipid, purine, and metabolism; the mucopolysaccharidoses and mucolipidoses; and some endocrine conditions. Some diseases that can be successfully treated and for which neonatal screening programs exist are presented.

Phenylketonuria. Autosomal recessive defect of phenylalanine hydroxylase (defective conversion of phenylalanine to tyrosine). Infants appear normal at birth. Vomiting and irritability develop by 2 months. Mental retardation is apparent by 4 to 9 months. Untreated, children have severe mental retardation, seizures, and imperfect hair pigmentation. With early institution of a phenylalanine-restricted diet, most children develop normally.

Maple syrup urine disease. Autosomal recessive defect in branched-chain amino acid metabolism (valine, leucine, isoleucine). Urine has a sweet odor. Infants appear normal at birth, but in the first week of life opisthotonus, intermittent increased muscle tone, and respiratory irregularity develop. Untreated, infants may die in early infancy, or may survive a few years with severe mental retardation and spasticity. With a diet restricted in branched-chain amino acids instituted in the first 2 weeks of life, most infants have a normal outcome. Treated infants are vulnerable to fulminant sepsis.

Galactosemia. Autosomal recessive deficiency of galactose-1-uridyl transferase (defective conversion of galactose-1-phosphate to UDP-galactose). Infants usually appear normal at birth. Listlessness, jaundice, vomiting, diarrhea, and failure to gain weight appear in the first week of life. By age 2 weeks, hypotonia, cataracts, and hepatosplenomegaly develop. Untreated, infants develop mental retardation and die prematurely of liver cirrhosis. With a lactose-free diet most infants have a normal IQ but may have visual-perceptual deficits.

Hypothyroidism. Infants with neonatal hypothyroidism tend to be postterm, macrosomic (birth weight > 4 kg), and may have prolonged jaundice, large posterior fontanel, skin mottling, decreased motor activity, and abdominal distention with umbilical hernia. By age 2 months there is generalized hypotonia, a husky, grunting cry, widely open sutures and fontanel, and retarded osseous development. If not treated early, mental retardation, deaf-mutism, and spasticity result. Even if the condition is treated early, residual learning and speech disorders and cerebellar deficits are common.

Evaluation. A metabolic disease is often suspected when developmental delay becomes evident in late infancy. The following studies can be helpful: serum and urine metabolic screen, urine organic acid screen, ammonia, lactate and pyruvate values, ophthalmologic examination (cataracts), CT or MRI, skeletal films (bone age, osseous defects), lysosomal enzyme studies, and tissue biopsy (skin, muscle, peripheral nerve, and bone marrow).

REF: Menkes JH: *Textbook of child neurology*, ed 4, Philadelphia, 1990, Lea & Febiger.

METASTASES   (see Tumor)

MICROCEPHALY   (see also Child Neurology, Craniosynostosis, Degenerative Diseases of Childhood, Hypoxic-Ischemic Encephalopathy)

Microcephaly refers to head circumference greater than 2 standard deviations below the mean for age, sex, and race. Small skull size almost always reflects small brain size (except in craniosynostosis), and there is a high correlation with mental retardation. Microcephaly can be primary or secondary. Primary microcephaly is associated with conditions affecting neuronal maturation and migration from 4 to 20 weeks of gestation. Secondary microcephaly occurs with CNS injuries after 7 months of gestation. Thus microcephaly is associated with genetic factors, intrauterine infections (Cytomegalovirus, toxoplasmosis, and rubella), chemical agents (alcohol and anticonvulsants), anoxic injury, metabolic disorders, and exposure to ionizing radiation (especially between 4 and 20 weeks of gestation).

Evaluation of microcephaly includes a maternal history (fetal exposure to transplacental infections, toxins, or asphyxia), indirect ophthalmoscopy (chorioretinitis), CT or MRI scan (CNS structural anomaly), and chromosomal and metabolic evaluation. In an older infant with microcephaly previous head circumference measurements are necessary to determine the pattern of head growth.

MICTURITION SYNCOPE   (see Syncope)

MIGRAINE   *(see Headache)*

MITOCHONDRIAL MYOPATHY   *(see Myopathy)*

MONONEUROPATHY MULTIPLEX   *(see Neuropathy)*

MORO REFLEX   *(see Child Neurology)*

MOTOR NEURON DISEASE   *(see also Hypotonic Infant, Muscle Disorders)*

CLASSIFICATION OF MOTOR NEURON DISEASE

I. Inherited.
   A. Spinal muscular atrophy (SMA).
      1. Type I: Infantile (Werdnig-Hoffmann disease).
      2. Type II: Late (benign) infantile.
      3. Type III: Juvenile (Kugelberg-Welander disease).
      4. Type IV: Adult.
         a. Limb girdle.
         b. Fascioscapulohumeral.
         c. Scapuloperoneal.
         d. Peroneal.
         e. Ophthalmoplegia plus.
         f. Other.
      5. Hexosaminidase deficiency.
   B. Familial amyotrophic lateral sclerosis (ALS).
   C. Juvenile progressive bulbar palsy (Fazio-Londe syndrome).
   D. ALS-like syndrome in hexosaminidase deficiency.
II. Acquired.
   A. Acute: Acute anterior poliomyelitis (polio, coxsackie virus, other enteroviruses).
   B. Chronic.
      1. ALS.
      2. Anterior horn cell degeneration in the following:
         a. Spinocerebellar degeneration.
         b. Creutzfeldt-Jakob disease.
         c. Huntington's disease.
         d. Parkinsonism.
         e. Shy-Drager syndrome.
         f. Joseph disease.
         g. Paraneoplastic syndromes.

Amyotrophic lateral sclerosis (ALS) is a chronic, progressive, de-generative disease of unknown origin characterized on pathologic study by progressive loss of motor neurons in the spinal cord, brainstem, and motor cortex. The neuronal loss may occur at one or several levels.

On clinical examination patients have upper or lower motor neuron symptoms and signs in bulbar or spinal innervated muscles, or both (see Table 41).

Frequently weakness and atrophy of one muscle group is present, which then spreads to all extremities and to the bulbar muscles. Fasciculations are common. There is weakness of the muscles of mastication and palate with dysphagia and hypophonic dysarthria. Ophthalmoparesis is rare. Sphincter disturbance may occur late in the course. Upper motor neuron findings in the form of spasticity and hyperreflexia develop. Most cases progress to the typical picture of ALS with generalized upper and lower motor neuron findings. Death usually results from recurrent aspiration pneumonia and respiratory insufficiency.

Prognosis is related to the onset of bulbar involvement. Life expectancy is usually less than 1.5 to 2 years after bulbar involvement, especially if mainly involved with lower motor neuron. With predominantly spinal involvement (especially upper motor neuron), survival is longer; 20% survive for longer than 5 years. Overall survival in ALS averages 1 to 3 years. Most cases are sporadic. Some cases are familial, usually occurring among the Chamorro people of Guam and in the Kii peninsula in Japan, and may be associated with dementia and parkinsonism. Mutations in the superoxide dismutase gene have been associated with the familial form. Age at onset is usually between 40 and 70 years, peaking in the sixth decade.

Diagnostic evaluation includes EMG, which reveals wide-spread denervation with fibrillation potentials, positive waves, fasciculation potentials, and, occasionally, giant motor unit potentials. Sensory

TABLE 41
Classification of Motor Neuron Disease by Initial Presentation

	Spinal Cord	Brainstem
Lower motor neuron (atrophic)	Spinal muscular atrophy	Progressive bulbar palsy
Upper motor neuron (spastic)	Primary lateral sclerosis	Progressive pseudobulbar palsy

nerve conduction studies are normal. Cervical spine and craniocervical junction lesions can be ruled out with MRI. CSF is normal. Muscle biopsy specimen demonstrates denervation, but biopsy is usually not required. Anti GM_1 antibodies should be looked for (especially in patients with predominant lower motor neuron features), since plasmapheresis may help these patients.

Management is centered around supportive measures, patient and family education, good pulmonary toilet, and nasogastric or gastrostomy feeding.

Acute anterior poliomyelitis is due to destruction of spinal cord and brainstem motor neurons by the polio virus. Cerebral cortex and deep gray nuclei may also be involved. The virus initially infects and multiplies in the pharynx and the gastrointestinal tract.

On clinical examination the GI infection and viremia are usually asymptomatic or only mildly symptomatic, followed in several days by fever, headache, calf pains, meningeal signs, and asymmetric paralysis. The sensory system is usually spared. Paralysis usually progresses over 3 to 5 days. Bulbar involvement carries a worse prognosis.

Incidence of poliomyelitis has dropped as a result of the attenuated and killed polio vaccines from about 50,000 cases per year in the mid-1950s to an occasional case per year, usually in persons who have not been vaccinated or were inadequately vaccinated.

Laboratory findings include peripheral leukocytosis, slightly to moderately elevated CSF protein level with a lymphocytic pleocytosis, and fourfold rise between acute and convalescent viral titers. The virus may be isolated from blood, pharynx, stool, or CSF.

Treatment is supportive, with mechanical ventilation if needed.

REF: Rowland LP et al: *Neurology* 42:1101–1102, 1992.

Sanders KA et al: *Neurology* 418–420, 1993.

MOVEMENT DISORDERS   *(see Asterixis, Athetosis, Chorea, Choreoathetosis, Dyskinesia, Dystonia, Huntington's Disease, Myoclonus, Neuroleptics, Parkinson's Disease, Progressive Supranuclear Palsy, Rigidity, Tourette's Syndrome, Tremor, Wilson's Disease)*

MOYA-MOYA

From the Japanese words meaning "puff of smoke," *moyamoya* refers to the angiographic appearance of small collateral vessels arising from the circle of Willis in association with the gradual occlusion of large cerebral vessels. Moya-Moya may occur as an isolated finding or may be associated with arteriovenous malformations or aneurysms. Moya-Moya may become evident as cerebral infarction or hemorrhage, headache, or seizure, especially in children and young adults. With progression, hemiparesis, altered mental state, and movement disorders may occur. Conditions associated with Moya-Moya include Down's syndrome, neurocutaneous syndromes (tuberous sclerosis, neurofibromatosis, and Sturge-Weber syndrome), sickle cell disease, Fanconi's anemia, cyanotic congenital heart disease, pituitary tumor, type 1 glycogenosis, radiation therapy, vasculitis, and leptospirosis. Familial cases have been described. Although it may be more common in Oriental persons, Moya-Moya occurs throughout the world. There is no specific treatment, although surgical revascularization has been attempted in a limited number of cases.

MULTIPLE SCLEROSIS (see Demyelinating Disease)

Multiple sclerosis (MS) is the most common demyelinating disease. The diagnosis is made on clinical grounds; using established criteria, MS can be classified as clinically definite, laboratory-supported definite, clinically probable, or possible. For diagnostic purposes symptomatic attacks should have objective dysfunction and last a minimum of 24 hours, occur in different locations in the CNS involving primarily white matter, and be separated by a period of at least 1 month. Onset of the disease is usually between the ages of 10 and 50 years. The course is typically relapsing and remitting or chronic and (> 6 months) progressive. Clinically definite MS is diagnosed when there have been two attacks and there is clinical evidence of two separate lesions.

The most common initial symptoms are limb weakness, optic neuritis, paresthesias, diplopia, vertigo, and urinary difficulties. Signs and symptoms that occur later include upper and lower motor neuron weakness, spasticity, increased or depressed muscle stretch reflexes, pain, Lhermitte's sign, internuclear ophthalmoplegia, nystagmus, ataxia, impotence, hearing loss, affective disorders, and dementia. The Uhthoff phenomenon or sign is the worsening of a sign or symptom with exercise or increased temperature.

Radiologic and laboratory studies may support the clinical diagnosis. CT results are usually normal but can show areas of decreased attenuation in the white matter, areas of contrast enhancement, or both. MRI is far more sensitive than CT for detecting MS plaques. Focal enhancement with gadolinium is considered evidence of an "active" plaque. CSF may reveal a lymphocytic pleocytosis (usually less than 25 cells/mm^3) and normal or increased protein levels. Oligoclonal bands may be present in 80% of patients with clinically definite MS. Elevated levels of CSF-free kappa light chains are highly specific for MS. Elevated IgG:albumin ratio and index are indicative of intrathecal antibody synthesis and are increased in 92% of patients with clinically definite MS. The level of myelin basic protein is elevated during flares of disease activity but is also elevated in other CNS diseases. Visual, auditory, and somatosensory-evoked potentials may reveal abnormalities in their respective pathways. Cystometrics may show an uninhibited, spastic, or flaccid bladder or sphincter dyssynergia.

The incidence of MS increases with latitude. Risk for development of the disease correlates with the latitude at which one lived before the age of 15 years. There is a familial predisposition for its development; women are more commonly affected than men, and whites more so than blacks.

General management includes avoidance of heat and excessive fatigue. Fever and hot weather can decrease conduction and exacerbate symptoms. A small, spastic bladder can be treated with oxybutynin, propantheline, or imipramine. Sphincter dyssynergia and a spastic bladder often coexist and are treated with phenoxybenzamine or diazepam, or both. A large, flaccid bladder is treated with Valsalva or Credé maneuvers, catheterization (intermittent or permanent), or pharmacologic agents such as bethanechol and phenoxybenzamine. Surgical placement of an artificial sphincter or urinary diversion may be useful.

Spasticity is treated with baclofen, diazepam, or dantrolene sodium (see Spasticity).

Trigeminal neuralgia symptoms and tonic spasms respond to carbamazepine. Inappropriate laughing or crying are reduced with amitriptyline.

Interferon beta-1b at a dose of 8 million units SC (0.25 mg) qod lowers the relapse rate and burden of enhancing ("active") plaque areas in long-term trials of relapsing and remitting MS. Side effects of beta-interferon include depression, elevated liver function tests, depressed lymphocyte counts, and flu-like symptoms. A variety of other immunosuppressive therapies have been tested, but none have been shown to alter the course of the disease. Short-term, high-dose IV corticosteroid therapy is generally recommended for acute, disabling attacks. Administration of IV methylprednisolone followed by a short course of oral prednisone may lower the frequency of MS after an attack of isolated optic neuritis.

REF: Beck RW et al: N Engl J Med 329:1764–1769, 1993.

Fowler CJ et al: J Neurol Neurosurg Psych 55:986–989, 1992.

Kupersmith et al: Neurology 44:1-4, 1994.

Matthews WB, ed: McAlpine's multiple sclerosis, ed 2, New York, 1991, Churchhill, Livingstone.

MUSCLE DISORDERS (TABLE 42) *(see also Muscular Dystrophy, Myopathy)*

MUSCLE FIBER TYPES (TABLE 43)

MUSCLE TESTING *(see also Myotome)*

Bedside examination of the muscles involves assessment of *bulk, tone, and strength.* In certain neurologic diseases *fatigue* of muscular response may be important. Subtle weakness may not be demonstrated by action against resistance but may be revealed with provocative postures or movement, such as pronator drift or arm rolling. Quantitative measures of force generation by specific muscle groups may be helpful in the context of rehabilitation and physical or occupational therapy (see Table 44).

MUSCULAR DYSTROPHY

Muscular dystrophy (MD) refers to a group of genetically determined, progressive, degenerative myopathies.

Duchenne muscular dystrophy (DMD) is the most common, most severe MD. Inheritance is X-linked recessive. Early developmental milestones such as sitting are normally attained. Clinical manifestations occur in the second year of life with difficulty standing and walking. Patients have a waddling gait with lumbar lordosis and often stand on their toes because of shortening of calf muscles. By approximately 10 years of age patients no longer climb stairs or stand from the floor independently. By 12 years of age most are confined to a wheelchair. Once the patient is in a wheelchair, contractures and kyphoscoliosis

Text continued on p. 254.

TABLE 42
Syndromic Classification of Muscle Diseases

I. Acute (evolving in days) or subacute (weeks) paretic or paralytic disorders of muscle.*
  A. Rarely fulminant myasthenia gravis or myasthenic syndrome from a "mycin" antibiotic or hypokalemia.
  B. Idiopathic polymyositis and dermatomyositis.
  C. Viral polymyositis.
  D. Acute paroxysmal myoglobinuria.
  E. "Alcoholic" polymyopathy.
  F. Familial (malignant) hyperpyrexia precipitated by anesthetic agents.
  G. Malignant neuroleptic syndrome.
  H. First attack of episodic weakness may enter into differential diagnosis (see below).
  I. Botulism.
  J. Organophosphate poisoning.
II. Chronic (i.e., months to years) weakness or paralysis of muscle, usually with severe atrophy.
  A. Progressive muscular dystrophy.
    1. Sex-linked recessive.
      a. Duchenne.

C. Chronic thyrotoxic and other endocrine myopathies.
D. Chronic, slowly progressive, or relatively stationary polymyopathies.†
  1. Central core and multicore diseases.
  2. Rod-body and related polymyopathies.
  3. Mitochondrial and centronuclear polymyopathies.
  4. Other congenital myopathies (reducing-body, fingerprint, zebra-body, fiber-type atrophies, and disproportions).
  5. Glycogen storage disease.
  6. Lipid myopathies (carnitine deficiency myopathy and undefined lipid myopathies).
III. Episodic weakness of muscle.
  A. Familial (hypokalemic) periodic paralysis.
  B. Normokalemic or hyperkalemic familial periodic paralysis.
  C. Paramyotonia congenita (von Eulenberg).
  D. Nonfamilial hyperkalemic and hypokalemic periodic paralysis (including primary hyperaldosteronism).

b. Becker.
c. Benign with early contractures (Dreifuss-Emery).
d. Scapuloperoneal.
2. Autosomal recessive.
a. Scapulohumeral (limb-girdle).
b. Autosomal recessive dystrophy of childhood (Erb).
c. Congenital.
3. Autosomal dominant.
a. Facioscapulohumeral (Landouzy-Dejerine).
b. Scapuloperoneal.
c. Late-onset recessive (Erb).
d. Distal—adult onset.
e. Distal—childhood onset.
f. Ocular (Hutchinson-Fuchs)
g. Oculopharyngeal (Victor-Hayes-Adams).
h. Myotonic dystrophy
B. Chronic polymyositis or dermatomyositis (may be subacute).
1. Idiopathic.
2. With connective tissue disease.
3. With occult neoplasm.
4. Inclusion body myositis.

E. Acute thyrotoxic myopathy (also thyrotoxic periodic paralysis).
F. Conditions in which weakness fluctuates.
1. Myasthenia gravis, immunologic type.
2. Myasthenia associated with:
a. Lupus erythematosus.
b. Polymyositis.
c. Rheumatoid arthritis.
d. Nonthymic carcinoma.
3. Familial and sporadic nonimmunologic types of myasthenia.
4. Myasthenia resulting from antibiotics and other drugs.
5. Lambert-Eaton syndrome.
G. Exercise intolerance.
1. Myoadenylate deaminase deficiency.
2. Ca-adenosine triphosphate deficiency.
3. Hypothyroidism.
4. "Fibromyositis" syndrome.
5. Hypoparathyroidism.
6. Glycogenosis (debranching enzyme deficiency).
IV. Disorders of muscle presenting with myotonia, stiffness, spasm, and cramp.

Continued.

TABLE 42—cont'd
Syndromic Classification of Muscle Diseases

A. Myotonic dystrophy, congenital myotonia (Thomsen's disease), paramyotonia congenita, and Schwartz-Jampel syndrome.

B. Hypothyroidism with pseudomyotonia (Debré-Sémélaigne and Hoffmann syndromes).

C. Tetany.

D. Tetanus.

E. Black widow spider bite.

F. Myopathy resulting from myophosphorylase deficiency (McArdle's disease), phosphofructokinase deficiency, and other forms of contracture.

G. Contracture with Addison's disease.

H. Idiopathic cramp syndromes.

I. Myokymia and syndromes of continuous muscle activity.

V. Myalgic states.‡

A. Connective tissue diseases (rheumatoid arthritis, mixed connective tissue disease, Sjogren's syndrome, lupus erythematosus, polyarteritis nodosa, scleroderma, polymyositis).

B. Localized multifocal fibrositis (myogelosis).

F. Bornholm disease and other forms of viral polymyositis.

G. Anterior tibial syndrome.

H. Other.
  1. Hypophosphatemia.
  2. Hypothyroidism.
  3. Psychiatric illness (hysteria, depression).

VI. Localized muscle mass(es).

A. Rupture of a muscle.

B. Muscle hemorrhage.

C. Muscle tumor.
  a. Rhabdomyosarcoma.
  2. Desmoid.
  3. Angioma.
  4. Metastatic nodules.

D. Monomyositis multiplex.
  1. Eosinophilic type.
  2. Other.

E. Localized and generalized myositis ossificans.

F. Fibrositis (myogelosis).

G. Granulomatous infections.

C. Trichinosis.
D. Myopathy of myoglobinuria and McArdle's disease.
E. Myopathy with hypoglycemia.

1. Sarcoidosis.
2. Tuberculosis.
3. Wegener's granulomatosis.
H. Pyogenic abscess.
I. Infarction of muscle in the diabetic.

From Adams RA, Victor M: *Principles of neurology.* ed 5 *New York,* 1993, McGraw-Hill.

TABLE 43
Characteristics of Muscle Fiber Types

Characteristic	Type 1	Type 2a	Type 2b
Speed	Slow	Fast	Fast
Metabolism	Oxidative	Oxidative-glycolytic	Glycolytic
Fatigue resistance	+	+	−

TABLE 44
Grading of Muscle Strength

Grade	Strength
0	No perceptible contraction.
1	Trace contraction is observed, but no movement is achieved.
2	Movement is achieved in horizontal plane but not against gravity.
3	Movement is achieved against gravity but not against additional resistance.
4−	Movement is achieved against slight resistance.
4	Movement is achieved against moderate resistance.
4+	Movement is achieved against large resistance but is less than expected, given patient age and fitness.
5	Intact strength.

Aids to the examination of the peripheral nerves, ed 3, East Sussex, 1986, Balliere Tindall.

develop. Death usually occurs in the third decade of life as a result of respiratory insufficiency and infection. Examination results depend on stage. Initially weakness is proximal, with hips more involved than shoulders. Muscles are hard and rubbery. Pseudohypertrophy of the calves is usually present. Deep tendon reflexes are normal initially but disappear early in the disease. Average IQ is 85. Eighty percent of patients have ECG abnormalities that include tall right precordial R waves and precordial Q waves. Arrhythmias and cardiac failure are rare. Elevated levels of creatine kinase (CK) (may be in the thousands) and myoglobin are always seen in early stages of disease and fall as the disease progresses, but normal values are never attained. Results of muscle biopsy are characteristic; the specimen shows fibrosis, circular fibers, groups of basophilic fibers, and "opaque" fibers. Electromyography (EMG) results show polyphasic potentials and increased recruitment. Results of nerve conduction studies are normal.

The defective gene is located in the p21 region of chromosome X. The product of this gene is a protein called dystrophin, which is absent or present at less than 3% of normal quantity in 95% of males with DMD. The normal function of dystrophin has yet to be elucidated The creatine kinase level is elevated in 50% to 70% of female carriers and may be falsely low during pregnancy. Diagnostic techniques, including analysis of antidystrophin antibody, studies of immunofluorescence patterns, direct analysis of the dystrophin gene, and quantification of dystrophin, may help in early identification of patients and carriers.

Treatment involves physical therapy, bracing, Achilles tendon releases, and pulmonary care. Prednisone therapy (0.75 mg/kg per day) may improve strength for at least 18 months; use of cyclosporine (5 mg/kg per day) may also result in increased muscular force generation. Other techniques such as gene therapy or myoblast transfer are still experimental.

Becker (slowly progressive) muscular dystrophy (BMD) is an X-linked dystrophinopathy closely resembling DMD. In patients the same proximal hip and shoulder weakness, calf hypertrophy, and tendency to walk on their toes develop. However, onset is later, the disease is less severe, and survival is prolonged. Most patients walk until at least 16 years of age. In BMD mental retardation is less common, there is less tendency to contractures, and skeletal deformities are less marked than in DMD. The serum CK level is elevated. Electrocardiography results are abnormal in 30% to 40% of patients and are less specific than in DMD. Biopsy results are similar to those for DMD, but specimens show less severe disease. Sixty percent of carriers have elevated CK levels. As in DMD, the same gene product of region Xp21, dystrophin, is defective. Although dystrophin is absent in DMD, it is often present in BMD but is often of abnormal size and in normal or decreased amount.

REF: Griggs RC et al: *Neurology* 43:520-527, 1993.

Hoffman EP et al: *N Engl J Med* 318:1363-1368, 1988.

Facioscapulohumeral (FSH) (Landouzy-Dejerine) dystrophy is autosomal dominant with strong penetrance but variable expression. Onset is variable, usually occurring during the second decade of life. The course is slowly progressive; patients usually lead a full, productive life.

Initial features include facial weakness, inability to purse the lips, and incomplete eye closure. Muscles of the upper extremities may be involved simultaneously with facial muscles. Scapular fixation is lost, and biceps and triceps are involved early; relative sparing of the forearm results in a "popeye" arm. Weakness of the hips and dorsiflexors may develop, making differentiation from scapuloperoneal dystrophy difficult. Intellect is normal. The heart is rarely involved. Levels of CK are normal or minimally elevated. If patients are unable to raise their arms above horizontal because of loss of scapular fixation, surgical fixation of the scapula to the posterior chest wall should be considered.

There is an infantile form of FSH dystrophy that becomes evident by 2 years of age, may involve total paralysis of the face and severe weakness of other muscle groups, and is commonly associated with nerve deafness.

Another variant of FSH dystrophy occurs in patients who have had lifelong mild facial weakness; sometime in middle life rapidly progressive weakness of the hip and shoulder muscles develops in these patients.

Scapuloperoneal dystrophy overlaps FSH dystrophy. Anterior tibial and peroneal muscles are affected in childhood, when a foot drop develops and is followed by shoulder weakness. Fifty percent of patients have facial weakness. Inheritance is autosomal dominant or X-linked recessive.

Humeroperoneal muscular dystrophy (Emery-Dreifuss disease) is an X-linked disorder; onset usually occurs in the second decade of life. Wasting and weakness of scapulohumeroperoneal distribution are present, with prominent early contractures of elbows, posterior neck, and Achilles tendon. Cardiac conduction abnormalities are a constant finding, sudden death is reported in some cases. Results of EMG may reveal neurogenic as well as myopathic features.

Limb-girdle dystrophy is a wastebasket term for a collection of illnesses having in common the presence of progressive shoulder and hip weakness. Some of these illnesses probably represent undiagnosed metabolic myopathies. Age of onset, progression of disease, and inheritance vary. Most commonly onset becomes evident during the second or third decade of life as hip weakness followed by shoulder weakness shortly thereafter. There may be marked atrophy of the biceps. The course is slowly progressive over decades. Patients may eventually be confined to a wheelchair, but skeletal abnormalities are rare. Levels of CK may be as much as 10 times higher than normal. Biopsy specimens show variation in fiber size, fiber splitting, and internal nuclei with "motheaten" fibers. Differential diagnosis includes spinal muscular atrophy, polymyositis, and metabolic myopathies.

Ocular myopathy is usually autosomal dominant. Onset is in the third decade of life, with ptosis that precedes weakness of eye muscles. The myopathy is slowly progressive, and diplopia is rare. Eventually other muscle groups become involved, most commonly the facial muscles. Ocular myopathy is the major manifestation of chronic progressive external ophthalmoplegia and Kearns-Sayre syndrome (see Myopathy [Metabolic]).

Oculopharyngeal dystrophy is usually autosomal dominant and is commonest in French Canadians and Spanish Americans. Onset is in the third to fourth decade of life, with asymmetric ptosis and ocular dystrophy. Dysphagia follows, and some degree of facial weakness develops. Weakness of hips and shoulders is common but mild. Dysphagia becomes incapacitating, with weight loss and saliva pooling. Muscle enzyme levels are usually normal, but may be three to four times higher than normal. Conduction defects may be evident on ECG. Results of EMG show small-amplitude polyphasic motor units. Biopsy specimens show pathognomonic intranuclear filamentous inclusions in muscle nuclei. Other microscopic changes include fibrosis, rimmed vacuoles, and variation in fiber size.

Hereditary distal myopathy is rare except in Sweden. Inheritance is autosomal dominant. Onset occurs between 40 and 60 years of age, and the course is slowly progressive. Weakness and wasting of distal upper and lower extremities are present; extensors are more involved than flexors. A homozygous form has been suggested that begins in early life, has a more rapid course, and leads to widespread muscle weakness.

Congenital muscular dystrophy is a rare, autosomal recessive muscular dystrophy with generalized weakness sparing the eye muscles, normal or absent reflexes, variably increased levels of serum CK, and normal results of EMG. Biopsy specimens show variation in fiber size, necrosis, swollen hyalinized fibers with extensive fibrosis, and fatty infiltration. The disease is often accompanied by severe brain malformations, including lissencephaly, agyria, pachygyria, and hydrocephalus. In children with brains that are normal on morphologic study, intelligence is normal and the disease has a long, stable clinical course.

Myotonic dystrophy (see Myotonia).

REF: Kimura J: *Electrodiagnosis in diseases of nerve and muscle*, ed 2, Philadelphia, 1989, FA Davis.

Sher JH: Muscular Dystrophy. In Adachi M, Sher JH, eds: *Current trends in neuroscience: neuromuscular disease*, New York, 1990, Igaku-Shoin.

MYASTHENIA GRAVIS

Myasthenia gravis (MG), a disease affecting the neuromuscular junction, is characterized by fluctuating weakness. There are both congenital and acquired forms. The latter, an autoimmune disorder, is much more common. Myasthenia gravis may begin at any age. Neonatal myasthenia affects newborns of mothers with MG (see Pregnancy). Women and girls are more commonly affected than men and boys, and the disease tends to develop in women and girls at an earlier age (peak incidence in females, 10 to 40 years of age; in males, 50 to 70 years of age). Acquired MG has an incidence of 2 to 10 per 100,000 and a prevalence of 4 in 100,000. Circulating antiacetylcholine receptor antibodies are responsible.

Acquired MG is classified as either ocular or generalized. Ocular myasthenia is characterized by ptosis and extraocular muscle weakness. Generalized myasthenia can affect ocular, bulbar, and limb muscles. Generalized myasthenia develops in the majority of patients with ocular myasthenia.

Diagnosis is made on clinical grounds and confirmed by the following tests:

1. Edrophonium (Tensilon) is an ultrashort-acting cholinesterase inhibitor. A complete test consists of IV administration of edrophonium 10 mg. Initially 2 mg is injected to check for side effects such as bradycardia, hypotension, or other arrhythmias. If tolerated, the remaining 8 mg is given in 2- to 3-mg increments. Atropine sulfate 1 mg should be immediately available as an antidote for any side effects. To maximize sensitivity and specificity, an objectively weak muscle should be selected for testing. Ptosis and major ocular muscle limitation are easily evaluated, but diplopia is subjective and not easily evaluated; limb weakness changes are harder to evaluate. False-positive results can occur. Another bedside test is the ice-pack test. Cooling the eyelids can result in an improvement of ptosis.
2. Confirmation of the diagnosis is made with elicitation of a decremental response to slow repetitive stimulation on the EMG and with serum antiacetylcholine receptor antibody titers.

Pretreatment evaluation should include the following:

1. Chest x-ray or CT scan of the chest to rule out thymoma.
2. Complete blood cell count; Erythrocyte sedimentation rate, Antinuclear antibodies, and anti-DNA values; evaluations of thyroid function; antistriatal muscle antibody titers; and PPD (especially if use of corticosteroids is being considered).
3. Pulmonary function testing, if indicated, to evaluate extent of involvement of respiratory muscles. Patients may have little generalized weakness, but respiratory compromise may develop.

Treatment varies with treatment centers. The mainstays of therapy are the following:

1. Anticholinesterases.
2. Corticosteroid or cytotoxic immunosuppressive drugs.
3. Thymectomy.
4. Plasma exchange.

Anticholinesterase agents are used for diagnostic purposes (the edrophonium test) and in conjunction with other therapies. Pyridostigmine (Mestinon) therapy is started at 30 to 60 mg q 3 to 4 hours. Dosage ranges from 60 to 240 mg PO q 3 to 6 hours. Available forms of pyridostigmine include 60-mg tablets, syrup 12 mg/ml, parenteral 5 mg/ml, IM or SC (dosage is 1 to 5 mg q 30 to 120 minutes). Also available is a 180-mg sustained release preparation that is recommended for bedtime use only. Side effects are due to the muscarinic binding and include excess salivation, abdominal cramping, and secretory diarrhea. Diarrhea can be controlled with anticholinergics. Cholinergic crises resulting from medication excess should be suspected in patients with respiratory failure. Symptoms include miosis, sialorrhea, diarrhea, bronchorrhea, cramps, and fasciculations. Treatment consists of withdrawal of anticholinesterases.

Controversy exists over indications for thymectomy. Thymectomy is mandatory if thymoma is present; and in most other cases is usually indicated. In some studies thymectomy has been shown to induce remission when performed early. The patient's status should be optimized by plasma exchange before thymectomy.

Some authorities recommend that corticosteroid therapy be reserved for use only after thymectomy fails. It is not recommended for ocular myasthenia except in extreme circumstances (see later discussion). The patient should be hospitalized when high-dose steroid therapy is initiated because such therapy may precipitate weakness. Some authorities recommend a course of plasmapheresis during initiation of corticosteroid therapy. Start therapy at a dosage of 1 to 1.5 mg/kg per day. This dosage should be maintained until remission is induced; then qod dosing should be used. Anticholinesterase use should be tapered first to verify remission. Corticosteroid use is then tapered over 6 to 12 months. If the patient has a relapse, tapering is stopped and the dose-response optimized.

Azathioprine has been used in conjunction with corticosteroids for its steroid-sparing effect, and it has been used alone. There may be a 6-month lag before azathioprine becomes effective.

Environmental conditions and medications exacerbating myasthenia should be avoided unless necessary, including muscle relaxants such as quinine and curare; antiarrhythmic drugs such as quinidine, procainamide, and propranolol; certain antibiotics; trimethadione; penicillamine; and excessive body heat.

Ocular MG might best be treated by merely patching an eye if the patient has double vision (provided the other eye has good motility), but it is reasonable to try a small dose of pyridostigmine. If the therapeutic effect remains suboptimal, further increases are not indicated when the weakness is limited to the eyes. Pyridostigmine often relieves a unilateral ptosis, only to unmask diplopia. In addition, it might make a large-angle diplopia into a more disconcerting small degree of diplopia. If diplopia is the problem and a low dose is ineffectual, the patient should wear a patch. If bilateral ptosis is the problem, ptosis crutches attached to spectacles by an optician may prove quite helpful. Corticosteroids are extremely beneficial in treating ocular myasthenia, but because of risk versus benefit considerations, steroids should be reserved for the following situations: severe cosmetic embarrassment, bilateral ophthalmoplegia with frozen eyes, severe bilateral ptosis that renders the patient functionally blind, and strong insistence by the patient despite being warned of the risk of long-term corticosteroid therapy. Thymectomy, immunosuppression, and plasmapheresis should be avoided in patients with pure ocular myasthenia gravis.

REF: Verma P: Treatment of acquired autoimmune myasthenia gravis: a topic review, *Can J Neurol Sci* 19:360–375, 1992.

MYELITIS   *(see Spinal Cord)*

MYELOGRAPHY

An imaging technique that combines conventional x-ray of the spine with injection of radiopaque dyes into the subarachnoid space and is indicated for the evaluation of spinal cord and root compression. Useful for detecting intradural and extradural defects resulting from tumors, as well as herniated disks. Myelography does not provide information about the cord itself, other than its shape and size.

Side effects of mitrizamide myelography include nausea, vomiting, headache, meningitis, seizures, and transient encephalopathy.

Myelography is rapidly being replaced by MRI as the diagnostic imaging procedure of choice for evaluation of the spinal cord, since MRI is noninvasive and allows for visualization of the spinal cord (such as intramedullary tumors and syrinx). Myelography, when combined with CT, can complement MRI in preoperative evaluation of abnormalities of the vertebrae or disks.

MYELOPATHY   *(see Radiation, Spinal Cord)*

MYOCLONUS

Brief arrhythmic or repetitive muscular contractions of cortical, reticular, or spinal origin; they are irregular in amplitude and frequency, asynchronous, and asymmetric in distribution. Clonus refers to monophasic rhythmic contractions and relaxations of a group of muscles (compare with Tremors). Precipitants of myoclonus include sensory stimuli, physical contact, and anxiety, which may modulate the intensity of the myoclonus.

Segmental and focal myoclonus can be rhythmic or arrhythmic, involving somatotopic areas such as head and neck (without palatal myoclonus) or limbs and torso (spinal myoclonus). It is associated with myelopathies resulting from infection, degenerative disease, osteoarthritis, neoplasm (especially colon carcinoma), and demyelination.

Palatal myoclonus: Rhythmic, synchronous contractions of the palate at an average rate of 120 to 130 per minute can be either bilateral or unilateral and may be associated with contractions of extraocular muscles, larynx, neck, diaphragm, trunk, or limb. Palatal myoclonus persists during sleep. There is hypertrophic degeneration of the contralateral inferior olive if the myoclonus is unilateral. The lesion can be anywhere within the Guillain-Mollaret triangle — red nucleus, inferior olivary nucleus, and contralateral dentate nucleus — and the connecting pathways (central tegmental tract and crossing dentatoolivary pathway). The movements disappear after damage to the pathways of corticobulbar or corticospinal motor neurons. Palatal myoclonus is seen in cerebrovascular disease, multiple sclerosis, and encephalitis and occasionally is idiopathic.

CLASSIFICATION

I. Physiologic (in persons with normal health).
  A. Sleep jerks (hypnic jerks).
  B. Anxiety-induced.
  C. Exercise-induced.
  D. Hiccough (singultus).
  E. Benign infantile myoclonus with feeding.
II. Essential myoclonus (no known cause and no other gross neurologic deficit).
  A. Hereditary (autosomal dominant).
  B. Sporadic.
III. Epileptic myoclonus (seizures predominate, and encephalopathy is absent, at least initially).
  A. Fragments of epilepsy.
    1. Isolated epileptic myoclonic jerks.
    2. Epilepsia partialis continua.
    3. Idiopathic stimulus-sensitive myoclonus.
    4. Photosensitive myoclonus.
    5. Myoclonic absences in petit mal.
  B. Childhood myoclonic epilepsies.
    1. Infantile spasms (West syndrome).
    2. Myoclonic astatic epilepsy (Lennox-Gastaut syndrome).
    3. Juvenile myoclonic epilepsy (Janz).
  C. Benign familial myoclonic epilepsy.
  D. Progressive myoclonus epilepsy: Baltic myoclonus (Unverricht-Lundborg).
IV. Symptomatic myoclonus (progressive or static encephalopathy dominates).
  A. Storage diseases.
    1. Lafora body disease.
    2. Lipidoses (such as GM_2 gangliosidosis, Tay-Sachs disease, and Krabbe's disease).
    3. Ceroid lipofuscinosis (Batten disease and Kuf disease).
    4. Sialidosis.
  B. Spinocerebellar degenerations.
    1. Ramsay Hunt syndrome.
    2. Friedreich's ataxia.
    3. Ataxia-telangiectasia.

C. Basal ganglia degenerations.
   1. Wilson's disease.
   2. Torsion dystonia.
   3. Hallervorden-Spatz disease.
   4. Progressive supranuclear palsy.
   5. Huntington's disease.
   6. Parkinson's disease.
D. Dementias.
   1. Creutzfeldt-Jakob disease.
   2. Alzheimer's disease.
E. Viral encephalitides.
   1. Subacute sclerosing panencephalitis.
   2. Encephalitis lethargica.
   3. Arboviral encephalitis.
   4. Herpes simplex encephalitis.
   5. Postinfectious encephalomyelitis.
F. Metabolic.
   1. Hepatic failure.
   2. Renal failure.
   3. Dialysis syndrome.
   4. Hypoglycemia.
   5. Infantile myoclonic encephalopathy (polymyoclonus) (with or without neuroblastoma).
   6. Nonketotic hyperglycemia.
   7. Multiple carboxylase deficiency.
   8. Biotin deficiency.
   9. Mitochondrial encephalomyopathy with ragged red fibers.
G. Toxic encephalopathies.
   1. Bismuth.
   2. Heavy metal poisonings.
   3. Methyl bromide and DDT.
   4. Drugs (levodopa, penicillin, amitriptyline, imipramine, morphine, meperidine, L-tryptophan plus monoamine oxidase inhibitor, lithium, and phenytoin).
H. Physical encephalopathies.
   1. After hypoxia (Lance-Adams syndrome).
   2. Posttraumatic.
   3. Heat stroke.
   4. Electric shock.
   5. Decompression injury.
I. Focal CNS damage.
   1. After stroke.
   2. After thalamotomy.

3. Tumor.
4. Trauma.
5. Palatal myoclonus.

TREATMENT

Treatment of myoclonus depends on the underlying pathology; however, the degree of disability determines whether treatment is warranted. The following drugs have been helpful, especially in segmental or focal myoclonus:

1. Clonazepam: 1 to 1.5 mg/day in divided doses with a gradual increase if necessary.
2. Valproic acid: The drug of choice for many of the myoclonic epilepsies but also used in essential myoclonus, posthypoxic myoclonus, and other secondary myoclonic conditions such as Huntington's disease with myoclonus. Initial dosage is 250 mg per day, increasing up to a usual therapeutic dosage of 1200 to 1400 mg per day.
3. 5-OH tryptophan: 100 mg per day in divided doses, increasing by 200 mg every 2 to 3 days up to a total of 1000 to 4000 mg per day; carbidopa, 75 to 150 mg per day, may be given to prevent extracerebral decarboxylation of 5-OH tryptophan to serotonin. This regimen is reported to help many patients with posthypoxic myoclonus and some with progressive myoclonic epilepsy.
4. Many other medications have been used, mostly anecdotally, including alcohol, estrogens, botulinum toxin (palatal myoclonus), tetrabenazine, trihexyphenidyl, and benztropine.

REF: Fahn S, Marsden CD, Van Woert MH. In Fahn S, Marsden CD, Van Woert MH, eds: *Advances in neurology, vol 43, Myoclonus*, New York, 1986, Raven.

MYOGLOBINURIA

Myoglobin in the urine is due to rhabdomyolysis that occurs within several hours of acute muscle necrosis.

CLASSIFICATION

I. Hereditary myoglobinuria.
   A. Enzyme deficiency known.
      1. Phosphorylase deficiency (McArdle's disease).

    2. Phosphofructokinase deficiency (Tarui disease).
    3. Carnitine palmityltransferase deficiency (DiMauro).
  B. Incompletely characterized syndromes.
    1. Excess lactate production (Larsson syndrome).
  C. Uncharacterized.
    1. Familial, no clear biochemical abnormality.
    2. Familial susceptibility to succinylcholine or general anesthesia ("malignant hyperthermia").
    3. Repeated attacks in an individual; no known biochemical abnormality.
II. Sporadic myoglobinuria.
  A. Exertional myoglobinuria in untrained individuals.
    1. Squat-jump and related syndromes, including "march myoglobinuria."
    2. Anterior tibial syndrome.
    3. Convulsions, high-voltage electric shock.
  B. Crush syndrome.
    1. Compression by fallen weights.
    2. Compression in prolonged coma.
  C. Ischemic myoglobinuria.
    1. Arterial occlusion.
    2. Ischemic element in compression and anterior tibial syndrome.
  D. Metabolic abnormalities.
    1. Metabolic depression.
      a. Barbiturate, carbon monoxide, narcotic coma.
      b. Diabetic acidosis.
      c. General anesthesia.
      d. Hypothermia.
    2. Exogenous toxins and drugs.
      a. Haff disease.
      b. Heroin, cocaine.
      c. Alcoholism.
      d. Toluene.
      e. Malayan sea-snake bite poison.
      f. Malignant neuroleptic syndrome.
      g. Plasmocid.
      h. Fluphenazine.
      i. Succinylcholine, halothane.
      j. Glycyrrhizate, carbenoxolone, amphotericin B.
    3. Other disorders.
      a. Chronic hypokalemia.

   b. Heat stroke.
   c. Toxic shock syndrome.
E. Myoglobinuria with progressive muscle disease.
F. Myoglobinuria resulting from unknown cause.

Diagnosis depends on further characterization of pigmenturia (myoglobin, hemoglobin, porphyrins) by spectrophotometry, electrophoresis, or immunoprecipitation. Myalgia or fever and malaise, or both, may be present. Serum muscle enzyme levels are elevated.

Complications include acute tubular necrosis with oliguria and azotemia, hyperkalemia, hypercalcemia, hyperuricemia, and uncommonly, respiratory failure.

Myoglobinuria is life threatening only if there is renal injury, which should be treated with mannitol or alkalinizing agents or both.

REF: Rowland LP: *Can J Neurol Sci* 11:1–13, 1984.

MYOKYMIA   *(see Brachial Plexus, Electromyography, Ocular Oscillations)*

MYOPATHY
CLASSIFICATION

   I. Inflammatory.
   II. Endocrine.
   III. Metabolic.
   IV. Toxic.
   V. Congenital.
   VI. Muscular dystrophies (see Muscular Dystrophy).
   VII. Myotonic disorders (see Myotonia)
   VIII. Periodic paralysis (see Periodic Paralysis)

   I. *Inflammatory myopathies* (see Table 45).

Polymyositis (PM) and *dermatomyositis* (DM) are inflammatory, usually sporadic, myopathies. Age distribution is bimodal, with peaks at 5 to 15 years of age and 50 to 60 years. Clinical presentation includes symmetric, painless, proximal greater than distal limb weakness that progresses over weeks to months. Dysphagia or respiratory muscle weakness can occur, more commonly with DM. There may be spontaneous exacerbations and remissions. On examination muscle wasting is absent until late in the course, and reflexes are normal. The typical "heliotrope" rash of DM consists of a lavender discoloration of the eyelids and malar areas. A scaly red rash appears over the metacarpophalangeal and proximal interphalangeal joints (Gottron's sign). In group IV there

TABLE 45
Classification of Polymyositis/Dermatomyositis

Group I	Primary, idiopathic polymyositis (PM)
Group II	Primary, idiopathic dermatomyositis (DM)
Group III	DM or PM associated with carcinoma
Group IV	Childhood DM or PM associated with a vasculitis
Group V	DM or PM with another associated collagen vascular disease (overlap syndrome)

Adapted from Bohan A, Peter JB: N Engl J Med 292:344, 1975.

is a generalized necrotizing vasculitis that may produce multiple infarctions of the GI tract, lungs, skin, nerves, and brain. In group V
the associated collagen vascular disorders include scleroderma, systemic
lupus erythematosus, rheumatoid arthritis, polyarteritis nodosa, and
Sjögren's syndrome. The level of creatine kinase (CK) is usually elevated. Electrocardiography (ECG) results may be abnormal, usually
with a conduction block. Electromyography results show increased
insertional activity, fibrillations, and short, low-amplitude
polyphasic motor unit potentials. Muscle biopsy specimens demonstrate interstitial and perivascular inflammation, muscular fiber atrophy, necrosis, regeneration, and characteristic "ghost fibers." Occult
malignancy should be excluded in older patients with PM or DM.
Treatment begins with the administration of prednisone, 60 to 100 mg
per day until weakness resolves (1 to 4 months), followed by a slow
taper. Fifty percent of patients respond to corticosteroid therapy. Cyclosporine, azathioprine, methotrexate, IV immunoglobulin, and plasmapheresis have benefited some patients.

   Inclusion body myositis consists of slowly progressive, painless, distal
greater than proximal muscle weakness and wasting. Onset is after the
age of 50 years. Men are affected twice as often as women. The level
of CK is normal or mildly elevated; EMG findings resemble those in
PM and DM. In addition to the inflammatory changes seen in PM
and DM, muscle biopsy specimens show characteristic basophilic
rimmed vacuoles and nuclear and cytoplasmic eosinophilic inclusions.
No treatment is available. This condition may mimic spinal muscular
atrophy on clinical examination.

   Sarcoid myopathy is characterized by noncaseating granulomata in
muscle as well as other organs. Only 50% of sarcoid patients have
muscle involvement on biopsy, and most of those are asymptomatic.

Chronic, proximal myopathy is the most common clinical muscle presentation. Women are affected four times as often as men. Corticosteroid therapy is the treatment of choice.

Polymyalgia rheumatica is characterized by muscle pain and stiffness that worsen with rest and abate with continued exercise. There is no muscle weakness. Onset is after the age of 55 years, and twice as many women as men are affected. Shoulder muscles are most commonly involved. Temporal arteritis may develop in 55% to 75% of patients. Erythrocyte sedimentation rate (ESR) is elevated, and anemia is often present. The level of CK, EMG results, and muscle biopsy specimens are usually normal. Treat with prednisone 30 to 50 mg per day for 2 months, then taper. Clinical response and ESR must be followed up during the taper.

REF: Dalakos MC: *N Engl J Med* 325:1487, 1991.

Walton J: *J Neurol Neurosurg Psych* 54:285, 1991.

II. *Endocrine myopathies.*

Fifty percent to 80% of patients with *Cushing's disease* and 2% to 21% of patients with chronic corticosteroid use have weakness. The distribution is proximal greater than distal, and legs are more involved than arms. Biopsy specimens show type 2 atrophy. To treat, decrease the steroid dose, change to alternate-day dosing, or change to a non-fluorinated steroid.

Adrenal insufficiency (Addison's disease). Twenty-five percent to 50% of patients have general weakness, muscle cramps, and fatigue that resolve with corticosteroid replacement. The results of EMG are usually normal, and the biopsy specimen is unremarkable. Hyperkalemic periodic paralysis (see Periodic Paralysis) can develop in patients with adrenal insufficiency.

Thyrotoxic myopathy develops in approximately 60% of thyrotoxic patients. There are weakness and wasting proximally or myalgias, or both; bulbar muscles are usually spared. Serum muscle enzyme levels are normal to low. Treat by restoring the euthyroid state. Thyrotoxic periodic paralysis resembles familial hypokalemic periodic paralysis (see Periodic Paralysis, Thyroid).

Hypothyroidism causes proximal weakness, fatigue, exertional pain, myalgias and stiffness, cramps, and occasionally, myoedema and muscle enlargement. Deep tendon reflex relaxation time is prolonged. Women are affected 10 times as often as men. The level of CK may be elevated. Treat by restoring the euthyroid state (see Thyroid).

Acromegaly (increased growth hormone): Fifty percent have paroxysmal muscle weakness, decreased exercise tolerance, and slight enlargement of muscles.

Hypopituitarism in adults causes severe weakness and fatigability with disproportionate preservation of muscle mass.

Hyperparathyroidism: Of these patients 25% have fatigue, proximal muscle weakness and atrophy, myalgias, and stiffness. Bulbar muscles are spared. Deep tendon reflexes are brisk. Levels of CK and aldolase are normal. Alkaline phosphatase and calcium levels are elevated, and the phosphorus level is low.

Hypoparathyroidism is usually not associated with significant weakness, but muscle cramping and tetany are common. Tapping the facial nerve causes muscular contraction (Chvostek's sign), and occluding venous return of the arm causes carpopedal spasm (Trousseau's sign).

Osteomalacia: In 50% of patients proximal muscle weakness, wasting, myalgias, and characteristic bony changes develop.

REF: Ruff R, Weissman J: *Neurol Clin* 6(3):575–592, 1988.

III. *Metabolic myopathy.*

Metabolic myopathy refers to muscle disease caused by abnormalities of glycogen or lipid metabolism or a defect of the respiratory chain. Intramuscular glycogen provides energy for short-term, strenuous exercise, whereas fatty acids provide energy for endurance exercise. Thus glycogenoses usually become evident as weakness or cramps, or both, on heavy or intense short-term exercise, whereas lipidoses become evident as poor endurance (Figures 26 and 27).

A. *Glycogenoses.*

Glycogenoses are most often autosomal recessive. Muscle biopsy specimen shows abnormal accumulation of glycogen. The specific enzyme abnormality is diagnosed by biochemical analysis of the affected tissue (muscle, leukocytes, skin, and the like). Glycogenoses in general show blunted or no rise in venous lactate levels with ischemic forearm exercise testing. Acid maltase deficiency is the exception.

Myophosphorylase deficiency (McArdle's disease) and *phosphofructokinase deficiency (PFK)* cause early exercise intolerance. Strenuous exercise results in muscle pain, contractures, and myoglobinuria.

Phosphoglycerate kinase deficiency resembles McArdle's disease and PFK deficiency on clinical study but is distinguished by lack of increased glycogen on biopsy and x-linked transmission.

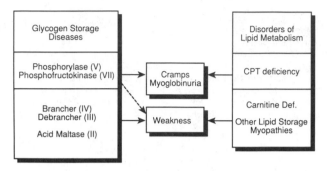

FIGURE 26
The two clinical syndromes associated with disorders of muscle glycogen and lipid metabolism. *Dotted line* represents less common clinical variant of phosphorylase and phosphofructokinase deficiencies. (Courtesy of the Continuing Professional Education Center, Princeton, NJ.)

Lactate dehydrogenase (LDH) deficiency and *phosphoglycerate mutase deficiency*, both autosomal recessive, also resemble McArdle's disease and PFK deficiency on clinical study. In distinction, both give a rise (although blunted) of lactate level with forearm exercise testing, during which LDH deficiency also has a rise in pyruvate level.

Acid maltase deficiency (Pompe's disease) results in generalized deposition of glycogen in all tissues. Quadriparesis in these patients is due to muscle, peripheral nerve, and CNS involvement. In the infantile type death occurs by 1 year of age. In the adult type there is proximal limb-girdle weakness with prominent respiratory involvement. Results of EMG may show electrical myotonia. Life expectancy is normal or slightly decreased. Inheritance is autosomal recessive.

Debranching enzyme deficiency (Forbes-Cori disease), also autosomal recessive, is characterized by abnormal glycogen accumulation in the heart, liver, spleen, and muscle. There is muscle wasting and weakness. Onset may be in infancy or adulthood.

Brancher enzyme deficiency is probably autosomal recessive. Amylopectin accumulates in the liver, spleen, and nervous system. The deficiency is associated with cirrhosis, hypotonia, areflexia, and muscle wasting and is fatal by age 5 years.

B. *Lipid metabolism myopathies.*

Primary carnitine deficiency occurs in two forms, myopathic and systemic. Both begin with progressive weakness during childhood or

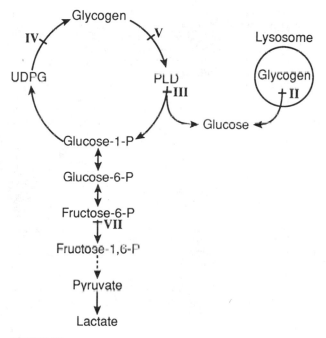

FIGURE 27
Scheme of glycogen metabolism and glycolysis, indicating the metabolic blocks in the five glycogenoses affecting muscle: *II,* acid maltase deficiency; *III,* debrancher deficiency; *IV,* brancher deficiency; *V,* phosphorylase deficiency; *VII,* phosphofructokinase deficiency. *PLD,* phosphorylase-limit dextrin; *UDPG,* uridine-diphosphate-glucose. (Courtesy of the Continuing Professional Education Center, Princeton, NJ.)

later. In the systemic form, in addition to weakness, there are recurrent episodes of hepatic encephalopathy. Muscle biopsy specimens and studies of histochemistry in both forms show abnormal lipid accumulation; biochemical analysis of muscle shows decreased carnitine content. Serum concentration of carnitine is normal in the myopathic form and decreased in the systemic form. Results of EMG show myopathic features. Prognosis in the systemic form is poor. death occurs in the late teens or early twenties. Most of the cases are sporadic, but there is evidence of autosomal recessive inheritance in some cases. Treatment with high-dose oral carnitine or prednisone may be effective. Secondary carnitine deficiency may occur in cirrhosis, renal dialysis, dystrophies, organic acidemia, mitochondrial myopathies, chronic illness, and parenteral nutrition.

Carnitine palmityltransferase (CPT) deficiency. Symptoms begin in childhood with weakness, myoglobinuria, and painful cramps (contractures) in response to prolonged exercise or fasting, or both. Strength between episodes is normal. Creatine kinase level rises during attacks. Forearm ischemic exercise testing shows normal rise in lactate level. Biochemical analysis of muscle and leukocytes shows markedly decreased CPT activity. Glycogen metabolism is normal; therefore the ability to perform intense exercise of short duration is not impaired. The deficiency is more common in males. Treatment with high-carbohydrate, low-fat diet may reduce the frequency of attacks.

Acyl coenzyme A (acyl-CoA) dehydrogenase deficiencies are lipid myopathies with variable proximal muscle weakness, metabolic acidoses, and episodic hypoglycemia with minimal ketonuria. Biopsy specimen shows lipid myopathy. One variety becomes evident in early childhood with the preceding symptoms, as well as cardiomegaly, hepatomegaly, and hypotonia.

Multisystem triglyceride storage disorder consists of congenital ichthyosis, hepatosplenomegaly, vacuolized granulocytes, and lipid myopathy. There may be nystagmus, retinal dysfunction, cataracts, corneal opacities, and sensorineural hearing loss.

REF: Carroll JE: *Neurol Clin* 6(3):563–574, 1988.

Servidei S, DiMauro S: *Neurol Clin* 7(1):159–178, 1989.

C. Mitochondrial disorders.
Abnormal mitochondrial function results in disorders of the CNS or muscle, or both. Defects of oxidative metabolism may involve pyruvate metabolism, Krebs cycle, or the respiratory chain. These defects typically result in lactic acidosis in blood and CSF. When the defect involves mitochondrial DNA, the muscle biopsy specimen usually contains abnormal mitochondria that are seen as ragged red fibers on trichrome stains.

Mitochrondrial myopathies result in weakness and exercise intolerance. In severe forms patients have profuse sweating and heat intolerance at rest without hyperthyroidism. The mitochondrial encephalomyopathies are primarily CNS disorders. They include the three clinical syndromes described in the next paragraph, whose common features include short stature, weakness, spongy degeneration of brain, dementia, and sensincural hearing loss (see Table 46).

Kearns-Sayre syndrome (KSS) becomes evident before 20 years of age with ophthalmoplegia, retinal degeneration, heart block, and weakness. The defect is a mitochondrial DNA deletion. Mitochondrial encephalopathy with lactic acidosis and strokelike episodes (MELAS) becomes evident in the first decade of life with episodic vomiting, recurrent hemiparesis or hemianopsia, and seizures. The defect is in complex I of the respiratory chain and is maternally inherited. Myoclonic epilepsy with ragged red fibers (MERRF) becomes evident before 20 years of age with myoclonus, seizures, and ataxia. These patients have a maternally inherited defect in complex IV of the respiratory chain.

Treatment consists of avoiding conditions that increase the body's energy demands (fasting, infection, overexertion, and extreme temperatures) as well as medications that inhibit respiratory chain function (phenytoin and barbiturates) and medications inhibiting mitochondrial protein synthesis (tetracycline and chloramphenicol). The administration of coenzyme Q may benefit some patients with KSS.

D. Adenylate deaminase deficiency affects 1% to 2% of the population. It is probably not a true myopathy but becomes evident with cramps.

REF: DeVivo DC, DiMauro S: *Int Pediatr* 5:112–120, 1990.

Tritschler HJ, Medori R: *Neurology* 43:280–288, 1993.

TABLE 46
Mitochondrial Syndromes

KSS	MELAS	MERRF
Ophthalmoplegia	Vomiting	Myoclonic epilepsy
Retinal degeneration	Strokelike episodes	Ataxia
Heart block	Seizures	Central hypoventilation
—	—	
CSF protein increase	Positive family history	Positive family history
Ataxia		

KSS, Kearns-Sayre syndrome; *MELAS,* mitochondrial encephalopathy with lactic acidosis and strokelike episodes; *MERRF,* myoclonic epilepsy with ragged red fibers.

IV. *Toxic myopathies.*

Alcohol myopathy takes two forms. There may be an acute attack of muscle pain, tenderness, swelling, weakness, and myoglobinuria after "binge" drinking. Thigh muscles are most commonly involved. The second form consists of a chronic, slowly progressive, proximal muscle weakness. The level of CK is slightly elevated. Results of biopsy are nonspecific.

Table 47 lists recognized toxins that cause a myopathy classified according to presence or absence of neuropathy or cardiomyopathy.

REF: Harris JB, Blain PG. In *Baillière's clinical endocrinology and metabolism*, 4:665-686, 1990.

Kuncl RW, Wiggins WW: *Neurol Clin* 6:593-621, 1988.

Urbano-Marquez A et al: *N Engl J Med* 320:409-415, 1989.

V. *Congenital myopathies.*

Symptoms are usually present from birth and include a "floppy infant" with hypotonia, decreased deep tendon reflexes, decreased spontaneous movement, muscular weakness, and often an abnormal consistency of muscle on palpation. Associated anomalies are variable and include scoliosis, high-arched palate, elongated facies, ophthalmoplegia, and pectus excavatum. Symptoms are nonprogressive or slowly progressive. The level of CK is often normal. Results of EMG show small-amplitude, polyphasic motor units. It is usually not possible to

TABLE 47
Recognized Toxins That Cause Myopathy

Myopathy With Neuropathy	Myopathy With Cardiomyopathy
Amiodarone (Cordarone)	Chloroquine (Aralen)
Chloroquine (Aralen)	Clofibrate (Atromid)
Clofibrate (Atromid)	Colchicine
Colchicine	Doxorubicin (Adriamycin)
Doxorubicin (Adriamycin)	Emetine, ipecac
Ethanol	Ethanol
Hydroxychloroquine (Plaquenil)	Hydroxychloroquine (Plaquenil)
Organophosphates	Metronidazole (Flagyl)
Vincristine (Oncovin)	

discern the specific types of myopathy on clinical basis alone; biopsy of a muscle specimen is necessary for classification.

Central core disease becomes evident as hypotonia, proximal weakness, delayed motor milestones; bulbar musculature is relatively spared. Biopsy specimens show a well-circumscribed circular region in the center of muscle fibers and a predominance of type I fibers.

Nemaline myopathy is usually associated with dysmorphic features and bulbar involvement (poor suck-and-swallow reflexes with a weak cry). The severe congenital type can result in respiratory failure and death. Biopsy specimens show a predominance of type I fibers and dark-staining rods originating from Z lines.

There are many other, less common congenital myopathies with specific abnormalities on biopsy, including myotubular myopathy, congenital fiber-type disproportion, multicore disease, fingerprint body myopathy, and sarcotubular myopathy.

REF: Banker BQ. In Engel AG, Banker BQ, eds: *Myology*, New York, 1986, McGraw Hill.

       Bodensteiner J: *Neurol Clin* 6:499–518, 1988.

MYOSITIS   *(see Myopathy)*

MYOTOMES   *(Table 48)*

MYOTONIA

Myotonia refers to a delay in muscle relaxation demonstrated after voluntary action (such as hand grip or forced eye closure) or percussion of the thenar or wrist extensor muscles *(percussion myotonia)*. Results of EMG show repetitive discharges with waxing and waning amplitude and frequency, giving a characteristic "dive bomber" sound. The myotonias result from several different abnormalities of muscle membrane and are treated with membrane-stabilizing drugs such as quinine, procainamide, phenytoin, or tocainamide. If potassium sensitivity is demonstrated, acetazolamide may be used. These medications treat myotonia with variable success but are often unable to improve associated weakness.

Myotonic dystrophy is the most common adult-onset muscular dystrophy (1 in 7500 persons). It becomes evident as weakness in excess of myotonia, particularly involving the face and distal limbs. Atrophy of the temporalis and masseter muscles causes the jaw to hang open, producing a characteristic "hatchet-head" and "fish-mouth" appear-

TABLE 48
Myotomes

Muscle	Nerve	Root
Levator scapulae	C3,4 and dorsal scapular	C3,4,5
Rhomboids (major and minor)	Dorsal scapular	C4,5
Supraspinatus	Suprascapular	C5,6
Infraspinatus	Suprascapular	C5,6
Deltoid	Axillary	C5,6
Biceps brachii	Musculocutaneous	C5,6
Brachioradialis	Radial	C5,6
Supinator	Radial	C5,6
Flexor carpi radialis	Median	C6,7
Pronator teres	Median	C6,7
Serratus anterior	Long thoracic	C5,6,7
Latissimus dorsi	Thoracodorsal	C6,7,8
Pectoralis major		
Clavicular head	Lateral pectoral	C5,6,7
Sternal head	Medial pectoral	C6,7,8, T1
Triceps brachii	Radial	C6,7,8
Extensor carpi radialis longus	Radial	C6,7
Anconeus	Radial	C7,8
Extensor digitorum	Radial	C7,8
Extensor carpi ulnaris	Radial	C7,8
Extensor indicis proprius	Radial	C7,8
Palmaris longus	Median	C7,8, T1
Flexor pollicis longus	Median	C7,8, T1
Flexor carpi ulnaris	Ulnar	C7,8, T1
Flexor digitorum sublimis	Median	C7,8
Flexor digitorum profundus	Median Ulnar	C7,8, T1
Pronator quadratus	Median	C8, T1
Abductor pollicis brevis	Median	C8, T1
Opponens pollicis	Median	C8, T1
Flexor pollicis brevis	Median	C8, T1
Lumbricals I and II	Median	C8, T1
First dorsal interosseous	Ulnar	C8, T1
Abductor digiti minimi	Ulnar	C8, T1

TABLE 48—cont'd
Myotomes

Muscle	Nerve	Root
Iliopsoas	Femoral	L2,3,4
Adductor longus	Obturator	L2,3,4
Gracilis	Obturator	L2,3,4
Quadriceps femoris	Femoral	L2,3,4
Anterior tibial	Deep peroneal	L4,5
Extensor hallucis longus	Deep peroneal	L4,5
Extensor digitorum longus	Deep peroneal	L4,5
Extensor digitorum brevis	Deep peroneal	L4,5, S1
Peroneus longus	Superficial peroneal	L5, S1
Internal hamstrings	Sciatic	L4,5, S1
External hamstrings	Sciatic	L5, S1
Gluteus medius	Superior gluteal	L4,5, S1
Gluteus maximus	Inferior gluteal	L5, S1,2
Posterior tibial	Tibial	L5, S1
Flexor digitorum longus	Tibial	L5, S1
Abductor hallucis brevis	Tibial (medial plantar)	L5, S1,2
Abductor digiti quinti pedis	Tibial (lateral plantar)	S1,2
Gastrocnemius lateral	Tibial	L5, S1,2
Gastrocnemius medial	Tibial	S1,2
Soleus	Tibial	S1,2

Italics in root column denote major root supply.

ance. Frontal balding, ptosis, and neck muscle atrophy add to this appearance. Other neurologic features include hypersomnia, dysarthria, dysphagia with nasal regurgitation, and cognitive dysfunction. Systemic features include cardiac conduction defects, impaired gastric motility, testicular atrophy, glucose intolerance resulting from decreased insulin sensitivity, early subcapsular cataracts, and increased risk associated with general anesthesia. The course is slowly progressive; death typically occurs in the sixth decade of life as a result of cardiac or respiratory complications. Muscle enzyme levels are often elevated. Muscle biopsy specimens show internal nuclei, type-I fiber atrophy, and ring fibers. "Anticipation," or earlier onset of more severe disease in successive generations, has been linked to an increasing number of repetitions of an unstable DNA sequence on chromosome 19 found in offspring of patients. Linkage analysis has been used for genetic counseling.

A congenital form of myotonic dystrophy associated with maternal inheritance becomes evident as generalized hypotonia and bulbar and respiratory weakness. Affected children have "shark mouth" and club feet, and 70% have mental retardation. Treatment is symptomatic for adult and congenital forms of disease.

Patients with myotonia congenita (Thomsen's disease is the autosomal dominant form; Becker's disease is the autosomal recessive form) typically complain of diffuse muscle stiffness (that is, myotonia) after resting, which relaxes with exercise. In paramyotonia congenita (Eulenberg's disease) the stiffness, often induced by cold, worsens with exercise (paradoxic myotonia). Muscles of the face and distal upper extremities are most often involved. Table 49 delineates the clinical features of the myotonias.

REF: Ptacek LJ, Johnson KJ, Griggs RC: *N Engl J Med* 323(7):482-489, 1993.

MYOTONIC DYSTROPHY   *(see Myotonia)*

MYXEDEMA   *(see Thyroid)*

NARCOLEPSY   *(see Sleep Disorders)*

NEGLECT

Neglect is the failure to report, respond to, or orient to novel and meaningful stimuli presented to the side opposite a brain lesion when this failure cannot be attributed to either simply sensory or motor dysfunction. Components of neglect include inattention or sensory neglect, motor neglect, spatial neglect, personal neglect, allesthesia and allokinesia, and anosognosia. Bedside tests for neglect include visual confrontation, double simultaneous stimulation, letter or figure cancellation, figure drawing, and line bisection. Lesions associated with neglect correlate with the type of neglect syndrome. Attentional system defects with sensory neglect are associated with right parietal lobe lesions. Motor neglect with varying degrees of akinesia and motor impersistence can be seen in frontal lesions. Defects in the representational system are often associated with right hemisphere lesions because the right hemisphere is important as an attentional system for left and right hemispace, whereas the left hemisphere is primarily important only for attention to right hemispace. Another explanation posits a

TABLE 49
Characteristics of the Myotonias

| | Myotonic Dystrophy | Myotonia Congenita | | Paramyotonia Congenita | Hyperkalemic Periodic Paralysis |
		Thomsen's Disease	Becker's Disease		
Inheritance	Autosomal dominant	Autosomal dominant	Autosomal recessive	Autosomal dominant	Autosomal dominant
Defect	Protein kinase	Chloride channel	Chloride channel	Sodium channel	Sodium channel
Gene locus	19q	7q	7q	17q	17q
Age of onset	Teens to twenties	Infancy to childhood	Childhood	Infancy	Childhood
Course	Slowly progressive	Nonprogressive	Rarely progressive	Variable weakness	Variable weakness
Presenting complaint	Distal weakness	Diffuse stiffness	Diffuse stiffness, weakness	Cold-induced stiffness	Episodic weakness
Other features	Systemic features; Typical facies	Absence of type II fibers	± Muscle hypertrophy; Absence of type II fibers	Paradoxic myotonia	May have cardiac arrhythmia

bihemispheric network of attentional systems, which is overrepresented in the right hemisphere.

REF: Heilman KH, Watson RT, Valenstein E. In Heilman KH, Valenstein E, eds: *Clinical neuropsychology*, ed 3, New York, 1993, Oxford University.

NERVE CONDUCTION STUDIES   *(see Electromyography)*

NEURALGIA   *(see also Zoster)*

Trigeminal neuralgia (tic douloureux) is characterized by paroxysmal, severe, lancinating, brief (<30 to 60 seconds), unilateral facial pain in the distribution of one or more branches of the trigeminal nerve (most commonly the second and third divisions). Paroxysms tend to occur in clusters. Trigger points set off by touching, chewing, talking, or swallowing are characteristic. Onset is after 40 years of age in 90% of patients, and the condition is more common in women (3:2). Results of neurologic examination, including trigeminal sensory and motor examination, are normal. The cause may be a redundant artery, multiple sclerosis, or idiopathic.

Secondary or symptomatic trigeminal neuralgia should be suspected with onset before age 40 years, with trigeminal sensory or motor abnormalities on examination, or with any other findings referable to the base of the skull or posterior fossa. Differential diagnosis includes posterior fossa mass lesions such as tumor (meningioma or acoustic neuroma), aneurysm, or arteriovenous malformations. Trigeminal neuroma and foraminal osteoma are other causes. Evaluation should include MRI with gadolinium and possibly arteriography.

Treatment of secondary trigeminal neuralgia is aimed at the underlying cause. Treatment of idiopathic trigeminal neuralgia is described in the following section.

MEDICAL TREATMENT

1. Carbamazepine is the drug of choice and is effective in 80% of patients. Start therapy at 200 mg per day, and increase gradually to 1 to 1.2 g per day in divided doses. Serum levels of 8-12 mg/ dl should be achieved.
2. Imipramine or amitriptyline starting at 25 to 50 mg orally at bedtime and gradually increasing to 150 mg.

3. Phenytoin 300 to 500 mg per day to achieve therapeutic levels (see Epilepsy).
4. Baclofen starting at 5 mg orally three times a day and increasing gradually to 20 mg orally four times a day.
5. Clonazepam starting at 0.5 mg orally twice a day and increasing slowly up to 10 mg per day in two or three divided doses.
6. Divalproex sodium 500 to 2000 mg per day in divided doses.
7. Pimozide starting at 0.5 to 1 mg per day, increasing the dose by 0.5 to 1 mg every several days up to 4 to 12 mg per day bid.
8. Combination approaches have utilized phenytoin with carbamazepine or imipramine. Baclofen has also been used with phenytoin or carbamazepine.
9. When pain has been controlled, medications should be tapered periodically because spontaneous remissions can occur.

SURGICAL TREATMENT

Surgical therapy is reserved for intractable pain unresponsive to drug treatment. Such therapy includes the following:

1. Local neurolysis and nerve block is associated with a risk of painful anesthesia and persistent paresthesias as well as recurrence.
2. Percutaneous radiofrequency coagulation of the trigeminal ganglion can be performed with the patient under local anesthesia. Painful anesthesia and recurrences are less common.
3. Trigeminal rhizotomy.
4. Microsurgical vascular decompression of the trigeminal root entry zone.

Glossopharyngeal neuralgia has much the same origin and pathogenesis as trigeminal neuralgia. Clinical features also are similar, although the pain may be more variable, with longer duration, and may be associated with autonomic dysfunction (salivation, lacrimation, bradycardia, and syncope). Distribution is to the throat, posterior one third of the tongue, tonsillar pillars, eustachian tube, and ear. Trigger points are variable and are most commonly associated with swallowing or touching particular areas in the distribution of the glossopharyngeal nerve and upper sensory fibers of the vagus nerve. Onset is after age 40 years; both sexes are affected equally. The differential diagnosis includes underlying causes such as oropharyngeal carcinoma, paratonsillar abscess, enlarged styloid process, or enlarged tortuous vertebral or posterior inferior cerebellar arteries. Evaluation is as for trigeminal neuralgia and should include a thorough ear, nose, and throat examination. Treatment is aimed at underlying causes of "symptomatic" neuralgias. Otherwise, carbamazepine or phenytoin, or both, may be used, although full response is seen in less than fifty percent of patients. Surgical therapy has included microsurgical decompression of the glossopharyngeal and vagal root entry zones and section of the glossopharyngeal nerve.

REF: Green MW, Selman JE: *Headache* 31:588, 1991.

Terrence CF, Fromm GH. In Olesen J, Tfelt-Hansen P, Welch KMA, eds: *The headaches*, New York, 1993, Raven.

NEUROCUTANEOUS SYNDROMES

Neurocutaneous syndromes, or phakomatoses (from the Greek *phakos*, lens-shaped, mole, or freckle), represent disordered development early in embryogenesis, which produces defects in multiple organ systems roughly according to germ cell layers. The syndromes may be divided into disorders affecting ectodermal derivatives (neural and cutaneous tissue) and those involving mesodermal tissue (vascular elements, widespread) or classified by mode of inheritance.

AUTOSOMAL DOMINANT INHERITANCE

Neurofibromatosis type 1 (NF-1, von Recklinghausen's disease) is a neuroectodermal disorder related to genetic abnormality on chromosome 17. The diagnosis requires at least two of the following:

1. Six or more café au lait spots greater than 5 mm in diameter.
2. Axillary or inguinal freckles.
3. Two neurofibromas of any type or one or more plexiform neurofibromas. (Neurofibromas occur along peripheral nerves and are made from Schwann's cells, fibroblasts, vascular elements, or pigmented cells. They are pedunculated, nodular, or diffuse but not encapsulated. A neurofibroma that extends into the surrounding tissue is a plexiform neurofibroma.)
4. Optic nerve or chiasmatic glioma.
5. Two or more Lisch nodules (pigmented hamartomas of the iris, best seen with slit lamp examination of the iris and more common in older patients).
6. First-degree relative with NF-1 by foregoing criteria.
7. Bony abnormalities such as thinning of cortical long bone or dysplasia of sphenoid.

Other associated features of NF-1 include presence of tumors (pheochromocytoma, Wilms' tumor, and leukemia), pseudoarthroses of radius and tibia, kyphosis, and endocrine dysfunction resulting from hypothalamic and pituitary compression caused by an optic glioma.

Neurofibromatosis type 2 (NF-2) is a genetic abnormality on chromosome 22. The diagnostic criteria include the following:

1. Bilateral eighth-nerve tumors.
2. Unilateral eighth-nerve tumor and a first-degree relative with NF-2.
3. A first-degree relative with NF-2 and two of the following: glioma, schwannoma, presenile posterior cataract, astrocytoma, neurofibroma of another type, plexiform neurofibroma, or retinal hamartoma.

Tuberous sclerosis (Bourneville's disease) has multiple manifestations, including generalized or partial complex seizures after 3 months of age that are occasionally associated with mental retardation or hemiparesis.

Neuroradiologic features are multiple subependymal nodular calcifications, cortical tubers, and ventricular dilation. Development of giant astrocytomas is relatively frequent. Cutaneous manifestations include facial angiofibroma (hamartomas of facial skin that usually appear after the age of five years), depigmented nevi, subungual fibromas, and shagreen patches (hamartomas in the dermis with the appearance of cobblestone pavement, commonly located in the posterior neck and lumbar back region). Other associated conditions include renal angiolipomas and cysts, cardiac rhabdomyomas, pulmonary cysts, and retinal hamartomas.

von Hippel-Lindau disease (VHD). Diagnostic criteria are met by a hemangioblastoma of the CNS (most commonly found in the cerebellum, medulla, spinal cord, or cerebral hemispheres) or retina and one additional characteristic lesion or a direct relative with the disease. Characteristic lesions include hypernephroma, renal cell carcinoma, pheochromocytoma, renal, pancreatic, or epididymal cysts, and islet cell tumors. Secondary polycythemia may occur because of an erythropoietic factor produced by a cerebellar or renal tumor. Retinal hemangioma may be the earliest sign and can appear in the first decade of life. Exudate from the hemangioblastoma may accumulate under the retina, causing detachment and blindness. Therefore individuals at risk for VHD should be examined periodically after 6 years of age to prevent blindness caused by retinal lesions. Treatment involves surgical removal of the hemangioblastoma or radiotherapy (if inoperable).

AUTOSOMAL RECESSIVE INHERITANCE

Xeroderma pigmentosa is a rare disorder resulting from a defect in cellular repair of light-damaged DNA. Accelerated aging in tissue exposed to solar light and degeneration of neurons result. Skin and eye manifestations usually occur within the first months of life. Neurologic findings are not present in all patients but may include microcephaly, ataxia, spasticity, and choreoathetosis. Peripheral nerve involvement results in hyporeflexia occasionally progressing to areflexia. The diagnosis is made by means of family history and laboratory tests showing deficient DNA repair in fibroblasts.

Chédiak-Higashi syndrome is a disorder of lysosomal abnormality resulting in large granulations in leukocytes, neurons, pigment cells, and platelets. Cellular immunity is deficient, and recurrent pyogenic infections include otitis media, bronchitis, pharyngitis, cellulitis, and subcutaneous abscesses. Leukemias are frequent in this syndrome. Neurologic symptoms occur in approximately 50% of patients and include mental retardation, seizures, cerebellar ataxia, increased intracranial pressure, and a chronic polyneuropathy with a "stocking-glove" type of sensory loss, weakness, and atrophy. The diagnosis is made by finding large granulations in leukocytes in peripheral blood or bone marrow or giant lysosomes in the cytoplasm of Schwann's cells.

Ataxia-telangiectasia becomes evident as progressive cerebellar ataxia, oculomotor apraxia, and choreoathetosis beginning in childhood. Telangiectasias of the conjunctiva, ears, and flexor surfaces appear later. Systemic manifestations include decreased IgA and IgE, increased alpha-fetoprotein, recurrent pulmonary infections, and development of reticuloendothelial tumors.

NONHEREDITARY NEUROCUTANEOUS DISEASES

Neurocutaneous melanosis occurs predominantly in white patients and is characterized by large pigmented nevi that are light to dark brown. Melanin-containing cells in the pia may develop into intracranial or intraspinal melanomas. Hydrocephalus may result from obstruction of the arachnoid villi. Patients rarely live beyond 20 years of age.

Sturge-Weber syndrome (meningofacial angiomatosis with cerebral calcifications) is a sporadic congenital malformation of the cephalic venous microvasculature resulting in neurologic, cutaneous, and optic symptoms. On pathologic study there are venous angiomas with tortuous vessels involving the face, leptomeninges, and choroid, in addition to calcification of layers 2 and 3 of the parieto-occipital cortex. Neurologic manifestations include unilateral seizures, cerebral hemiatrophy with hemiparesis, hemisensory deficits, visual-field defects, and mental abnormalities. Cutaneous lesions vary in extent from a small "port-wine nevus" on the upper eyelid to those involving the entire face and other parts of the body. Ocular manifestations include congenital glaucoma.

Other syndromes grouped among the neurocutaneous syndromes include Klippel-Trenaunay-Weber syndrome (limb hypertrophy and hemangiomas), Osler-Weber-Rendu syndrome (hemorrhagic telangiectasias), Wyburn-Mason syndrome (facial angioma, retinal arteriovenous malformations, cerebrovascular anomalies, and seizures), incontinentia pigmenti (bullous lesions of skin, micropolygyria, microcephaly, and mental retardation), hypomelanosis of Ito (skin whorls, mental retardation, seizures, and ocular deficits), Fabry's disease (papular eruption, painful sensory neuropathy, and stroke), and linear nevus syndrome (linear yellow papules, mental retardation, and seizures).

NEUROFIBROMATOSIS (see Neurocutaneous Syndromes)

NEUROLEPTICS

Neuroleptics include several classes of compounds whose primary common feature is blockade of dopamine receptors, although all of them have other effects at other receptors, such as anticholinergic activity. An exception is clozapine, which blocks serotonin receptors and has little dopamine receptor blockade. The primary clinical use of neuroleptics is in the treatment of psychosis and agitation. Neuroleptics are also used for control of hyperkinetic movement disorders (chorea, tics, and dystonia), for suppressing nausea, for control of vertigo, neuralgic pain, and acute and refractory migraines, and for treating the abdominal pain of porphyric crises.

Aliphatic phenothiazines such as chlorpromazine (Thorazine) are strongly sedating. Potent α-adrenergic antagonism results in postural hypotension. Antiemetic and anticholinergic effects are significant. Extrapyramidal and dystonic symptoms occur with medium frequency.

Piperidine phenothiazines such as thioridazine (Mellaril) and mesoridazine (Serentil) have a relative potency similar to that of the aliphatic compounds. Sedative and α-adrenergic antagonism are less than with aliphatic compounds. Antiemetic effects are negligible. This class has a low incidence of extrapyramidal and dystonic side effects.

Piperazine phenothiazines, such as prochlorperazine (Compazine), trifluoperazine (Stelazine), perphenazine (Trilafon), and fluphenazine (Prolixin), have the highest relative potency and the strongest antiemetic effects. They also have the highest incidence of extrapyramidal and dystonic symptoms. Sedation and α-adrenergic antagonism are minimal.

The pharmacologic features of butyrophenones such as haloperidol (Haldol) closely resemble those of the piperazines. They have strong dopaminergic-blocking effects and a high incidence of extrapyramidal and dystonic symptoms. Relatively less orthostatic hypotension and sedation occur than with lower potency neuroleptics.

Pimozide (Orap), a diphenylbutylpiperidine, is similar in effect to haloperidol and is used in the United States primarily for the treatment of Tourette's syndrome.

The thioxanthenes resemble the phenothiazines. Thiothixene (Navane) resembles the piperazines, with greater dystonic and extrapyramidal side effects. Chlorprothixene (Taractan) resembles chlorpromazine, with greater sedative and autonomic effects and fewer extrapyramidal and dystonic effects.

Intermediate-potency neuroleptics include the dihydroindolones such as molindone (Moban), which have moderately frequent extrapyramidal and dystonic side effects. The dibenzoxazepines such as loxapine (Loxitane) also have moderate sedative, anticholinergic, and extrapyramidal effects.

Clozapine (Clozaril) is a newly developed neuroleptic that is unique in that it does not cause significant extrapyramidal effects. It is used primarily in the treatment of patients who do not respond to or cannot tolerate other neuroleptics. It may also be of value in the treatment of agitation in patients with Parkinsonism who have preexisting, significant motor impairment. It may also be of value in the treatment of Huntington's disease. Side effects include orthostatic hypotension, sedation, and lowered seizure threshold. Clozapine also causes agranulocytosis in 1% to 2% of patients; therefore its use must be accompanied by weekly monitoring of the complete blood cell count.

Risperidone (Risperdol) is a promising new agent which has dopaminergic and serotonergic receptor binding, and a low incidence of extrapyramidal effects.

EXTRAPYRAMIDAL SIDE EFFECTS

Dystonia may occur early (1 to 3 weeks) in the course of neuroleptic therapy or after a single parenteral injection. It may consist of generalized torsion dystonia, opisthotonos, torticollis, retrocollis, oculogyric crisis, trismus, or focal appendicular dystonia. Dystonia is more common in younger patients, especially children or adolescents, and in black males. It usually resolves spontaneously within 24 hours of stopping use of the drug but may be terminated within minutes with benztropine (Cogentin) 1 mg IM or IV or diphenhydramine (Benadryl) 50 mg IV; oral therapy may be continued for 24 to 48 hours.

Parkinsonian symptoms of stiffness, "cog-wheeling," tremor, and shuffling gait are dose related and may begin as early as a few days to 4 weeks after starting therapy. The neuroleptic dosage should be decreased, or an anticholinergic agent may be added. Anticholinergic agents in use include benztropine 0.5 to 4.0 mg bid, biperiden (Akineton) 2.0 mg qd to tid, and trihexyphenidyl (Artane) 2 to 5 mg tid. Anticholinergics carry the risk of precipitating anticholinergic delirium, which may mimic psychotic symptoms; therefore prophylactic use should be limited to patients at high risk for extrapyramidal symptoms.

Akathisia is a subjective sensation of motor restlessness with an urge to move around that generally occurs within several weeks of starting neuroleptic therapy. It improves on decreasing the dose of neuroleptic or adding β blockers or benzodiazepines. Neuroleptic dose should not be increased to treat this form of "agitation," which may mimic the initial psychotic symptoms.

Tardive dyskinesia, consisting of oral-lingual-facial-buccal movements or other choreoathetoid or ballistic movements, may occur after prolonged neuroleptic therapy. Its incidence may be decreased by using neuroleptics only when indicated, keeping doses as low as possible and duration of therapy as short as possible, and early detection through careful monitoring. The more advanced the dyskinesia, the less likely is resolution. Primary treatment consists of tapering and withdrawing the neuroleptic. Treatment with reserpine 0.25 mg per day, increasing by 0.25 mg per day to 1 to 5 mg per day in divided doses, with care to avoid orthostatic hypotension, may help. Neuroleptics themselves have no role in the treatment of tardive dyskinesias.

A *withdrawal syndrome*, seen particularly in children and consisting of choreic movements, may occur when long-term administration of neuroleptics is suddenly stopped. The syndrome usually resolves within 6 to 12 weeks but can be avoided by restarting the drug therapy and tapering more slowly.

The *neuroleptic malignant syndrome* is rare but often (20% to 30%) fatal. Hyperthermia, hypertonia of skeletal muscles, fluctuating consciousness, and autonomic instability are characteristic. Laboratory findings include elevated creatine kinase level, leukocytosis, and liver function abnormalities. The differential diagnosis includes heat stroke (neuroleptics may potentiate by decreasing sweating), malignant hyperthermia associated with anesthesia, idiopathic acute lethal catatonia, drug interactions with monoamine oxidase inhibitors, and central anticholinergic syndromes. Treatment begins with discontinuing the neuroleptic and providing cooling blankets, antipyretics, and IV hydration.

Dantrolene sodium 0.8 to 10 mg/kg per day IV has been used. Bromocriptine, 2.5 to 10 mg PO tid, amantadine, and levodopa with carbidopa have also been used effectively.

Neuroleptics lower the seizure threshold and may precipitate seizures. Their use in patients with epilepsy is not contraindicated unless seizure control is a significant problem. Clozapine and loxapine seem to lower the seizure threshold most, and molindone, the least.

REF: Kaplan HI, Sadock BJ, eds: *Synopsis of psychiatry*, ed 6, Baltimore, 1991, Williams & Wilkins.

NEUROMUSCULAR JUNCTION *(see Electromyography, Lambert-Eaton Myasthenic Syndrome, Myasthenia Gravis)*

NEUROPATHY
CLINICAL CLASSIFICATION

I. Polyneuropathies.
  A. Acute, predominantly motor neuropathy with variable sensory involvement.
    1. Acute inflammatory demyelinating polyradiculoneuropathy (Guillain-Barré syndrome).
    2. Polyneuropathy associated with:
      a. Diphtheria.
      b. Porphyria (see Porphyria).
      c. AIDS.
      d. Thallium.
      e. Triorthocresyl phosphate, dapsone.
  B. Acute motor neuropathy.
    1. Diabetic multiple mononeuropathy (asymmetric proximal diabetic neuropathy, diabetic amyotrophy).
  C. Acute asymmetric sensorimotor polyneuropathy (multiple mononeuropathy or mononeuritis multiplex).
    1. Polyarteritis nodosa.
    2. Wegener's granulomatosis.
    3. Diabetes.
    4. AIDS.
    5. Other angiopathies, vasculitides.
  D. Subacute symmetric sensorimotor neuropathy.

1. Toxic.
    a. Heavy metals (arsenic, mercury, thallium).
    b. Drugs.
        (1) Antibiotics (clioquinol, ethambutol, isoniazid, ni-trofurantoin, streptomycin, dideoxycytodine).
        (2) Antineoplastic (vinca alkaloids, cisplatin, chlor-ambucil, methotrexate, daunorubicin).
        (3) Cardiovascular (clofibrate, disopyramide, hydral-azine).
        (4) Other (gold salts, colchicine, phenylbutazone, methaqualone, penicillamine, chloroquine, disul-firam, cyclosporin A).
    c. Industrial chemicals (triorthocresyl phosphate, acry-lamide, methyl bromide, n-hexane, methyl-n-butyl ketone, b-amino-propionitrile).
2. Nutritional deficiency (vitamin B_{12}, niacin [pellagra], thi-amine [beriberi], pyridoxine, vitamin E).
3. Uremia.
4. Chronic alcoholism (nutritional deficiency).
5. Early chronic relapsing demyelinating polyneuropathy.
E. Subacute to chronic, predominantly sensory neuropathy.
    1. Diabetes.
    2. Drugs (chlorambucil, metronidazole, ethambutol, pyri-doxine, phenytoin [rare], propylthiouracil).
    3. Leprosy.
    4. Paraneoplastic.
    5. AIDS.
F. Subacute to chronic, predominantly motor neuropathy.
    1. Diabetes (proximal diabetic motor neuropathy ["amyotro-phy"]).
    2. Lead.
G. Chronic sensory motor neuropathy.
    1. Diabetes (mixed sensory-motor-autonomic neuropathy).
    2. Associated with multiple myeloma.
    3. Other dysproteinemias (macroglobulinemia, cryoglobu-linemia, ataxia-telangiectasia).
    4. POEMS syndrome, that is, polyneuropathy, organome-galy (lymphadenopathy, splenomegaly, or hepatomegaly), endocrinopathy (usually hypogonadism or hypothyroid-ism), monoclonal gammopathy, and skin changes.
    5. Paraneoplastic.
    6. Uremia.
    7. Leprosy.

8. Amyloidosis.
9. Chronic inflammatory demyelinating polyradiculoneuropathy (CIDP).
10. Sarcoidosis.
H. Hereditary motor and sensory neuropathies (HMSN), types I to III.
I. Hereditary sensory and autonomic neuropathies (HSAN), types I to IV.
J. Hereditary neuropathies with known or suspected metabolic defects.
   1. Fabry's disease (α-galactosidase deficiency, X linked).
   2. Metachromatic leukodystrophy (aryl sulfatase A deficiency, autosomal recessive).
   3. Refsum's disease (phytanic oxidase deficiency, autosomal recessive).
   4. Adrenomyeloneuropathy (x linked).
   5. Tangier disease (hypo-α-lipoproteinemia, autosomal recessive).
   6. Krabbe's disease (globoid cell leukodystrophy, galactosyl ceramidase deficiency; autosomal recessive).
K. Other hereditary neuropathies.
   1. Familial amyloid neuropathy.
   2. Hereditary predisposition to pressure palsies.
   3. Giant axonal neuropathy.
   4. Friedreich's ataxia.
II. Mononeuropathies.
   1. Trauma (fractures and dislocations, penetrating injuries, and pressure palsies).
      a. Brachial plexus (fracture of clavicle or humerus, birth trauma, traction injuries).
      b. Axillary nerve (as for brachial plexus; also, IM injections, shoulder subluxation).
      c. Radial nerve (fracture of head of humerus, compression at the radial groove ["Saturday night palsy" and "bridegroom's palsy"]).
      d. Ulnar nerve (fracture of radius or ulna).
      e. Median nerve (carpal tunnel syndrome, anterior interosseous syndrome).
      f. Sciatic nerve (fracture of pelvis (sacro-iliac joint), fracture of acetabulum, IM gluteal injections).
      g. Femoral nerve (fracture of femur, lithotomy position).
      h. Lateral femoral cutaneous nerve (meralgia paresthetica).

    i. Tibial nerve (fracture of tibia or fibula).
    j. Common or superficial peroneal nerve (pressure palsy
       at fibular head resulting from crossed legs or after
       weight loss).
 2. Entrapment (see Carpal Tunnel Syndrome, Ulnar Neu-
    ropathy).
 3. Carcinomatous infiltration.
 4. Vasculitis.
 5. Leprosy.

CLINICAL FEATURES OF SELECTED NEUROPATHIES
Hereditary Motor and Sensory Neuropathies (HMSN), Types I to III

Hereditary neuropathies are common and may occur in subtle forms. Careful family history taking and examination of family members (including foot examination for pes cavus and EMG) are important in diagnosis. The differential diagnosis of HMSN types includes Friedreich's ataxia, hereditary distal spinal muscular atrophy, and chronic inflammatory demyelinating polyneuropathy (CIDP), which has slight asymmetries in involvement of different peripheral nerves, as opposed to the hereditary types, which demonstrate uniform involvement.

HMSN I. Hypertrophic form of Charcot-Marie-Tooth disease (peroneal muscular atrophy, Roussy-Lévy syndrome). Inheritance is autosomal dominant with variable penetrance, rarely autosomal recessive. Onset is usually in the second decade of life but may be later. In many patients findings are subtle and the disease is undiagnosed. Slowly progressive distal weakness and atrophy are present with little sensory loss. The lower extremities are more involved than the upper. Palpably thickened nerves occur in 50% of cases. Total areflexia is common. Foot deformity (pes cavus, calluses, and hammer toes) results from unopposed flexor action of the posterior compartment muscles and may be the only clinical finding. Life span is usually normal, with only rare wheelchair confinement. Nerve conduction velocities are decreased by 40% to 75%. Compound muscle action potentials are dispersed and low in amplitude. Electromyographic study reveals chronic denervation. Abnormalities on EMG may precede and be more extensive than clinical involvement. The CSF is usually normal. On pathologic study there are hypertrophic ("onion bulb") changes and myelinated axon loss resulting from chronic demyelination and remyelination.

HMSN II. Neuronal form of Charcot-Marie-Tooth disease (peroneal muscular atrophy). Inheritance is as in HMSN I, except that onset is slightly later. HMSN II is distinguished from HMSN I by the absence of hypertrophic changes, later age of onset, slower progression, less involvement of upper extremities, and greater involvement of lower extremities (atrophy of ankle flexors). Nerve conduction velocities are normal or slightly slowed, but amplitudes are severely diminished. Electromyographic study reveals spontaneous activity and greater denervation changes. CSF is usually normal. On pathologic study there are no hypertrophic changes, and demyelination is mild; axonal number is decreased in distal myelinated nerves.

HMSN III. Dejerine-Sottas disease (hypertrophic neuropathy of childhood, congenital hypomyelination neuropathy). Inheritance is autosomal recessive. Onset is congenital or in infancy. The congenital form is more severe. Motor milestones are initially delayed and then lost. Walking occurs after 15 months of age and as late as 3 to 4 years of age. Best motor performance occurs late in the first or early in the second decade of life. Patients are confined to a wheelchair by the end of the second decade of life. Severe progressive weakness and atrophy are initially distal but eventually affect proximal muscles. There are severe sensory loss and sensory ataxia. Skeletal deformities (short stature, kyphoscoliosis, and hand and foot deformities) are more severe and frequent than in HMSN I or II. Motor nerve conduction velocities are extremely slow, and sensory nerve action potentials are unrecordable. CSF protein level is elevated. On pathologic study, in addition to hypertrophic changes, myelin sheaths are thin or absent.

X-linked HMSN is similar to HMSN I on clinical study but shows an X-linked pattern of inheritance. Symptoms usually develop in boys from 5 to 15 years of age.

Other, complex, poorly characterized forms of HMSN show pyramidal tract signs, optic atrophy, spinocerebellar degeneration, or deafness as well as neuropathy.

Hereditary Sensory and Autonomic Neuropathies (HSAN) Types I to IV

HSAN I. Dominantly inherited sensory neuropathy (hereditary sensory neuropathy of Denny-Brown). Inheritance is autosomal dominant. Onset is in the second to third decade of life. There is progressive distal lower-extremity dissociated sensory loss; pain and temperature are relatively more involved. There is distal hyporeflexia. Autonomic function is normal, except for impaired distal sweating. Painless ulcerations and foot deformities may be present. Mild distal lower-extremity weakness and atrophy are late findings. Upper-extremity sensory loss is mild. Life expectancy is normal. Nerve conduction studies of the lower extremity reveal decreased sensory amplitudes and normal or mildly decreased sensory conduction velocities; results of motor nerve conduction studies are normal. On pathologic study axonal degeneration causes decreased numbers of small myelinated fibers and unmyelinated fibers. Differential diagnosis includes diabetic neuropathy, hereditary amyloidosis (prominent autonomic dysfunction), and syringomyelia.

HSAN II. Infantile and congenital sensory neuropathy (Morvan's disease). Inheritance is autosomal recessive. HSAN II is similar to HSAN I on clinical study, except that onset is in infancy and involvement of all sensory modalities is equal, severe, and proximal as well as distal. The lips and tongue may be affected. Strength is normal. Painless ulcerations and fractures are common. There is distal areflexia. Sensory nerve action potentials are unrecordable; results of motor nerve conduction studies are normal. On pathologic study the number of all myelinated axons is severely decreased, with moderately decreased numbers of unmyelinated fibers and some segmental demyelination and remyelination.

HSAN III. Familial dysautonomia (Riley-Day syndrome). Inheritance is autosomal recessive, and the neuropathy occurs primarily in Ashkenazi Jews. Onset of symptoms is usually shortly after birth, with episodic cyanosis, vomiting, unexplained fever, poor suck, and an increased susceptibility to infection. Characteristic blotching of the skin is present, and fungiform papillae on the tongue is absent. Autonomic symptoms include decreased lacrimation, hyperhidrosis, fluctuating body temperature, and episodic hypotension (usually postural). There is a dissociated sensory loss with predominant involvement of pain and temperature, causing corneal ulcerations, painless skin lesions, and deformed joints. Areflexia is generalized. Strength, sweating, and sphincter function are normal. Intelligence is usually normal. Prognosis is generally poor, but occasionally individuals survive to middle age. Sensory nerve action potentials are severely diminished; results of motor nerve conduction studies may be mildly abnormal. Peripheral nerves show marked depletion of unmeylinated fibers.

HSAN IV. Congenital sensory neuropathy. Inheritance is autosomal recessive. This rare disorder is characterized by congenital anhidrosis, generalized insensitivity to pain and temperature, mental retardation, and episodic pyrexia.

Diabetic Neuropathy

A clinical or subclinical disorder of the somatic or autonomic peripheral nervous system that occurs in patients with diabetes mellitus without other causes for peripheral neuropathy. Proposed etiologic factors include localized endoneurial hypoxia, chronic hyperglycemia, episodic hypoglycemia, polyol accumulation, myoinositol deficiency, and impaired axonal transport. Microangiopathy and infarction have been proposed as the mechanism for diabetic multiple mononeuropathies. The following diabetic neuropathy syndromes are recognized:

Symmetric Polyneuropathies. *Distal sensory polyneuropathy* is the most common symmetric polyneuropathy. Onset is usually insidious but may occur immediately after an episode of diabetic coma or hypoglycemia. Usually, clinical manifestations reflect involvement of all fiber types. Occasionally, however, a large- or small-fiber pattern is more prominent. The large-fiber pattern becomes evident as paresthesias in the feet and loss of distal reflexes, position sensation, and vibratory sensation. The small-fiber pattern is loss of thermal and pinprick sensation associated with burning pain. Autonomic neuropathy often accompanies the small-fiber pattern. On pathologic study distal axonal loss is present with variable degrees of segmental demyelination. Nerve conduction studies show reduced sensory action potential amplitude and variable slowing of motor nerve conduction velocity (related to degree of demyelination). Results of EMG show denervation, despite little or no weakness.

Autonomic neuropathy becomes evident in symptoms that include abnormal pupillary reaction, postural hypotension, abnormalities of heart rate, peripheral edema, anhidrosis, abnormalities of reflex vasoconstriction, abnormal gastrointestinal motility, diarrhea, atonic bladder, and impotence. Sudden death may occur as a result of lack of reaction to hypoglycemia or cardiorespiratory arrest.

Symmetric proximal lower-extremity motor neuropathy ("amotrophy") becomes evident as slowly progressive, symmetric weakness, which is distinct from asymmetric "amyotrophy" (discussed with the focal diabetic neuropathies). Initial manifestations include lower back and proximal lower-extremity pain; progressive proximal weakness, loss of patellar reflexes, and atrophy follow. Sensation is spared, but a distal sensory polyneuropathy may coexist. Initial results of EMG show reduced motor unit recruitment; evidence of denervation appears later. Prognosis for recovery varies but is generally worse with insidious onset of symptoms. Control of hyperglycemia may promote recovery.

Focal and Multifocal Diabetic Neuropathies. *Trunk and limb mononeuropathy* (including mononeuropathy multiplex) occurs acutely, most often in the ulnar, median, radial, femoral, lateral cutaneous, thoracic, and peroneal nerves. These lesions often occur at the same sites as entrapment neuropathies. It is important to exclude other causes such as radiculopathy. It may not be possible to distinguish between a diabetic mononeuropathy and an entrapment syndrome.

Prognosis is good. *Cranial neuropathies* most commonly affect the extraocular muscles (see Ophthalmoplegia) and may be associated with facial pain or headache. Third-nerve lesions show rapid onset and pupillary sparing, whereas aneurysmal compression typically has an unresponsive pupil.

Asymmetric proximal lower-limb motor neuropathy is the unilateral form of "amyotrophy." Onset of unilateral pain and proximal weakness is sudden, progressing over 1 to 2 weeks. The patellar reflex is lost, and proximal atrophy eventually develops. Although the cause remains uncertain, prognosis is good.

Inflammatory Demyelinating Polyneuropathies

Guillain-Barré ([GBS], Guillain-Barré-Strohl syndrome, acute inflammatory demyelinating polyradiculoneuropathy [AIDP]) is probably immunologically mediated, involving both cellular and humoral responses, but no single autoantigen has been identified.

Typical clinical presentation includes paresthesias in the distal extremities followed by lower-extremity weakness. The weakness then ascends to involve the arms and face. Bilateral sciatica is common. Initial examination shows symmetric limb weakness, absent or greatly diminished deep tendon reflexes, and minimal sensory loss. Progression that involves respiration, eye movements, swallowing, and autonomic function occurs in severe cases. For 1 to 3 weeks weakness progresses before stabilization and then recovery. Severity of symptoms varies among individual cases. In severe cases complications of pneumonia, sepsis, adult respiratory distress syndrome, pulmonary embolus, and cardiac arrest are responsible for most severe disease and death.

Guillain-Barré syndrome is often preceded by an infection, usually viral. Important associated infections include human immunodeficiency virus (HIV), Epstein-Barr virus, cytomegalovirus, and *Campylobacter jejuni* enteritis. Underlying systemic diseases such as systemic lupus erythematosus, Hodgkin's disease, and sarcoidosis are occasionally associated with GBS. Vaccinations may also precede GBS.

Confirmatory test findings include CSF protein levels greater than 55 mg/dL with little or no pleocytosis ("albuminocytologic dissociation") 1 week after onset of symptoms. Level of CSF protein is often normal during the first few days of the illness. Results of nerve conduction studies show signs of demyelination early, before CSF protein changes. Differential diagnosis includes spinal cord disease, myasthenia gravis, neoplastic meningitis, vasculitic neuropathy, paraneoplastic neuropathy, botulism, heavy-metal intoxication, poliomyelitis, tick paralysis, and porphyria.

There are several GBS variants. These share signs of diminished reflexes, demyelination pattern on nerve conduction studies, and elevated CSF protein level. Variant syndromes include *Fisher syndrome* (ophthalmoplegia, ataxia, and areflexia with little associated weakness), weakness without paresthesias and sensory loss, and pharyngeal-cervical-brachial weakness, paraparesis, and sensory and pure ataxia.

Plasma exchange significantly alters the progression and severity of GBS, decreasing the need for mechanical ventilation by approximately 50%. The efficacy of intravenous immunoglobulin treatment (IV Ig) is probably comparable with that of plasmapheresis but is less documented. IV Ig given daily at 0.4 g/kg for 2 weeks is the preferred treatment for patients in unstable condition. Corticosteroids are inefficacious in GBS.

Chronic inflammatory demyelinating polyradiculoneuropathy ([CIDP]), chronic relapsing dysimmune polyneuropathy) is similar to GBS but shows a protracted, often relapsing course, pronounced sensory involvement, response to corticosteroid treatment, and greater association with systemic disease.

Worsening of symptoms for longer than 2 months, with subacute onset and fluctuation of symptoms over years, is characteristic of CIDP. Sensory involvement often accompanies proximal extremity and neck flexor weakness and diminished reflexes. Corticosteroids, plasmapheresis, immunosuppressive drugs and IV Ig can be used to treat CIDP. Treatment regimens include prednisone 100 mg per day for 4 weeks, tapering gradually over 1 year to a dose of 10 to 20 mg qod. Plasma exchange is usually given in three to five exchanges over 1 to 2 weeks. Plasmapheresis with lower-dose prednisone may be tried as initial therapy. IV Ig given at 0.4 g/kg per day for 5 days is efficacious, according to some but not all studies. Immunosuppressive drugs are used only in cases refractory to other treatments.

Underlying systemic diseases causing a syndrome indistinguishable from CIDP include monoclonal gammopathies, lymphoma, connective tissue disease (polyarteritis nodosa, cryoglobulinemia, and systemic lupus erythematosus) polyneuropathies associated with anti-myelin–associated glycoprotein (MAG), Lyme disease, HIV infection, and sarcoidosis.

GENERAL PRINCIPLES OF TREATMENT

  I. Patient education and counseling.
 II. Genetic counseling.
III. Withdrawal of medications suspected of causing neuropathy.
IV. Withdrawal from exposure to toxins.

    V. Correction of nutritional and vitamin deficiencies.
    VI. Treatment of alcoholism.
    VII. Blood glucose control in diabetic neuropathies.
    VIII. Specific drug therapies.
        A. Chelating agents in lead neuropathy.
        B. Hematin infusions in acute intermittent porphyria.
        C. Long-term prednisone in CIDP.
        D. Phytanic acid (reduced) diet in Refsum disease.
    IX. Plasmapheresis in AIDP and other autoimmune disorders.
    X. Pain control.
        A. Improve control of blood glucose level in diabetic neuropathies.
        B. Simple analgesics such as aspirin and acetaminophen.
        C. Phenytoin and carbamazepine (achieve anticonvulsant levels [see Epilepsy]).
        D. Tricyclic drugs (amitriptyline and imipramine).
        E. Transcutaneous electrical nerve stimulation.
    XI. Meticulous foot care.
    XII. Orthotic devices and splints.
    XIII. Surgical correction of entrapment neuropathies.
    XIV. Physical and occupational therapy.

REF: Dyck PJ, Thomas PK: *Peripheral neuropathy*, ed 3, Philadelphia, 1993, WB Saunders.

        Ropper AH: N *Engl J Med* 326:1130–1136, 1992.

        Schaumburg HH, Berger AR, Thomas PK: *Disorders of peripheral nerves*, ed 2, Philadelphia, 1992, FA Davis.

NICOTINIC ACID *(see Nutritional Deficiency Syndromes)*

NMR *(see Magnetic Resonance Imaging)*

NUTRITIONAL DEFICIENCY SYNDROMES

Vitamin A deficiency may complicate disorders of fat malabsorption like sprue, biliary atresia, and cystic fibrosis and produces night blindness (nyctalopia). Vitamin A excess can cause pseudotumor cerebri.

Thiamine (B_1) deficiency occurs most commonly in chronic alcoholism but may complicate other conditions associated with poor nutritional status, such as hyperemesis of pregnancy, malignancy, dialysis, prolonged intravenous feeding, or refeeding after starvation. Neurologic manifestations include *Wernicke-Korsakoff syndrome, sensorimotor polyneuropathy*, and *optic neuropathy* (usually retrobulbar) (see *Alcoholism*). Treatment consists of thiamine therapy, 50 to 100 mg daily, administered parenterally if GI absorption is unreliable, as in alcoholics. Thiamine should be given before IV glucose or refeeding to avoid exacerbating the effects of thiamine deficiency in patients with unknown nutritional histories.

Pyridoxine B$_6$ deficiency in children causes recurrent *seizures* refractory to conventional anticonvulsants. It is due to inadequate dietary intake or an autosomal recessive disorder known as pyridoxine dependency. It usually becomes evident within a few days of birth with severe seizures, which cease after administering 50 to 100 mg of IV pyridoxine, and requires lifelong supplementation of 2 to 30 mg/kg per day of pyridoxine.

Pyridoxine deficiency in adults is rarely caused by deficient diets but is caused by medications such as isoniazid, hydralazine, or penicillamine, which interfere with pyridoxine activity. The deficiency causes a *sensorimotor polyneuropathy* prevented by concomitant supplementation of 50 mg pyridoxine qd PO.

Pyridoxine overdose causes a *sensory neuropathy* characterized by diminished reflexes, impaired position and vibration sense, and sensory ataxia; strength and pain and temperature sensation are relatively spared.

B$_{12}$ (cyanocobalamin) deficiency is almost always due to malabsorption; causes include pernicious anemia, gastrectomy, ileal diseases such as tropical sprue, regional enteritis and bacterial overgrowth, and rare, inherited metabolic conditions. Neurologic manifestations include *subacute combined degeneration*, that is, a myelopathy involving the posterior columns and lateral corticospinal tracts; *dementia; sensorimotor polyneuropathy*; and *optic neuropathy* (usually retrobulbar). Laboratory evaluation includes complete blood cell count; serum levels of cyanocobalamin, and folate; urinary homocystine and methylmalonic acid levels; and the Schilling test. Treatment consists of IM injections of 100 μg daily or 1000 μg twice weekly for 2 weeks, followed by weekly injections of 1000 μg for another 2 to 3 months. If the B$_{12}$ deficiency results from malabsorption, the patient should be placed on lifelong maintenance therapy of monthly 1000 μg injections. Oral repletion may also be effective if GI absorption is normal.

Folate deficiency is due to poor intake (alcoholism or pregnancy), malabsorption (small-intestine–like inflammatory bowel disease), or drug antagonism (for example, phenytoin). Whether postnatal folate deficiency causes neurologic disease remains controversial; syndromes attributed to folate deficiency include *subacute combined degeneration* of the spinal cord, *sensorimotor polyneuropathy*, and *dementia*. Treatment consists of 1 mg of folate orally per day. Low-folate diets have been associated with CNS dysraphic states (spina bifida and anencephaly), and supplementation with 0.4 mg per day early in the first trimester of gestation may be preventative.

Niacin (nicotinic acid) deficiency causes *pellagra*, which is characterized by the triad of dermatitis, diarrhea, and dementia. Pellagra is endemic to areas where corn, a poor source of niacin, is the staple food and the intake of meat, which contains the niacin precursor tryptophan, is low. The major neurologic manifestation is an *encephalopathy* or *dementia*. Polyneuropathy, *optic neuropathy* or *myelopathy* may also occur. Treatment consists of 50 mg of oral niacin several times per day.

Vitamin D deficiency causes rickets and osteomalacia and may be associated with hypocalcemia. Long-term therapy with phenytoin, phenobarbital, or primidone may result in vitamin D deficiency and osteomalacia. Treatment is vitamin replacement.

Vitamin E deficiency occurs (1) in patients with severe fat malabsorption resulting from chronic cholestatic diseases, especially biliary atresia, intestinal resection, cystic fibrosis, and Crohn's disease, and (2) as part of inherited metabolic diseases like abetalipoproteinemia (Bassen-Kornzweig syndrome) and familial isolated vitamin E deficiency. The hallmark of vitamin E deficiency is *spinocerebellar degeneration* variably associated with a *peripheral neuropathy*, resulting in areflexia, ataxia, and impaired position and vibration sense. In this regard it appears similar to Friedreich's ataxia on clinical study. *Pigmentary retinitis* (with night blindness), *nystagmus, ophthalmoplegia*, and *proximal muscle weakness* may also occur. Treatment is with very high-dose oral vitamin E.

REF: Kayden JH: *Neurology* 43:2167–2169, 1993.

So YT et al. In Bradley WG et al, eds: *Neurology in clinical practice*, Boston, 1991, Butterworth-Heinemann.

NYSTAGMUS   *(see also Vertigo, Calorics, Optokinetic Nystagmus, Ocular Oscillations)*

A biphasic ocular oscillation in which at least one phase is slow. The direction may be horizontal, vertical, diagonal, or rotational.

There are two general types, jerk and pendular. In jerk nystagmus the slow phase is always centripetal and the fast (saccadic) phase returns the eye to the target. The nystagmus direction is defined as the direction of the fast component. In pendular nystagmus the oscillations are of equal velocity in both directions. When examining a patient with nystagmus, observe changes in amplitude and frequency with change in gaze direction. Nystagmus is of value in indicating dysfunction somewhere in the posterior fossa, that is, vestibular system (including the end organ), brainstem, or cerebellum.

Congenital nystagmus is present at birth or noted in early infancy at the time of development of visual fixation, and it persists throughout life. Some cases are familial. It may accompany primary visual defects and is a cardinal feature of albinism. It is almost always binocular, of similar amplitude in both eyes, and uniplanar (usually horizontal). It increases with attempts to fixate, decreases with convergence, disappears in sleep, often has a "null" position, and may have "inversion" of the optokinetic reflex. There may be associated head oscillations that are not compensatory or head tilt or turn that helps bring the eyes to the null position. Being present from infancy, it is not associated with oscillopsia.

Latent nystagmus is a form of congenital nystagmus. There is no nystagmus with binocular vision, but when one eye is occluded, jerk nystagmus develops in both eyes, with the fast phase toward the viewing eye. Latent nystagmus can be elicited by the intention of viewing with one eye. *Manifest latent nystagmus* occurs in patients with amblyopia, strabismus, or other eye disease who fixate monocularly. The fast phase is in the direction of the fixating eye.

Acquired nystagmus in infants may be due to progressive bilateral visual loss in early childhood, CNS disease, or spasmus nutans. Spasmus nutans is a syndrome of nystagmus, head nodding, and anomalous head positions. The nystagmus is pendular, rapid, of small amplitude, and usually bilateral but can differ in each eye; it may be monocular in a horizontal, rotary, or vertical direction. The nystagmus may vary with the direction of gaze. It begins in infancy (4 to 18 months of age) and spontaneously remits within 1 to 2 years after onset. There are usually no associated neurologic abnormalities. Some cases are familial.

Acquired pendular nystagmus is usually horizontal but may be vertical, diagonal, elliptic, or circular and may be associated with head tremor. There may be marked dissociation between the two eyes. It is associated with vascular or demyelinating lesions of the brainstem or cerebellum. In demyelinating disease it usually indicates a cerebellar lesion. Rarely, it is associated with visual dysfunction.

Vestibular nystagmus (see also Calorics, Vertigo) results from dysfunction of the vestibular end-organ, nerve, or brainstem connections and from acute lesions of the cerebellar flocculus. It is usually present in primary position, increases with gaze toward fast phase, and decreases with gaze toward the slow phase (with central lesions it may reverse direction). Vertigo usually coexists. The hallmarks of peripheral lesions are that the nystagmus can be suppressed by fixation and is accentuated when fixation is removed. For further differentiation of peripheral from central vestibular nystagmus, see Vertigo

Gaze-evoked nystagmus, the most common form of nystagmus, is elicited by attempting to maintain an eccentric eye position. If this cannot be maintained, the eyes drift back toward primary position. Quick corrective phases then bring the eyes back to the eccentric position. The fast phase is in the direction of gaze. Gaze-evoked vertical nystagmus almost always occurs with the horizontal type. There may be a torsional component to the nystagmus. With severe intoxications nystagmus may be horizontal pendular in primary position. Drugs are the most common cause of bidirectional gaze-evoked nystagmus. Offending agents include anticonvulsants, barbiturates, tranquilizers, ethanol, and phenothiazines. If the patient is not receiving any medications, gaze-evoked nystagmus indicates vestibulocerebellar, brainstem, or cerebral hemispheric dysfunction; neuromuscular fatigue, or muscular weakness. More precise localization requires assessment of the associated signs and symptoms.

Downbeat nystagmus occurs in primary position, increases in down gaze and lateral gaze, and may be accentuated by convergence. It is highly suggestive of a dysfunction at the craniocervical junction affecting posterior midline cerebellum and underlying medulla. When downbeat nystagmus is seen in cerebellar disease, other cerebellar eye signs are usually present, most commonly impaired vertical smooth pursuit and vertical vestibulo-ocular reflex. For differential diagnosis see Table 50.

Upbeat nystagmus occurs in primary position and is usually secondary to lesions at the pontomesencephalic and pontomedullary junctions. Drug intoxication is an uncommon cause. Other causes are listed in Table 50.

Physiologic (end-point) nystagmus occurs in normal individuals in the extremes of horizontal or upward gaze. It is a small-amplitude, variably sustained jerk nystagmus that is often dissociated (more marked in the abducting eye).

See-saw nystagmus consists of one eye intorting and rising while the opposite eye extorts and falls. Repetition in alternating directions produces a see-saw effect. It can occur in all fields of gaze but may be

TABLE 50
Causes of Vertical Nystagmus

Upbeat Nystagmus
Cerebellar degenerations and atrophies
Multiple sclerosis
Infarction of medulla or cerebellum
Tumors of the medulla, cerebellum, or midbrain
Wernicke's encephalopathy
Brainstem encephalitis
Behçet's syndrome
Meningitis
Leber's congenital amaurosis or other congenital disorder of the
    anterior visual pathways
Thalamic arteriovenous malformation
Congenital
Organophosphate poisoning
Tobacco
Associated with middle ear disease
Transient finding in otherwise normal infants

Downbeat Nystagmus
Cerebellar degeneration, including familial periodic ataxia and
    paraneoplastic degeneration
Craniocervical anomalies, including Arnold-Chiari malformation,
    Paget's disease, and basilar invagination
Infarction of brainstem or cerebellum
Dolichoectasia of the vertebrobasilar artery
Multiple sclerosis
Cerebellar tumor, including hemangioblastoma
Syringobulbia
Encephalitis
Head trauma
Anticonvulsant medication
Lithium intoxication
Alcohol, including cerebellar degeneration
Wernicke's encephalopathy
Magnesium depletion
Vitamin B_{12} deficiency
Toluene abuse
Congenital
Midbrain infarction
Increased intracranial pressure and hydrocephalus
Transient finding in otherwise normal infants

Leigh RJ, Zee DS: *The neurology of eye movements,* ed 2, Philadelphia, 1991,
FA Davis.

limited to primary position or downward gaze. It is seen with diencephalic dysfunction, frequently caused by parasellar tumors expanding within the third ventricle. The pathogenesis is unknown but believed to involve the interstitial nucleus of Cajal.

Periodic alternating nystagmus is a horizontal jerk nystagmus that periodically changes directions. Typically it beats for 90 seconds in one direction, then is in a neutral phase for about 10 seconds, and then beats 90 seconds in the opposite direction. It may persist during sleep. It may be congenital or may be due to craniocervical junction abnormalities or brainstem and cerebellar disease, it frequently becomes evident after visual loss.

Rotary (torsional) nystagmus occurs around the globe's anteroposterior axis and is seen in medullary disease. In vestibular disease a rotational component is usually combined with a prominent horizontal or vertical nystagmus.

Dissociated nystagmus refers to a significant asymmetry in either amplitude or direction between the two eyes. It occurs in internuclear ophthalmoplegia (see Ophthalmoplegia), in pendular nystagmus in patients with multiple sclerosis, and in a variety of posterior fossa lesions.

Rebound nystagmus is a transient nystagmus that develops on return to primary gaze after maintaining an eccentric gaze. The fast phase is in the opposite direction of prior gaze. It occurs most frequently in cerebellar disease.

Circular or elliptic nystagmus is a form of pendular nystagmus (horizontal and vertical pendular oscillations 90 degrees out of phase) with a continuous oscillation in a fine, rapid, circular, or elliptic pattern.

Diagonal (oblique) nystagmus occurs when simultaneous, pendular, horizontal, and vertical components are in phase or 180 degrees out of phase.

Nystagmus in myasthenia gravis may manifest as a gaze-evoked nystagmus in any direction with asymmetry between the two eyes. Muscle fatigue is seen as an increase in the nystagmus. Such nystagmus of the abducting eye occurring with impaired adduction of the contralateral eye constitutes the "pseudointernuclear ophthalmoplegia" of myasthenia gravis.

Voluntary "nystagmus" consists of bursts of rapid, conjugate, horizontal oscillations that are actually voluntarily produced back-to-back saccades. They can rarely be sustained for more than 10 to 30 seconds at a time.

Lid nystagmus is of three types. Upward jerking of the eyelids synchronous with vertical ocular nystagmus is nonlocalizing. Rapid twitching of the eyelids synchronous with the fast phase of horizontal ocular nystagmus induced by lateral gaze may occur with the lateral medullary syndrome. Lid nystagmus induced by convergence (Pick's sign) is associated with medullary lesions.

Convergence-retraction nystagmus is caused by lesions of the mesencephalon that involve the posterior commissure, classically, pineal tumors as part of Parinaud's syndrome.

Treatment of symptomatic nystagmus relies on physical and pharmacologic methods. Congenital nystagmus can be treated with prisms, surgery, and contact lenses. Baclofen may benefit acquired periodic alternating nystagmus. Trihexyphenidyl may be useful for pendular nystagmus in multiple sclerosis. Botulinum toxin A is under investigation.

REF: Dell'Osso LF et al. In Duane TD, Jaeger EA, eds: *Clinical ophthalmology*, Philadelphia, 1988, Lippincott.

Leigh RJ, Zee DS: *The neurology of eye movements*, ed 2, Philadelphia, 1991, FA Davis.

OBTURATOR NERVE   *(see Peripheral Nerve, Pregnancy)*

OCCIPITAL LOBE

The occipital lobe extends from the parieto-occipital fissure on the medial surface of the brain to the lateral surface, where it merges with the parietal and temporal lobes. Its function is mainly concerned with visual perception and recognition. Clinical syndromes associated with occipital lesions include visual field defects, cortical blindness, visual anosognosia (Anton's syndrome), visual agnosias, achromatopsia, metamorphopsias, illusions, and hallucinations. Causes include infarcts of the middle or posterior cerebral artery, tumors, or other mass lesions. Visual symptoms referable to the occipital lobe occur commonly in migraine. Occipital lobe epilepsy may present with visual phenomena and postictal blindness may also occur.

OCULAR OSCILLATIONS   *(see also Nystagmus, Optokinetic Nystagmus)*

The following abnormal oscillatory eye movements are distinct from nystagmus because of waveform differences.

Ocular bobbing consists of intermittent downward jerks of both eyes, followed by a slow drift to primary position. It is seen with extensive destructive lesions of the pons but also occurs with pontine compression, obstructive hydrocephalus, or metabolic encephalopathy. *Ocular dipping* is an inverse movement (slow downward, fast upward) with less reliable localization.

Ping-pong gaze denotes slow, horizontal, conjugate drift of the eyes that alternates every few seconds and is associated with bilateral hemispheric dysfunction.

Ocular myoclonus refers to pendular vertical oscillations seen with brainstem lesions and often accompanied by rhythmic movements of the palate and other midline structures.

The term *saccadic oscillations* includes several specific entities. *Saccadic dysmetria* can produce oscillation when overshooting saccades are followed by one or more corrective saccades. *Square-wave jerks*, seen most prominently in cerebellar disorders and progressive supranuclear palsy, and *macro square-wave jerks*, seen in multiple sclerosis and olivopontocerebellar atrophy, are saccades that interrupt fixation with normal intersaccadic intervals.

Flurries of rapid eye movements without an intersaccadic interval are termed *ocular flutter* if purely horizontal and *opsoclonus* if multidirectional. Both can be secondary to viral infection, drug effects, or tumor or can occur in paraneoplastic syndromes such as neuroblastoma in children or with anti-Purkinje's cell antibodies in adults (mostly women with gynecologic tumors).

Superior obliquo myokymia is a monocular torsional oscillation of small-amplitude, high-frequency contractions of a monocular superior oblique muscle. It causes oscillopsia, diplopia, or visual blurring. Although sometimes seen with brainstem disease, it is usually idiopathic and may respond to carbamazepine therapy.

Spasmus nutans is an ocular oscillation accompanied by head nodding and torticollis. It appears before 18 months of age and remits spontaneously, usually by age 3 years. The abnormal eye movements are usually dysconjugate and vary in direction. Although usually benign, this entity must not be confused with signs of intracranial tumor; the presence of poor feeding, optic atrophy, or raised intracranial pressure should be investigated by neuroimaging studies.

REF: Abel LA. Ocular oscillations: congenital and acquired. In Daroff R, Neetens A, eds: *Neurological organization of ocular movement*, Berkeley, 1990, Kugler.

Leigh RJ, Zee DS: *The neurology of eye movements*, ed 2, Philadelphia, 1991, FA Davis.

OLFACTION

The sense of smell is mediated by the first cranial nerve. It is the only sensory modality without a thalamic relay. Complaints may include anosmia, hyposmia, parosmia, or loss of appreciation of flavors in food. Smell is tested on clinical examination by means of nonirritating aromatic compounds such as oil of wintergreen, cloves, coffee, almond oil, or lemon oil. The stimulus is presented to one nostril with the other occluded. The ability to appreciate the presence of a substance, even if not properly identified, is evidence that anosmia is not present. Unilateral anosmia is more often due to a structural lesion than to a diffuse process. Causes of anosmia or hyposmia include the following:

1. Infection: Rhinitis, sinusitis, basilar meningitis, frontal abscess, osteomyelitis (Frontal or ethmoidal), viral hepatitis, syphilis, influenza.
2. Toxic or metabolic disorders: Pernicious anemia, zinc deficiency, lead and calcium intoxication, diabetes mellitus, hypothyroidism.
3. Neoplasms: Frontal tumor, olfactory groove or sphenoid meningioma, radiation therapy.
4. Trauma to cribriform plate.
5. Congenital: Olfactory agenesis (Kallmann's syndrome) and septo-optic dysplasia (De Morsier's syndrome).
6. Other: Hydrocephalus, amphetamine and cocaine abuse, aging, smoking, trigeminal lesions (causing mucosal atrophy), anterior cerebral artery disease, polyps, multiple sclerosis, Alzheimer's disease, and Parkinson's disease.

Hyperosmia is seen in hysteria, migraine, hyperemesis gravidarum, cystic fibrosis, Addison's disease, and strychnine poisoning.

Olfactory hallucinations can occur with neoplasms or vascular disease involving the inferomedial temporal lobe, near the hippocampus or uncus. "Uncinate" fits are so called because of the presence of olfactory or gustatory hallucinations as part of complex partial or simple partial seizures; these may be triggered or even be arrested by olfactory stimulation. Anosmia is not present in such cases.

REF: Shiffman: N Engl. J Med 308:1275-1279; 1337-1343, 1983.

OLIVOPONTOCEREBELLAR ATROPHY *(see Parkinsonism, Spinocerebellar Degeneration)*

ONDINE'S CURSE *(see Sleep)*

OPHTHALMOPLEGIA *(see also Eye Muscles, Gaze Palsy, Myasthenia Gravis, Graves' Ophthalmopathy)*

If extraocular muscle testing reveals misalignment of the visual axes, first determine whether this is due to a nerve palsy or some other cause of impaired motility.

I. Causes of impaired ocular motility other than a nerve palsy.
   A. Concomitant strabismus.
   B. Graves' ophthalmopathy.
   C. Myasthenia gravis (and other pharmacologic or toxic causes of neuromuscular blockade).
   D. Convergence spasm.
   E. Old blow-out fracture of the orbit with entrapment myopathy.
   F. Restrictive ophthalmopathy (Brown's superior oblique tendon sheath syndrome).
   G. Orbital inflammatory disease (pseudotumor).
   H. Orbital masses and neoplasms.
   I. Orbital infections.
   J. Brainstem disorders causing abnormal prenuclear inputs (internuclear ophthalmoplegia, skew deviation).
   K. Ocular myopathies.
   L. Chronic progressive external ophthalmoplegia (Kearns-Sayre syndrome).
   M. Congenital syndromes.

II. Causes of abducens (cranial nerve VI) palsies.
   A. Nuclear (associated with ipsilateral horizontal gaze palsy).
      1. Developmental anomalies (Möbius syndrome, some Duane's syndromes).
      2. Infarction.
      3. Tumor (pontine glioma, cerebellar tumors).
      4. Wernicke-Korsakoff syndrome.
   B. Fascicular.
      1. Infarction.
      2. Demyelination.

      3. Tumor.
- C. Subarachnoid.
    1. Aneurysm or anomalous vessels (anterior inferior cerebellar artery, basilar artery).
    2. Subarachnoid hemorrhage.
    3. Meningitis (infectious, neoplastic).
    4. Sarcoid.
    5. Cerebellopontine angle tumor (acoustic neuroma, meningioma).
    6. Clivus tumor (chordoma, nasopharyngeal carcinoma).
    7. Trauma.
    8. Surgical complication.
    9. Postinfectious.
- D. Petrous.
    1. Infection or inflammation of mastoid or petrous tip.
    2. Trauma (petrous fracture).
    3. Thrombosis of inferior petrosal sinus.
    4. Increased intracranial pressure (pseudotumor cerebri, supratentorial mass).
    5. Following lumbar puncture.
    6. Aneurysm.
    7. Persistent trigeminal artery.
    8. Trigeminal schwannoma.
- E. Cavernous sinus and superior orbital fissure.
    1. Aneurysm.
    2. Thrombosis.
    3. Carotid cavernous fistula.
    4. Dural arteriovenus malformation.
    5. Tumor (pituitary adenoma, meningioma, nasopharyngeal carcinoma).
    6. Pituitary apoplexy.
    7. Sphenoid sinusitis (mucormycosis).
    8. Herpes zoster.
    9. Granulomatous inflammation (sarcoid, Tolosa-Hunt syndrome).
- F. Orbital: Tumor.
- G. Uncertain localization.
    1. Infarction (diabetes, hypertension).
    2. Migraine.
- III. Causes of trochlear nerve palsies.
    - A. Nuclear and fascicular.
        1. Developmental anomalies.

      2. Hemorrhage.
      3. Infarction.
      4. Trauma.
      5. Demyelination.
      6. Surgical complications.
  B. Subarachnoid.
      1. Trauma.
      2. Tumor (pineal, tentorial meningioma, trochlear schwan-
         noma, ependymoma, metastases).
      3. Surgical complication.
      4. Meningitis (infectious, neoplastic).
      5. Mastoiditis.
  C. Cavernous sinus and superior orbital fissure: As for CN VI
     palsies.
  D. Orbital.
      1. Trauma.
      2. Ethmoiditis.
      3. Ethmoidectomy.
  E. Uncertain localization: Infarction (diabetes, hypertension).
IV Causes of oculomotor nerve palsies
  A. Nuclear and fascicular.
      1. Developmental anomaly.
      2. Infarction.
      3. Tumor.
  B. Subarachnoid.
      1. Aneurysm (posterior communicating artery).
      2. Meningitis (infectious, syphilitic, neoplastic).
      3. Infarction (diabetes).
      4. Tumor.
      5. Surgical complication.
  C. Tentorial edge.
      1. Increased intracranial pressure (uncal herniation, pseu-
         dotumor cerebri).
      2. Trauma.
  D. Cavernous sinus and superior orbital fissure.
      1. As for CN VI palsies.
      2. Infarction (diabetes, hypertension).
  E. Orbital: Trauma.
  F. Uncertain localization.
      1. Mononucleosis and other viral infections.
      2. Following immunization.
      3. Migraine.

4. Cyclic oculomotor palsy of childhood.
5. Guillain-Barré syndrome.

Combined ophthalmopareses from third, fourth, and sixth cranial nerve involvement most commonly occur with base of skull infiltrations, cavernous sinus or superior orbital fissure lesions, and generalized neuropathies. Proptosis, chemosis, and vascular engorgement suggest orbital or cavernous sinus involvement. Base of skull problems include extension of nasopharyngeal carcinoma, sarcoidosis, lymphoma, clivus chordoma, pituitary apoplexy, meningeal carcinoma, and cavernous sinus thrombosis.

Chronic progressive external ophthalmoplegia (CPEO) is a slowly progressive, painless, symmetric ophthalmoplegia without fluctuations or remissions. Ptosis and orbicularis oculi weakness usually accompany the external ophthalmoplegia. The pupils are spared, and there are no orbital signs. Fibrotic changes of the extraocular muscles may occur over time, causing a superimposed restrictive ophthalmopathy. CPEO has multiple causes. One such cause, Kearns-Sayre syndrome, is due to a mitochondrial cytopathy: it has childhood onset without a family history, ataxia, retinal pigmentary degeneration, short stature, cardiac conduction defects often leading to Stokes-Adams attacks, increased cerebrospinal fluid protein, spongiform changes of the cerebrum and brainstem, and muscle mitochondrial abnormalities.

Painful ophthalmoplegias may be due to diabetes, aneurysm, tumors, (primary and metastatic), Tolosa-Hunt syndrome (inflammatory process such as granulomas, affecting cavernous sinus and surrounding structures), herpes zoster, cavernous sinus thrombosis, carotid cavernous fistula, ophthalmoplegic migraine, arteritis, carcinomatous meningitis, or fungal infection.

Internuclear ophthalmoplegia (INO) is characterized by slow, incomplete adduction or complete inability to adduct past midline and nystagmus of the opposite abducting eye. INO is caused by a lesion of the medial longitudinal fasciculus (MLF) between mid-pons and the oculomotor nucleus ipsilateral to the impaired adduction. Subtle defects are best solicited by observing the fast phases of optokinetic nystagmus. If the patient has bilateral INO, nystagmus on upward gaze and a skew deviation may be present. The most frequent cause of INO in young adults (especially when bilateral) is multiple sclerosis. Vascular causes tend to be more common in older patients. Rarely, intrinsic or extra-axial brainstem tumors are the cause. Myasthenia gravis should be excluded as a cause of very similar appearing "pseudo-INO."

One and one-half syndrome refers to a gaze palsy in one direction and an INO in the other (see Gaze Palsy). This condition results from combined lesions of the MLF and the more ventral, ipsilateral abducens nucleus or paramedian pontine reticular formation (PPRF). The only intact horizontal movement is abduction of the contralateral eye. Acutely the patient may appear exotropic, with nystagmus in the deviated eye. Causes include brainstem ischemia (most common), multiple sclerosis, tumor, or hemorrhage. As with INO, myasthenia must be considered if there are no long tract or sensory signs.

REF: Glaser JS: *Neuro-ophthalmology*, ed 2, Philadelphia, 1990, Lippincott.

Leigh RJ, Zee D: *Neurology of eye movements*, ed 2, Philadelphia, 1991, FA Davis.

OPSOCLONUS   (see Ocular Oscillations, Paraneoplastic Syndromes)

OPTIC CHIASM   (see Pituitary, Visual Fields)

OPTIC NERVE

The signs and symptoms of the optic nerve dysfunction include a decreased sense of brightness, diminished visual acuity, afferent pupillary defects, color desaturation, and characteristic visual field defects—central, centrocecal, arcuate, or altitudinal scotomas; these findings may accompany all the disorders described below except acute papilledema. Disc swelling may be present (papilledema, "anterior" optic neuropathy, or "papillitis" in the case of optic neuritis) or absent ("posterior" or "retrobulbar" neuropathy or neuritis) in optic nerve disease. Optic atrophy indicates optic nerve fiber loss resulting from chronic or past optic nerve disease.

Papilledema is disc swelling caused by increased intracranial pressure. Fundoscopic manifestations include disc hyperemia, venous dilation, blurred disc margins with haziness of the retinal vessels, splinter hemorrhages, and absent venous pulsations (these are absent in 20% of individuals and their presence aids only in excluding papilledema). Papilledema is usually bilateral; unilateral papilledema associated with contralateral optic atrophy sometimes occurs with subfrontal masses (Foster Kennedy syndrome). Acute papilledema may produce enlargement of the blind spot and transient visual obscurations with sudden changes of position but otherwise spares vsion. Chronic papilledema may cause constriction of the visual fields and nerve bundle defects.

Optic neuritis refers to the inflammation of the optic nerve. It usually becomes evident between the ages of 15 and 45 years as acute unilateral visual loss and increased periorbital pain with eye movement;

disc swelling occurs in 50% of affected adults. Visual acuity usually returns to near-normal levels within 2 to 3 months. Most cases are associated with a demyelinating disorder or are idiopathic. Other causes include viral or postviral syndromes, contiguous inflammation (such as sinusitis or meningitis), sarcoidosis, tuberculosis, syphilis, "autoimmune" neuritis, and paraneoplastic neuritis. Administration of IV methylprednisolone followed by oral prednisone hastens recovery, but a regimen of oral prednisone alone may increase the risk of recurrences and is contraindicated. The former regimen may also prevent the occurrence of multiple sclerosis after isolated optic neuritis.

Ischemic optic neuropathy refers to infarction of the optic nerve. It becomes evident in adults over 60 years of age as acute unilateral visual loss and disc swelling (retrobulbar form is rare); recovery rate is poor. The common "idiopathic" form is characterized by an association with hypertension and diabetes mellitus, a normal erythrocyte sedimentation rate (ESR), and steroid unresponsiveness. The rarer "arteritic" form is characterized by associated headaches, weight loss, fever, arthralgias, myalgias, jaw claudication, and scalp tenderness; an elevated ESR; and steroid responsiveness (see Vasculitis).

Toxic and *nutritional optic neuropathies* become evident as slowly progressive bilateral visual loss and are usually retrobulbar. Causes include toxins (for example, ethambutol, isoniazid, chloramphenicol, streptomycin, lead, and methanol), vitamin deficiencies (B_{12}, thiamine, niacin, and riboflavin), and tobacco-alcohol amblyopia, seen with heavy tobacco and alcohol use (probably nutritional and responds to vitamin supplementation).

Other causes of optic neuropathies include *compressive lesions* such as primary optic nerve tumors (gliomas and perioptic meningiomas), *infiltration* (sarcoidosis, leukemia, lymphoma, plasmacytomas, and histiocytosis), *carcinomatous meningitis*, *radiation* (seen 1 to 3 years after parasellar or sinus radiation therapy), *Leber's hereditary optic neuropathy*, and *trauma*.

REF: Beck RW: *Neurology* 42:1133-1135, 1992.

   Breen LA, ed: *Neurol Clin* 9(1):131–145, 1991.

   Miller NR: *Walsh and Hoyt's clinical neuro-ophthalmology*, ed 4, Baltimore, 1982, Williams & Wilkins.

OPTOKINETIC NYSTAGMUS

The optokinetic system is an ocular motor subsystem that enhances the ability to stabilize images on the retina, thus allowing adequate visual acuity. When the head moves for an extended period, the vestibular response decays because of the mechanical properties of the labyrinthine sense organs. Only retinal information remains as the input resulting in compensatory eye movements. When the proper conditions are reproduced in the laboratory with movement of the entire visual surround, *optokinetic nystagmus* (OKN) is generated: slow components of nystagmus that match eye velocity with visual surround velocity, and fast components that reset eye position.

At the bedside a true optokinetic stimulus is usually not possible. Stimulation with hand-held moving stripes induces nystagmus reflecting smooth-pursuit eye movement function (slow components) and saccadic system integrity (fast components). The examiner looks for the presence of both components of nystagmus and for symmetry in both horizontal and both vertical directions. Some clinical conditions are well demonstrated by observation of the bedside OKN response, as follows:

1. Presence of optokinetic nystagmus proves that visual function is at least partially intact and is relevant in examining infants and in patients with suspected psychogenic blindness.
2. Frontal lobe lesions often produce abnormalities of saccades but spare pursuit. The eyes tonically deviate in the direction of the moving target, and the fast phases may be absent or impaired when the target moves toward the side of the lesion.
3. Deep parietal lesions may impair pursuit toward the side of the lesion, causing an abnormal slow component of OKN when the target moves toward the side of the lesion. There may be an amplitude asymmetry between the two directions.
4. Extensive hemispheric lesions may impair both pursuit and saccades. Movement of the target toward the side of the lesion may produce deficits in both slow and fast components.
5. Occipital or temporal lesions usually spare OKN. If the OKN response is asymmetric, deep parietal involvement is probable.
6. Moving the OKN target away from the field of action of an individual eye muscle prompts saccades in the appropriate direction and may help define a muscle paresis. Look for differences between paired muscles, for example, the left lateral rectus and the right medial rectus: the paretic eye moves more slowly and lags behind.
7. Internuclear ophthalmoplegia may be demonstrated by horizontal movement of the target, resulting in dysconjugate saccades when fast components of OKN require action of the affected medial rectus muscle.

8. Downward movement of the OKN target may help demonstrate convergence retraction nystagmus (see Nystagmus).

9. Congenital nystagmus may be accompanied by "inverted" OKN, in which the fast components are in the direction of target movement.

REF: Leigh RJ, Zee DS: *The neurology of eye movements*, ed 2, Philadelphia, 1991, FA Davis.

ORBIT   *(see Graves' Ophthalmopathy, Opthalmoplegia, Ptosis)*

PAGET'S DISEASE   *(see Craniocervical Junction)*

Paget's disease, a disorder of local bone remodeling, usually develops after 40 years of age and becomes evident as pain at rest or motion. Back pain may occur as a result of the bony changes, but compression fracture is also possible. The bony changes may lead to lumbar stenosis or thoracic cord compression. Skull involvement can lead to headache or cranial nerve abnormalities (hearing loss, vision loss, diplopia, or facial weakness). With more severe skull involvement, basilar invagination and odontoid process dislocation may occur, with resultant brainstem compression or obstructive hydrocephalus. Diagnosis is based on typical radiographic changes and increased 24-hour urine hydroxyproline excretion. Alkaline phosphatase level is often elevated. Therapy includes calcitonin, biphosphonates, and plicamycin. Nonsteroidal anti-inflammatory medications can reduce bone pain.

PAIN

Pain is produced by the stimulation of peripheral nocicepters or afferent nerve fibers. The perception of pain is modulated by many factors, including previous behavioral experiences, strong emotions, drugs, and hypnosis. This modulation suggests a neural mechanism that modifies either the transmission of pain or the emotional reaction to it, or both.

Cutaneous afferent nociceptive fibers enter the dorsal horn of the spinal cord, where they may ascend or descend 1 to 2 segments as Lissauer's tract. Primary afferents terminate in the superficial layers of the dorsal horn in an area known as the substantia gelatinosa. Second-order neurons decussate and ascend rostrally as the lateral and anterior spinothalamic tracts. The spinothalamic tract projects to the ventral posterolateral nucleus of the thalamus, which then sends its projections to other diencephalic structures, the brainstem reticular activating system, the limbic system, and the primary somatosensory cortex. In addition to the ascending pain system, there is a descending modulation system with origins in the brainstem periaqueductal gray and projections to the raphe nucleus. Projections from the raphe nucleus project directly to the ventral and dorsal horns of the spinal cord, including the substantia gelatinosa, and act to inhibit nociception. Serotonin is the main transmitter in this system. The locus ceruleus also acts as a descending modulating system, using norepinephrine as its transmitter. Prominent within the pain modulating systems is the opiate receptor system and endogenous opioid peptides, which exist throughout the nervous system, as well as in the periaqueductal gray and raphe nucleus. Opiate drugs given systemically act on the brainstem and limbic system.

Acute pain follows an injury and generally resolves with healing. It has a well-defined temporal onset and is often associated with objective physical signs of autonomic activity such as tachycardia, hypertension, and diaphoresis. Chronic pain persists beyond expected healing time and often cannot be related to a specific injury. It may not have a well-defined onset, does not respond to treatments aimed at the presumed origin or cause, and is not associated with signs of autonomic activity; the patients do not "look" like they are in pain.

Reflex sympathetic dystrophy and *phantom limb pain* are unique chronic pain syndromes. Reflex sympathetic dystrophy is characterized by burning pain, hyperesthesia, swelling, hyperhidrosis, and trophic skin and bone changes. It is treated with sympathetic denervation and aggressive physical therapy. Phantom limb pain differs from the usual nonpainful sensory illusion that the lost limb is still present. Phantom limb pain is refractory to most treatments, although local anesthetic injections have limited success.

Chronic (noncancer) pain requires an integrated multidisciplinary approach directed at both physical and psychologic rehabilitation. The goal is to control the factors that increase pain. All therapies, especially drugs, should be given on a time-contingent basis, not as necessary (prn). The patient thus is not rewarded for having pain by getting medication. This approach serves to reduce the total amount of drug required daily. Each drug must be given an adequate trial. Start with simple analgesics, increase the dose or frequency before changing drugs, and when changing, use equianalgesic doses. Avoid excessive sedation.

Pharmacologic management of pain utilizes treatment directed at specific sites along the pain pathways. Peripherally, aspirin and non-steroidal anti-inflammatory agents produce analgesia by preventing the formation of prostaglandin from arachidonic acid metabolism. Prostaglandin sensitizes tissues to the pain-producing effects of bradykinin and other substances resulting from tissue injury. These medications are effective in treatment of mild to moderate pain, especially bone pain. These substances also potentiate the effects of narcotic analgesics. Capsaicin, a derivative of hot peppers, acts by depleting nociceptors of substance P, rendering the skin insensitive to pain. A treatment trial requires 2 to 4 weeks of daily topical application, three to four times per day, to the affected area. Tricyclic antidepressants (TCAs) may act via influencing the biogenic amine system, affecting levels of serotonin, norepinephrine, and dopamine. Patients with pain are often locked into a pain-depression-insomnia cycle, and TCAs can affect each of these aspects of pain. The TCAs are effective in a variety of chronic pain conditions, including chronic low back pain, headache, neuropathy, and neuralgias. Anticonvulsants act to suppress spontaneous neuronal firing. They are useful in the management of chronic pain states such as trigeminal neuralgia, postherpetic neuralgia, diabetic neuropathy, and postamputation pain.

Narcotic analgesics are used to treat severe, acute pain and chronic cancer pain. When using narcotics, start with the lowest dose needed to obtain analgesia and titrate to pain relief or to the appearance of unacceptable side effects. Whereas prn dosing for several days allows for the determination of total daily dose, thereafter give narcotic analgesics on a fixed dosing schedule. Add nonnarcotic drugs to increase analgesia. Tolerance to narcotics usually becomes evident as a reduction in duration of analgesia and the need for higher doses. Treat this situation by increasing the dose or by using an alternative drug (start with one half of the equianalgesic dose). The narcotic conversion nomograms can guide conversion between narcotics (Figures 28 and 29). For example, 30 mg of oral methadone is equivalent to approximately 20 mg of parenteral morphine. Physical dependence occurs if the patient receives prolonged therapy in high doses, and patients experience withdrawal symptoms with abrupt narcotic cessation. Physical dependence is not to be confused with psychological dependence, which is a behavioral syndrome of drug craving.

Other pharmacologic interventions include the use of corticosteroids in the treatment of cancer, especially when cancer is due to bony metastasis; neuroleptics in dysesthetic pain; and dextroamphetamine for potentiating narcotic analgesia and reducing narcotic-induced sedation. Antihistamines (hydroxyzine) and neuroleptics can also be used to decrease nausea associated with narcotic use.

Other treatment modalities used in pain management include trigger-point injections; epidural, intrathecal, and sympathetic blockade; ganglionolysis; cordotomy; transcutaneous and percutaneous electrical stimulation; dorsal column stimulation; and relaxation techniques, including biofeedback and hypnosis.

REF: Bach S, et al: *Pain* 1988; 33:297.

Portenoy RK: *CA Cancer J Clin* 1988; 38:327-392.

Schwartzmann RJ, McLellan TL: *Arch Neurol* 1987; 44:555.

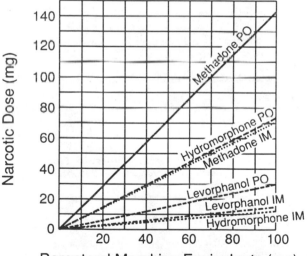

FIGURE 28
Narcotic conversion nomogram: high-potency narcotics. (From Grossman SA, Scheidler VR: *World Health Forum* 8:525, 1987.)

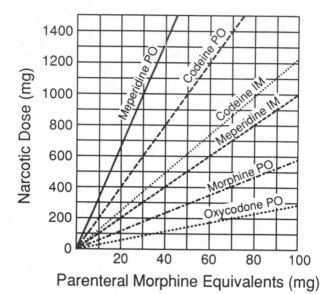

FIGURE 29
Narcotic conversion nomogram: low-potency narcotics. (From Grossman SA, Scheidler VR: *World Health Forum* 8:525, 1987.)

PAPILLEDEMA   *(see Intracranial Pressure, Optic Nerve, Pseudotumor Cerebri)*

PARALYSIS AGITANS   *(see Parkinson's Disease)*

PARANEOPLASTIC SYNDROMES

Paraneoplastic syndromes are remote effects of cancer that occur in 7% to 15% of patients with systemic cancer. In more than 50% of patients the paraneoplastic syndrome precedes diagnosis of the primary cancer. Paraneoplastic or nonmetastatic nervous system disease can occur by metabolic, nutritional, or hormonal derangement causing encephalopathy; by coagulation disturbance leading to nonbacterial thrombotic endocarditis, disseminated intravascular coagulation, infarction, or hemorrhage; by opportunistic infection producing meningoencephalitis or myelitis; or by possible autoimmune-mediated injury. Pathologic findings include vascular, inflammatory, and immunologic changes. Some paraneoplastic syndromes, presumably of immunologic origin, are associated with specific antibodies (see Table 51). Most paraneoplastic syndromes progress independently of the underlying cancer, and only rarely does treatment of the primary disorder affect the course of the syndrome.

The paraneoplastic syndromes include the following.

I. Brain and cranial nerves.
   A. Cerebellar degeneration.
      1. Anti-Yo.
      2. Atypical autoantibodies.
      3. Antibody-negative.
   B. Opsoclonus-myoclonus.
      1. Anti-Ri.
      2. Antibody-negative.
      3. With cerebellar degeneration.
   C. Limbic encephalopathy and other dementias.
      1. Anti-Hu.
      2. Antibody-negative.
   D. Brainstem encephalitis.
      1. Upper brainstem (for example, parkinsonism).
      2. Lower brainstem (with hearing loss, dysphagia).
   E. Retinal degeneration.
      1. Anti-visual paraneoplastic syndrome (VPS).
      2. Antibody-negative.
   F. Optic neuritis.
II. Spinal cord and dorsal root ganglia.
   A. Myelitis or encephalomyelitis.
   B. Necrotizing myelopathy.
   C. Sensory neuronopathy.
      1. Anti-Hu.
      2. Antibody-negative.
   D. Subacute motor neuronopathy.
   E. Motor neuron disease.
III. Peripheral nerves.
   A. Subacute or chronic sensory or sensorimotor peripheral neuropathy.
   B. Guillain-Barré syndrome.
   C. Mononeuritis multiplex and vasculitic neuropathy (microvasculitis).
   D. Brachial neuritis.

TABLE 51
Autoantibodies in Paraneoplastic Syndromes

Antibody	Syndrome	Associated Neoplasms	Histochemistry
Anti-Hu	Sensory neuropathy; encephalomy-elitis; limbic encephalitis	Small cell lung carcinoma; ? Prostate	Nuclei of CNS neurons
Anti-Ri	Opsoclonus or myoclonus	Breast; small cell lung; ovary; neu-roblastoma (children)	Nuclei of CNS neurons
Anti-VPS	Visual paraneoplastic syndrome (VPS)	Small cell lung	Retinal ganglion cells
Anti-Yo	Cerebellar degeneration	Ovary; breast; ?lung	Purkinje's cell cyto-plasm
LEMS	Lambert-Eaton myasthenic syndrome (LEMS)	Small cell lung; ?leukemia; neuro-blastoma (children)	Voltage-gated calcium channels of periph-eral nerve terminals

Adapted from Posner JB, Furneaux HM: Paraneoplastic syndromes. In Waksman BH, ed: *Immunologic mechanisms in neurologic and psychiatric disease*, New York, 1990, Raven.

E. Autonomic neuropathy.
   1. Anti-Hu.
   2. Antibody-negative.
F. Peripheral neuropathy with islet cell tumors.
G. Peripheral neuropathy associated with paraproteinemia.
IV. Neuromuscular junction and muscle.
   A. Lambert-Eaton myasthenic syndrome (LEMS).
   B. Myasthenia gravis.
   C. Dermatomyositis or polymyositis.
   D. Acute necrotizing myopathy.
   E. Carcinoid myopathy.
   F. Myotonia.
   G. Cachectic myopathy.
   H. Neuromyopathy.

REF: Posner JB, Furneaux HM: Paraneoplastic syndromes. In
        Waksman BH, ed: *Immunologic mechanisms in neurologic and
        psychiatric disease*, New York, 1990, Raven.

        Rosenfeld MR, Dalmau J: *Semin Neurol* 13:291-298, 1993.

        Schor NF: *J Child Neurol* 7:253-258, 1992.

PARATHYROID   *(see Electrolytes—Calcium)*

PARATONIA   *(see Rigidity)*

PARIETAL LOBE

The parietal lobe contains the primary somatosensory and association cortices dealing with integration of multiple sensory modalities. It also contributes fibers to the pyramidal tracts. Parietal lobe syndromes depend on the laterality of the lesion. Hemisphere-independent parietal syndromes include contralateral cortical sensory loss, incongruent homonymous hemianopsia, contralateral hemiparesis (especially associated with hemiatrophy if onset is in childhood), impaired ipsilateral optokinetic nystagmus, sensory hallucinations, and simple sensory seizures. Dominant parietal syndromes include aphasia, alexia, Gerstmann's syndrome, tactile agnosia, and apraxia (ideomotor and ideational). Nondominant parietal lobe lesions lead to neglect syndromes, anosognosia, topographic memory loss, constructional apraxia, "dressing apraxia," and acute confusional states. Bilateral parietal lesions are associated with visual agnosia, Balint's syndrome, Anton's syndrome, color agnosia, and catatonia.

PARINAUD'S SYNDROME   *(see Gaze Palsy, Ischemia)*

PARKINSONISM   *(see also Parkinson's Disease)*

Many disorders besides idiopathic Parkinson's disease (PD) become evident as akinetic-rigid syndromes with features of "parkinsonism," that is, varying combinations of akinesia, rigidity, tremor, and postural instability. These disorders are frequently distinguished from PD by the presence of supranuclear palsy, cerebellar signs, Babinski's signs, early severe dementia, orthostatic hypotension, and a history of definite encephalitis, repeated head trauma, neuroleptic treatment, or lack of response to levodopa. Because of additional neurologic features, they are sometimes called secondary parkinsonism or parkinsonism-plus syndromes.

1. *Progressive supranuclear palsy* (PSP, Steele-Richardson-Olszewski syndrome) is characterized by supranuclear ophthalmoplegia (usually beginning with paresis of downgaze, then upgaze, followed by horizontal gaze), axial rigidity, pseudobulbar palsy, marked bradykinesia, and dementia. Onset of the disease is later than in PD. Nonspecific visual complaints are a common presenting feature. Early gait difficulties are prominent because of axial rigidity and visual-vestibular impairment. The typical finding on CT or MRI is brainstem and midbrain atrophy. The majority of patients do not improve on a regimen of levodopa.

2. *Striatonigral degeneration* is difficult to distinguish from PD; features helpful for differential diagnosis are hyperreflexia, extensor plantar responses, and early onset of falling. Most patients with striatonigral degeneration do not improve on a regimen of levodopa.

3. *Shy-Drager syndrome* encompasses the syndrome of parkinsonism with a prominent autonomic component (orthostatic hypotension, syncope, incontinence, and sexual impotence). Autonomic dysfunction can either precede or follow the onset of the akinetic-rigid syndrome. Occasionally, cerebellar or pyramidal signs occur. Treatment with levodopa can worse parkinsonism; fludrocortisone and indomethacin may ameliorate orthostasis (see Autonomic Dysfunction).

4. *Olivopontocerebellar atrophy* is a heterogeneous disorder, often with usually autosomal dominant inheritance, but sporadic cases occur. Cerebellar ataxia is the initial symptom in the

majority of patients, followed by an extrapyramidal syndrome; signs of involvement of other systems vary. Striatonigral degeneration, Shy-Drager syndrome, and olivopontocerebellar atrophy are also considered by some authorities to be different manifestations of a more generic disorder termed "multiple system atrophy."

5. *Corticobasal ganglionic degeneration* is characterized by akinetic-rigid syndrome, often with dystonia, myoclonus, ideomotor and ideational apraxia, cortical sensory loss, the alien limb phenomena, and dementia. Onset is frequently asymmetric.

6. *Other primary degenerative diseases* include the juvenile form of Huntington's disease, Wilson's disease, Hallervorden-Spatz disease, and neuroacanthocytosis.

7. *Diseases that come to medical attention with dementia* (Alzheimer's disease (AD), diffuse Lewy body disease (DLBD), and Pick's disease). Patients with AD have higher frequency of extrapyramidal symptoms than do persons without dementia, but dementia always precedes parkinsonism (see Alzheimer's Disease). Diffuse Lewy body disease is characterized by the presence of cortical Lewy bodies; differentiation from AD is difficult. Early onset of dementia followed by parkinsonism with prominent postural instability, gait disturbances, and visual hallucinations has been suggested as a diagnostic criterium. Levodopa may be beneficial in DLBD.

8. *Vascular parkinsonism* resulting from lacunar infarcts of the basal ganglia, vasculitis, or amyloid angiopathy is a rare cause of parkinsonism. It may account for patients with lower-body parkinsonism with gait disturbances and minimal upper-limb involvement.

9. *Toxins and drugs:* MPTP, manganese, mercury, methanol, carbon monoxide, cyanide, neuroleptics, lithium, alpha-methyldopa, and metoclopramide.

10. *Postencephalitic* (encephalitis lethargica, other viral encephalitides, and AIDS).

11. *Head injury* with midbrain hemorrhage and dementia pugilistica.

12. *Hydrocephalus*, both communicating and noncommunicating.

REF: Riley D, Fogt N, Leigh RJ: *Neurology* 44:1025-1029, 1994.

Stacy M, Jankovic J: *Neurol Clin* 10:341-359, 1992.

PARKINSON'S DISEASE   (see also Parkinsonism)

Parkinson's disease (PD, paralysis agitans, idiopathic Parkinson's disease) is a common neurodegenerative disease of unknown origin. Prevalence of the disease increases with age and in persons older than 65 years of age is estimated to be 1 per 100. Juvenile and familial cases have been described; more men than women are affected. On pathologic study there is neuronal loss in the substantia nigra (especially pars compacta), and Lewy bodies (eosinophilic inclusion bodies) are present in the substantia nigra and other brainstem nuclei.

The onset of symptoms is insidious. The cardinal features are tremor, rigidity, bradykinesia, and postural disturbances. In typical cases tremor is a rest tremor of 4 to 6 Hz; muscle tone is increased, with "cogwheel" or "lead pipe" rigidity; gait is slowed and festination (uncontrolled acceleration of gait) may develop; and posture is stooped, with flexion of arms. Loss of postural stability falls generally occur in the later stages of PD. *Bradykinesia* describes slowness and fatiguing of movements and often is accompanied with masked face, loss of associated movements (arm swings), and monotonous, hypophonic speech. Cognitive decline manifests in 30% to 60% of patients (see Dementia), and many patients have depression. Autonomic dysfunction is also common (orthostatic hypotension or erectile dysfunction) and may be related to PD and its treatment.

Conventional criteria for diagnosis of PD are based on the presence of bradykinesia and either rigidity or typical rest tremor. Diagnosis is further supported by unilateral onset and good response to levodopa (see later discussion). Although in the majority of patients diagnosis is not difficult, the presence of atypical features may cause uncertainty. Other disorders that become evident as akinetic-rigid syndrome must be considered (see Parkinsonism).

Levodopa (L-DOPA) is the major therapeutic agent providing effective symptomatic relief in the majority of patients. The best time for initiating levodopa treatment is controversial because side effects and motor fluctuations may be related to the duration of treatment. A regimen of levodopa is most commonly started when functional disability interferes with patient's daily activities. Levodopa is usually combined with carbidopa or benserazide, inhibitors of peripheral dopa decarboxylase that decrease peripheral conversion of levodopa to dopamine, thereby reducing the side effects of postural hypotension and nausea. The carbidopa-levodopa (Sinemet) preparation comes in the following combinations: 10/100, 25/100, 25/250, and a controlled-release form of 50/200. The usual starting dosage is 25/100 bid or tid, and the lowest dose that provides significant improvement should be used. Side effects of the carbidopa-levodopa preparation are dyskinesias (athetosis, chorea, dystonia, and myoclonus), visual hallucinations, sleep disturbances, confusion, and psychotic states. Patterns of dose-related dyskinesias include dyskinesias at the beginning and end of each dose, and those observed only at peak of each dose. Lowering the dose improves side effects at the expense of worsening the PD symptoms. Motor fluctuation ("on-off") and end-of-dosage deterioration can be improved by increased frequency of dosing, by decreasing the dose of levodopa-carbidopa, or by dietary adjustments. Medication should be taken at least 30 minutes before or 1 hour after meals because reduction of competing protein improves absorption and transport of levodopa. Controlled-release preparation (Sinemet controlled-release 50/200) prolongs the plasma and brain half-life and can be useful in treatment of motor fluctuations. Because of the decreased bioavailability of Sinemet CR, slightly higher dose (20% to 30%) of levodopa is needed, but dose frequency can be cut to half.

Selegiline (L-Deprenyl), a selective inhibitor of monoamine oxidase B, has been suggested to prevent progression of PD resulting from neuroprotective action, but it also influences dopamine metabolism, making it difficult to distinguish neuroprotection from symptomatic relief. Selegiline can be used as monotherapy in mild PD and as an adjunct in reducing motor fluctuations. Selegiline in de novo patients with PD at a dosage of 5 mg bid (morning and noon doses) may provide satisfactory symptomatic efficacy and delay the need to start levodopa treatment. Selegiline is usually well tolerated.

Dopaminergic agonists are also used in the treatment of PD. Combination with the levodopa-carbidopa preparation can be used to reduce side effects of levodopa in more advanced stages of PD because these agents act directly on dopamine receptors and do not require metabolic transformation in the brain. Random motor oscillations between doses ("on-off") may be improved by combination of levodopa and dopaminergic agonists. Bromocriptine (Parlodel) can be also used as monotherapy in early PD in dosages starting at 1.25 mg qhs up to 10 to 30 mg per day divided in three doses. Pergolide (Permax) is another dopaminergic agonist; initial dose is 0.05 mg per day and is titrated up to a dosage of 2 to 3 mg daily in three doses. Side effects are similar to those for levodopa, but psychiatric symptoms are usually more common than dyskinesia. Rare side effects include pleuropulmonary fibrosis and erythromelalgia (tender, edematous, and red extremity).

Amantadine blocks re-uptake of dopamine, some patients respond to a dosage of 100 mg bid, but long-term benefit is limited. Side effects are confusion, nausea, and livedo reticularis.

Anticholinergic agents used in therapy of PD are benztropine (initial dosage is 0.5 mg bid, increasing up to a dose of 4 to 6 mg per day) and trihexyphenidyl (1 mg bid, increasing up to a dose of 6 to 10 mg daily). These agents are most helpful in reducing tremor without altering bradykinesia. Side effects are dry mouth, blurred vision, urinary retention, hypotension, and confusion. Patients with dementia should be receive cautious treatment with these agents because anticholinergic effect may further impair cognitive deficit. Sudden withdrawal may worsen the parkinsonism.

Neural and adrenal medullary transplants may benefit occasional patients but are associated with significant perioperative morbidity and are not currently recommended as standard therapy in PD.

Parkinson's disease is progressive, and management of end-stage patients is challenging. These patients frequently fail to respond to the antiparkinsonian drugs and become functionally dependent in activities of daily living. Frequent falls and poor or absent postural reflexes may leave the patient bed-bound. Dementia with periods of agitation sometimes necessitates treatment with neuroleptics or clozapine. Other adjunctive treatments used to improve the parkinsonism include the following:

1. Limited drug holidays for 7 to 10 days have the aim of restoring dopaminergic responsiveness, but hospital admission is required and these are of limited value.
2. Low-protein diet during the day facilitates absorption of levodopa and its entry into brain. These patients frequently need extensive nursing care and physical therapy.

REF: Calne DB: N Engl J Med 329:1021-1027, 1993.

Hughes AJ et al: Arch Neurol 50:140-148, 1993.

Jankovic J, Marsden CD, eds: Parkinson's disease and movement disorders, Baltimore and Munich, 1988, Urban & Schwarzenberg.

Koller WC, Hubble JP: Neurology 40(suppl 3):40-47, 1990.

PELLAGRA   (see Nutritional Deficiency Syndromes)

PERIODIC PARALYSIS   (see Myotonia)

Periodic paralysis refers to remitting and relapsing episodes of flaccid, painless weakness traditionally categorized according to the serum potassium level during the attack. However, the episodes are better classified by sensitivity to potassium and changes in its level rather than by its absolute value. They can be primary familial (autosomal dominant) forms or can result from other causes. Genetic forms of periodic paralysis associated with mutations in the α subunit of the skeletal muscle sodium-channel protein include hyperkalemic periodic paralysis and paramyotonia congenita. See Table 52 for a review of clinical features of the primary familial kalemic periodic paralysis.

Secondary hypokalemic periodic paralysis occurs in illnesses with potassium depletion, including hyperaldosteronism, chronic diarrhea, or chronic use of potassium depleting diuretics. A high incidence of hypokalemic periodic paralysis is associated with thyrotoxicosis in Oriental men.

Secondary hyperkalemic periodic paralysis is seen only with very high potassium levels, and cardiac abnormalities usually predominate. Causes include renal insufficiency, potassium-sparing diuretics, and adrenal insufficiency.

Normokalemic periodic paralysis has not been established as a distinct clinical entity. On clinical study it resembles hyperkalemic periodic paralysis and probably represents the approximately 20% of patients with normal potassium levels.

All forms of periodic paralysis may respond to acetazolamide therapy. Its mode of action includes kaliuresis but also induces metabolic acidosis, which may explain its benefit in hypokalemic periodic paralysis. Other kaliuretic diuretics (such as thiazides) may also be effective.

REF: Ebers GC et al: *Ann Neurol* 30:810-816, 1991.

PERIPHERAL NERVE
CLINICAL CLUES IN THE DIAGNOSIS OF FOCAL PERIPHERAL NERVE DISEASE

I. Upper extremity.
  A. With marked differences in strength between BICEPS and BRACHIORADIALIS (both innervated by C5-6 roots via *upper trunk*), think of:
    1. A lesion of the *lateral cord* or *musculocutaneous nerve* (if BICEPS is *weaker*).
    2. A lesion of the *posterior cord* or *radial nerve* (if BRACHIORADIALIS is *weaker*).
  B. With marked differences in strength between BICEPS and DELTOID, think of:

TABLE 52
Primary Familial Kalemic Periodic Paralysis

Characteristic	Hypokalemic	Hyperkalemic
Age of onset	10-20 yr, worse during third and fourth decades	Infancy/childhood
Inheritance	Autosomal dominant, 3 male: 1 female, often not expressed in female	Autosomal dominant, male = female
Duration of attacks	Hours to days	Usually <1 hr
Frequency of attacks	Several per week to years between attacks	Several per day to months between attacks
Clinical signs	Often occurs in early morning, begins with hip weakness and spreads over 1 hr from proximal to distal; can totally paralyze patient, ↓ DTRs, spares face, eyes, and respiratory muscles	Proximal > distal weakness, spreads over minutes, associated wiht myotonia of face, eyes, hands. Respiratory muscles may be involved
Laboratory findings	K^+ 1.5-3 mEq ECG changes of ↓ K+ EMG silent during attack	K ↑ in 80%, ± ↑CK ECG changes of ↑ K+ EMG silent during attack
Precipitating factors	Heavy exercise followed by rest or sleep, cold, emotion, heavy meal, alcohol, trauma, epinephrine, corticosteroids	Rest after exercise, cold, anesthesia, sleep, pregnancy
Provocative tests	Glucose ± insulin	Oral KCl
Treatment	KCl, acetazolamide, spironolactone	Acetazolamide, calcium gluconate

1. A lesion of the *lateral cord* or *musculocutaneous nerve* (if BICEPS is *weaker*).
2. A lesion of the *posterior cord* or *axillary nerve* (if DELTOID is *weaker*).

C. The *median nerve* sensory fibers to the hand pass via the upper brachial plexus, originating from:
   1. The C6 root to the thumb,
   2. The C6 and C7 roots to the index finger,
   3. The C7 root to the middle finger.

D. It is not possible to differentiate C8 from T1 radiculopathy because all INTRINSIC MUSCLES of the hand are innervated by C8 and T1 roots.

E. With an *ulnar nerve* lesion of the arm, elbow, or upper forearm, sensory loss usually involves palmar and dorsal aspects of the little and ring fingers. With an *ulnar nerve lesion* of the distal forearm or wrist, sensory loss involves only the palmar aspect of these fingers (due to sparing of the *dorsal ulnar sensory branch* that arises 6 to 7 cm above the wrist).

F. With *ulnar neuropathy*, sensory loss should not ascend above the wrist. With C8 T1 radiculopathy or *lower trunk plexopathy*, sensory loss can ascend to the entire medial aspect of the upper limb, following the distribution of the *medial cutaneous nerves* of the forearm and arm (both arising from the *lower trunk*).

G. With weakness and/or atrophy of the THENAR and HYPOTHENAR eminences, think of:
   1. C8-T1 radiculopathy.
   2. A *lower trunk* brachial plexopathy.
   3. Concomitant *ulnar* and *median* mononeuropathy (for example, carpal tunnel syndrome and ulnar neuropathy at the elbow). In this case, FLEXOR POLLICIS LONGUS should be intact (flexor of the distal phalanx of the thumb, located in the forearm and innervated by the *anterior interosseus branch of the median nerve*).

H. If there is suspicion of a *lower trunk* brachial plexopathy and/or C8-T1 radiculopathy, the presence of a second-order-neuron Horner's syndrome is supportive evidence.

I. When evaluating wrist drop, correct the wrist angle to the neutral position before testing finger flexors and extensors:
   1. If the BRACHIORADIALIS and TRICEPS are spared, the lesion is an isolated *posterior interosseous* mononeuropathy. In such cases there is no sensory loss.

2. If only the TRICEPS is spared, the *radial nerve* lesion is at the spiral groove.
3. If the TRICEPS is weak, the *radial nerve* lesion is at the axilla.
4. If, in addition to the TRICEPS, the DELTOID is weak, the lesion is not radial nerve, but rather a *posterior cord* brachial plexopathy (supplying *radial* and *axillary* nerves).

J. In the case of scapular winging,* the winging is caused by:
1. SERRATUS ANTERIOR weakness if:
   a. There is considerable winging at rest.
   b. There is medial translocation of the scapula (vertebral border closer to the midline).
   c. The shoulder appears lower on the affected side.
   d. Winging is accentuated by forward flexion of the humerus.
2. TRAPEZIUS weakness if:
   a. There is less winging at rest.
   b. There is lateral translocation of the scapula.
   c. The shoulder is definitely lower on the affected side.
   d. Winging is decreased by forward flexion of the humerus.
   e. Winging is increased by abduction of the humerus.

II. Lower extremity.
A. The *only L4-innervated* muscle below the knee is TIBIALIS ANTERIOR (L4-5, dorsiflexor of the ankle).
B. When evaluating foot drop (complete or incomplete), testing inversion of the ankle (TIBIALIS POSTERIOR) and flexion of the toes (FLEXOR DIGITORUM LONGUS) is very important. These muscles are innervated by L5 (and to a lesser extent S1) nerve roots via the *tibial nerve*. They are spared with *peroneal neuropathy* but are weak with L5 radiculopathy. Remember to correct the angle of the foot back to 90 degrees before testing eversion and inversion.
C. It is not possible to differentiate L2 from L3 radiculopathy because QUADRICEPS, ILIOPSOAS, and ADDUCTOR muscles are innervated by L2 *and* L3 roots.
D. The testing of THIGH ADDUCTORS (L2-4, *obturator nerve*) is essential in differentiating "pure" *femoral neuropathy* from

*Note that scapular winging can be falsely diagnosed in patients with poor posture or skeletal deformity. In addition, proximal weakness (such as myopathy or spinal muscular atrophy) can cause generalized shoulder girdle atrophy and "pseudowinging."

root or lumbar plexus involvement (THIGH ADDUCTORS are not involved in *femoral* neuropathy).

E. In proximal weakness of the lower extremity(ies), compare QUADRICEPS and THIGH ADDUCTORS with THIGH ABDUCTORS (GLUTEUS MEDIUS). If the weakness is significantly different, think of a selective root-plexus involvement rather than a myopathy (QUADRICEPS and THIGH ADDUCTORS are L2-4 and GLUTEUS MEDIUS is L5-S1).

Peripheral innervation is shown in Figures 30 to 37.

PERONEAL MUSCULAR ATROPHY   (see Muscular Dystrophy Neuropathy)

PERONEAL NERVE   (see Peripheral Nerve)

PET AND SPECT

Both positron emission tomography (PET) and single photon emission computed tomography (SPECT) are based on transaxial reconstruction of images derived from the distribution of administered radionuclides. A series of tomographic images are reconstructed by computer. Spatial resolution is significantly lower than that obtained with CT or MRI. PET methodology provides both qualitative and quantitative data (the latter require an arterial line for serial blood sampling), whereas SPECT provides only qualitative data. Both methods are safe, and actual radiation exposure is less than or equal to that received in many other routine radiologic procedures.

PET uses positron-emitting nuclides such as oxygen-15, fluorine-18, carbon-11, and nitrogen-13, which must be produced in a cyclotron. They have a short half life, enabling administration of relatively high doses of radioactivity but remaining within safe limits of radiation exposure. These radionuclides can be incorporated into biologically active compounds to measure biochemical, pharmacologic, and metabolic processes. Deoxyglucose labeled with fluorine-18 (FDG) is used to measure brain glucose metabolism. Compounds labeled with oxygen-15 are used to measure regional cerebral blood flow and volume and cerebral metabolic rates. Specific receptors such as dopamine or serotonin can be targeted with positron-emitting analogues of those monoamines.

Text continued on p. 338.

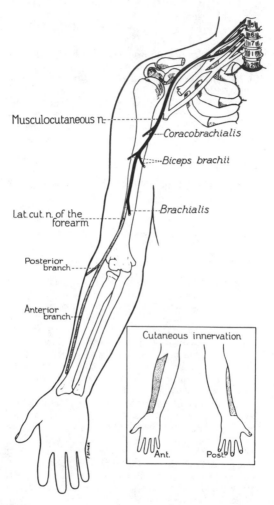

Musculocutaneous n.

Coracobrachialis

Biceps brachii

Brachialis

Lat. cut. n. of the forearm

Posterior branch

Anterior branch

Cutaneous innervation

Ant.

Post.

FIGURE 30
Musculocutaneous nerve. (From Haymaker W, Woodhall B: Peripheral nerve injuries: Principles of diagnosis, Philadelphia, 1953, WB Saunders.)

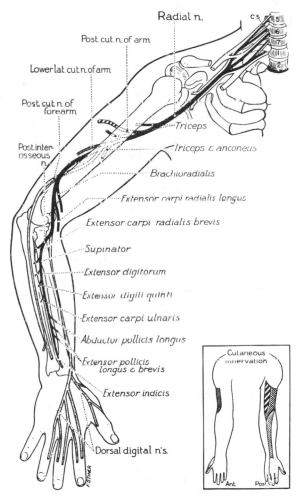

Radial n.

Post. cut. n. of arm

Lower lat. cut. n. of arm

Post. cut. n. of forearm

Post. inter-osseous n.

C 5

Triceps

Triceps & anconeus

Brachioradialis

Extensor carpi radialis longus

Extensor carpi radialis brevis

Supinator

Extensor digitorum

Extensor digiti quinti

Extensor carpi ulnaris

Abductor pollicis longus

Extensor pollicis longus & brevis

Extensor indicis

Dorsal digital n's.

Cutaneous innervation

Ant.   Post.

FIGURE 31
Radial nerve. (From Haymaker W, Woodhall B: *Peripheral nerve injuries: Principles of diagnosis,* Philadelphia, 1953, WB Saunders.)

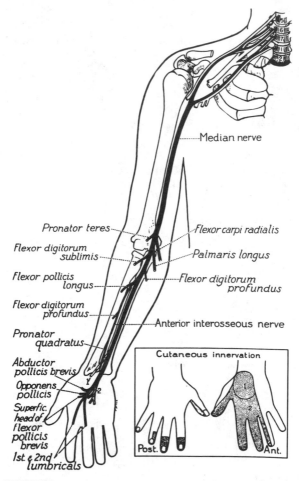

FIGURE 32
Median nerve. (From Haymaker W, Woodhall B: *Peripheral nerve injuries: Principles of diagnosis,* Philadelphia, 1953, WB Saunders.)

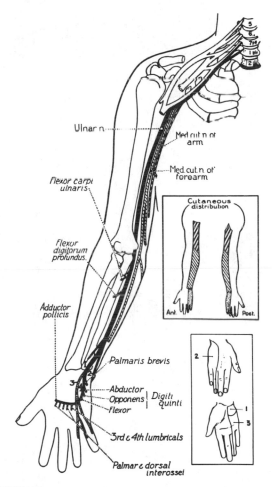

FIGURE 33
Ulnar and medial cutaneous nerves. (From Haymaker W, Woodhall B: *Peripheral nerve injuries: Principles of diagnosis*, Philadelphia, 1953, WB Saunders.)

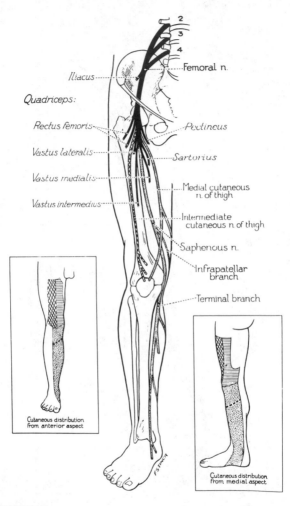

2
3
4

Femoral n.

Iliacus

Quadriceps:

Rectus femoris

Pectineus

Vastus lateralis

Sartorius

Vastus medialis

Medial cutaneous n. of thigh

Vastus intermedius

Intermediate cutaneous n. of thigh

Saphenous n.

Infrapatellar branch

Terminal branch

Cutaneous distribution from anterior aspect

Cutaneous distribution from medial aspect

FIGURE 34
Femoral nerve. (From Haymaker W, Woodhall B: *Peripheral nerve injuries: Principles of diagnosis*, Philadelphia, 1953, WB Saunders.)

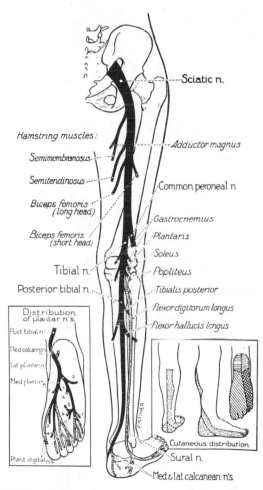

FIGURE 35

Sciatic, tibial, posterior tibial, and plantar nerves. (From Haymaker W, Woodhall B: *Peripheral nerve injuries: Principles of diagnosis,* Philadelphia, 1953, WB Saunders.)

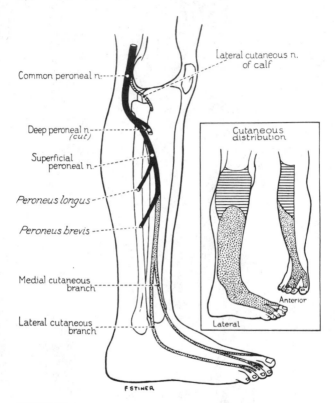

FIGURE 36
Superficial peroneal nerve. (From Haymaker W, Woodhall B: *Peripheral nerve injuries: Principles of diagnosis*, Philadelphia, 1953, WB Saunders.)

In clinical situations PET has utility in the evaluation of patients with refractory seizures of presumed focal origin. Detection of unilateral temporal hypometabolism using FDG is considered a highly specific procedure for localizing the epileptic focus. Gliomas can also be evaluated for malignant potential, and FDG uptake patterns can differ-

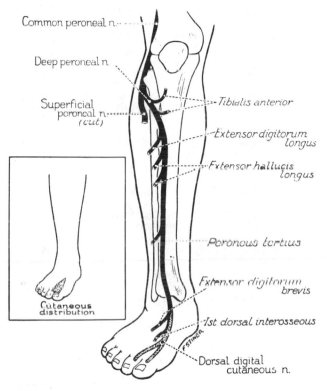

FIGURE 37
Deep peroneal nerve. (From Haymaker W, Woodhall B: *Peripheral nerve injuries: Principles of diagnosis,* Philadelphia, 1953, WB Saunders.)

entiate necrosis from tumor recurrence. Other uses for PET have been limited to research studies by the high cost, invasiveness, and need for extremely sophisticated technology.

SPECT utilizes gamma emitters, such as iodine-123 or technetium-99, attached to highly lipophilic substances that easily pass the blood-brain barrier by simple diffusion. Thus uptake, as measured by gamma camera, is proportional to regional blood flow. Gamma emitters have also been successfully labeled to various neurotransmitter analogues, allowing for localization and evaluation of receptor densities. Indications for studies are similar to those for PET. In contrast to PET, however, SPECT technology is widely available.

REF: Alavi A, Hirsch LJ: *Semin Nucl Med* 21:58-81, 1991.
        American Academy of Neurology: *Neurology* 41:163-167, 1991.

PHAKOMATOSES   *(see Neurocutaneous Syndromes)*

PHENOBARBITAL   *(see Epilepsy)*

PHENOTHIAZINES   *(see Neuroleptics)*

PHENYLKETONURIA   *(see Metabolic Disorders of Childhood)*

PHENYTOIN   *(see Epilepsy)*

PHOSPHORUS   *(see Electrolyte Disorders)*

PICK'S DISEASE   *(see Dementia)*

PITUITARY   *(see also Ophthalmoplegia, Visual Fields)*

Mass lesions occurring within the sella include pituitary adenomas, arachnoid cysts, and rarely, tumors of the neurohypophysis. Meningiomas, metastases, dermoids, teratomas, arachnoid cysts, and cholesteatomas may occur in any of several locations around the sella. Suprasellar masses include craniopharyngiomas, optic gliomas, chondromas, hypothalamic gliomas, supraclinoid carotid artery aneurysms, choroid plexus papillomas, and colloid cysts of the third ventricle. Parasellar lesions include cavernous carotid aneurysms, temporal lobe neoplasms, and gasserian ganglion neuromas. Chordomas and basilar artery aneurysms are seen in the retrosellar region. Infrasellar lesions include sphenoid sinus mucoceles, carcinomas, granulomas, and other nasopharyngeal tumors.

Pituitary adenomas may cause only endocrine symptoms if less than 10 mm in diameter (microadenoma). Larger tumors usually produce visual symptoms or headache, or both, with or without endocrine abnormalities, including variable hypopituitarism. Pituitary adenomas are usually classified on histologic study on the basis of immunoperoxidase stains used to identify specific hormones. Prolactin-secreting and nonfunctional adenomas (usually chromophobe adenomas) are the most common. The most common of these, the prolactinomas, usually become evident as amenorrhea or galactorrhea, or both, in females and decreased libido and impotence in males. Glycoprotein hormone-secreting tumors typically produce only symptoms of local mass effect and make up the majority of nonfunctioning adenomas. The less common growth hormone–secreting and adrenocorticotropic hormone (ACTH) secreting adenomas become evident as acromegaly and Cushing's syndrome, respectively, usually while small in size. Acromegaly may also be associated with entrapment neuropathies such as carpal tunnel syndrome and with diabetes. Cushing's syndrome may be associated with mental status changes, personality changes, and myopathy. Rarely, pituitary tumors secrete follicle-stimulating hormone (FSH) and, even less commonly, thyroid-stimulating hormone (TSH) or luteinizing hormone (LH).

Prolactinomas may rapidly expand during pregnancy. The differential diagnosis of hyperprolactinemia includes hypothalamic and infundibular lesions (loss of inhibitory control of prolactin secretion), renal failure, Chiari-Frommel syndrome, and drugs (phenothiazines, butyrophenones, benzodiazepines, reserpine, morphine, alpha methyldopa and isoniazid). Serum prolactin levels > 100 ng/ml (normal level, <15 ng/ml) are almost always due to tumor. Levels from 15 to 100 ng/ml may be due to tumor but are more commonly due to the other disorders listed previously, particularly drugs. MRI scan with gadolinium enhancement is the imaging test of choice. However, since microadenomas are sometimes undetected by MRI, endocrinologic testing is needed to confirm the diagnosis of small, hormone-secreting pituitary tumors if they are suspected on clinical examination.

Treatment of symptomatic prolactinomas primarily consists of bromocriptine because of the risk of tumor recurrence after surgical resection. Occasionally microadenomas resolve with medical treatment. Visual symptoms resulting from macroadenomas usually remit with bromocriptine use. Transsphenoidal microsurgical resection is required when bromocriptine is inefficacious or symptoms progress quickly. Extension into brain parenchyma requires an intracranial approach.

Corticosteroid coverage should be provided during surgery. Visual and endocrine function may improve after surgery and must be followed up regularly after surgery. Postoperative radiation therapy is used only for macroadenomas that do not respond to medical or surgical management. Transsphenoidal microsurgical resection is the primary treatment in growth hormone–secreting and ACTH-secreting tumors and in symptomatic glycoprotein hormone–secreting tumors.

Craniopharyngiomas, which may be distinguished from pituitary adenomas by the presence of calcifications (see later discussion), are treated by surgical removal and postoperative radiation therapy. There is a fairly high recurrence rate, even if resection seems complete. Stereotactic decompression of recurrent fluid-filled cysts may obviate the need for craniotomy in some cases.

Pituitary apoplexy refers to the sudden expansion of the pituitary gland, usually the result of hemorrhage into a preexisting adenoma. Sudden severe headache, variable ocular motor palsies, rapid loss of vision (chiasmal or optic nerve), evidence of dyspituitarism, and subarachnoid hemorrhage with associated changes in mental status are present. Features helpful in the difficult clinical distinction from aneurysmal subarachnoid hemorrhage are the presence of mixed oculomotor palsies or bilateral ophthalmoplegias and the presence of an afferent pupillary defect or chiasmal patterns of field loss. Diagnostic procedures include CT and MRI, which may show a pituitary mass containing blood; angiography to exclude an intracavernous aneurysm; and lumbar puncture. Baseline hormonal levels should be obtained before treatment, for subsequent determination of endocrine dysfunction. Treatment includes immediate high-dose IV corticosteroid therapy and prompt transsphenoidal decompression to prevent further vision loss.

Empty sella syndrome is the. major cause of asymptomatic sellar enlargement. The subarachnoid space extends into the sella through an incompetent diaphragm with flattening of the gland inferiorly and posteriorly. Empty sella syndrome may also follow pseudotumor cerebri, spontaneous regressive changes of pituitary adenomas, and surgery. Although usually asymptomatic, symptoms may occur, including headache, occasional mild endocrine abnormalities (exclude hypopituitarism), CSF rhinorrhea, and rarely, visual disturbances. If symptoms are present, pituitary tumor shuld be excluded with endocrine and neuro-ophthalmic evaluations and MRI. Differential diagnosis of an enlarged sella turcica in the absence of endocrinopathy includes nonsecreting adenoma, empty sella syndrome, and craniopharyngioma. Hypopituitarism, diabetes insipidus, and visual field defects are much less common in the empty sella syndrome. A ballooned sella without erosion is more characteristic of the empty sella. Suprasellar extension and calcification is more characteristic of craniopharyngioma.

REF: Klibanski A, Zervas NT: N Engl J Med 324:822-831, 1991.

PLASMAPHERESIS   (see Lambert-Eaton Myasthenic Syndrome, Myasthenia Gravis, Neuropathy)

PLEXUS   (see Brachial Plexus, Lumbosacral Plexus)

POLIO   (see Encephalitis, Motor Neuron Disease)

POLYARTERITIS NODOSA   (see Neuropathy, Vasculitis)

POLYMYALGIA RHEUMATICA   (see Myopathy, Vasculitis)

POLYMYOSITIS   (see Myopathy)

PONTINE SYNDROMES   (see Ischemia)

PORPHYRIA

The porphyrias are rare disorders of heme biosynthesis with neurologic, cutaneous, and other organ manifestations. They are classified as hepatic and erythropoietic. Neurologic symptoms occur in the hepatic porphyrias: acute intermittent porphyria (AIP), variegate porphyria (VP), hereditary coproporphyria (HC), and aminolevulinic acid (ALA) dehydratase deficiency (see Table 53). These disorders are autosomal dominant enzyme defects of the pathways of heme biosynthesis in the liver resulting in elevations in the levels and excess excretion of the porphyrins and the porphyrin precursors (Figure 38). Although the enzyme defects are well characterized, the pathogenesis of neurologic dysfunction is not known. It has been postulated that the δ-ALA and porphobilinogen (PBG) are directly neurotoxic. Other possibilities include abnormalities of heme metabolism in neurons and interference with serotonergic metabolism.

The first step in the pathway catalyzed by δ-ALA synthase results in the formation of ALA and is the rate-limiting step. Heme exerts

TABLE 53
Characteristics of the Hepatic Porphyrias

Type of Porphyria	Enzyme Defect	Increased Erythrocyte Porphyrins	Urine	Feces
Acute intermittent porphyria	PBG deaminase	None	↑ ALA, PBG	None
Variegate porphyria	Protoporphyrinogen oxidase	None	↑ ALA, PBG, COPRO	COPRO, PROTO
Hereditary coproporphyria	Coproporphyrinogen oxidase	None	↑ ↑ COPRO	↑ ↑ COPRO
ALA dehydratase deficiency	ALA dehydratase	Protoporphyrin	ALA	None

ALA, Aminolevulinic acid; COPRO, coproporphyrin; PBG, porphobilinogen; PROTO protoporphyrin.

Glycine + Succinyl CoA → ALA → PBG → Hydroxy-
                     1   2   3 methylbilane

$$4 \nearrow \text{Uro'gen III} \rightarrow \text{Copro'gen III} \rightarrow \text{Proto'gen IX} \rightarrow \text{Protoporphyrin IX} \rightarrow \text{HEME}$$
                       5   6   7   8

$$4 \searrow \text{Uro'gen I} \rightarrow \text{Copro'gen I}$$
                       5

Enzymes

1, Aminolevulinic acid (ALA) synthase.
2, ALA dehydratase.
3, Porphobilinogen (PBG) deaminase.
4, UROgen III synthase.

5, UROgen decarboxylase.
6, COPROgen oxidase.
7, PROTOGEN oxidase.
8, HEME synthetase.

FIGURE 38
The Heme synthesis pathway.

control at this step via three different mechanisms: (1) repression of synthesis of new enzyme, (2) interference of transfer of the enzyme from cytosol to mitochondria, and (3) direct inhibition of enzyme activity. Processes that deplete the regulatory pool of heme by inducing cytochrome p450 or increasing the turnover of hemoglobin drive the heme synthesis pathway. For example, dilantin induces the cytochrome p450 system and starvation increases the turnover of hemoglobin. Both processes deplete the heme pool, thereby removing repression of ALA synthetase.

Depending on the specific enzyme deficiency, an excess of intermediates from preceding steps in the pathway are excreted in urine and stool; the pattern of porphyrin precursors in the urine, feces, and serum characterizes the type of porphyria. Diagnosis is complicated by the variable intensity of porphyrin excretion in affected individuals, and drug-induced porphyrinuria in some normal individuals leads to occasional false-positive results (see Table 54). Lead poisoning can result in elevation of ALA and porphyrin levels. Special handling of specimens obtained for porphyria is necessary. Specimens from twenty-four-hour urine collection should be kept refrigerated in a dark container. Specimens from twenty-four-hour stool collection must be kept frozen and in a light-free container.

Acute intermittent porphyria is the most common of these rare disorders. Prevalence is estimated at 5 to 10 per 100,000 in the United States. Up to 90% of persons with the enzyme deficiency are asymptomatic. It lacks cutaneous manifestations, since the PBG is not a porphyrin. Variegate porphyria occurs mainly in South Africa but has occurred worldwide; hereditary coproporphyria and ALA dehydratase deficiency are very rare.

Clinical manifestations include the following:

1. Dysautonomia that becomes evident as abdominal pain out of proportion to clinical findings, nausea, vomiting, diarrhea or constipation, tachycardia, orthostatic hypotension, hypertension, diaphoresis, and urinary retention.
2. A motor > sensory polyneuropathy or mononeuritis multiplex often occurs, as well as an ascending flaccid paralysis resembling Guillain-Barré syndrome, which may result in fatal respiratory failure. Cranial nerves may be involved.
3. Headaches.
4. Seizures.
5. Psychosis.
6. Delirium.
7. Back and extremity pain are not unusual.

TABLE 54
Drugs and Acute Porphyria

Drugs That May Precipitate an Attack of Acute Intermittent Porphyria

Alcohol	Meprobamate
Barbiturates	Methsuximide
Carisoprodol	Methyldopa
Chloramphenicol	Methyprylon
Chlordiazepozide	Pentazocine
Chloroquine	Phenylbutazone
Dichloralphenazone	Phenytoin
Ergots	Progesterones
Estrogens	Pyralones
Eucalyptol	Sulfonamides
Glutethimide	Sylfonal
Griseofulvin	Testosterones
Imipramine	Tolbutamide
	Trional

Drugs That Do Not Exacerbate Acute Intermittent Porphyria

Ascorbic acid	Nitrofurantoin
Aspirin	Opiates
Atropine	Penicillins
B vitamins	Phenothiazines
Chloral hydrate	Promethazine
Corticosteroids	Propranolol
Digoxin	Rauwolfia alkaloids
Diphenhydramine	Scopolamine
Guanethidine	Streptomycin
Methanamine mandelate	Tetracyclines
Meclizine	Tetraethylammonium bromide
Neostigmine	

Treatment consists of avoiding precipitating factors such as drugs that activate heme biosynthesis (see Table 54), weight loss, or even skipping meals. Other prophylactic measures include high-carbohydrate diet and propranolol therapy. Acute attacks are treated initially with IV glucose, 10 to 20 g per hour; severe attacks may require IV hematin, 4 mg/kg over 10 to 12 minutes every 12 hours. Phenothiazines may be used to treat psychiatric symptoms. Abdominal symptoms respond to chlorpromazine. Opiates are used for treatment of pain. Treatment of seizures is perplexing, since all currently available anticonvulsants are porphyrinogenic, although benzodiazepines may be less likely to induce porphyria. Bromides, which are no longer available, did not have porphyrinogenic effects. New anticonvulsants that are not metabolized by the liver may be useful in this clinical setting.

REF: Kappas A, Sassa S, Galbraith RA, Nordmann Y: *The Porphyrias*. In Scriver CR et al, eds: The metabolic basis of inherited disease, ed 6, New York, 1989, McGraw Hill.

POSITRON EMISSION TOMOGRAPHY   *(see PET AND SPECT)*

POSTINFECTIOUS ENCEPHALOMYELITIS   *(see Demyelinating Disease, Encephalitis)*

POTASSIUM   *(see Electrolyte Disorders, Periodic Paralysis)*

PREGNANCY

A variety of neurologic disorders may begin or be modified by pregnancy. Conversely, the course and outcome of pregnancy can be affected by the presence of a neurologic disorder. These disorders are best considered by disease category, as follows.

I. Neuropathy.
    A. *Endometriosis:* Endometrial implants may occur along the cauda equina, roots, lumbosacral plexus, or sciatic nerve.
    B. *Bell's palsy:* Incidence increases threefold during pregnancy; the majority of cases occur in the third trimester and the first two puerperal weeks.
    C. *Carpal tunnel syndrome:* May occur transiently during pregnancy, regressing after delivery. Weakness and wasting are unusual.
    D. *Meralgia paresthetica:* Midlateral thigh numbness, tingling, or stinging pain, which is exacerbated by extending the hip when standing and relieved by sitting down. It is due to the entrapment of the lateral femoral cutaneous nerve of the

thigh. Treatment includes avoidance of excessive weight gain and, if severe, local anesthetic infiltration. It resolves within 3 months after delivery.

E. *Recurrent brachial plexus neuropathy:* May be familial or associated with menarche, pregnancy, or early puerperium. Becomes evident as severe, persistent pain and rapid onset of weakness in the arm and shoulder. As the pain diminishes, weakness increases and wasting of the shoulder girdle ensues. Improvement begins in 4 to 8 weeks; functional recovery occurs in 90% of patients within 4 years.

F. *Guillain-Barré syndrome:* Incidence and course are unaffected by pregnancy. Pregnancy is not complicated, except for possibly increased incidence of premature labor in third trimester in severe cases.

G. *Chronic inflammatory demyelinating polyradiculopathy* (CIDP): May begin during pregnancy; the relapse rate is three times greater during a pregnancy year, mostly occurring during the third trimester and postpartum period.

H. *Gestational distal polyneuropathy:* A symmetric axonal neuropathy associated with malnutrition consequent to hyperemesis.

I. *Acute intermittent porphyria:* Pregnancy may induce crisis in some patients. Most relapses occur early; more serious are those (15%) that occur in the second and third trimester or are complicated by hypertension, hyperemesis, eclampsia, and pre-existing renal disease. These cases are associated with prematurity and high rates of fetal and maternal mortality.

J. *Charcot-Marie-Tooth* disease may worsen during pregnancy.

K. *Obstetric palsies:* Compression of a peripheral nerve or nerve trunk may be caused by the fetal head, forceps, trauma, hematoma during cesarean section, or improper positioning in leg holders. The most common maternal obstetric palsy is peroneal compression, followed by femoral neuropathy, obturator neuropathy, and rarely, sciatic neuropathy or lumbosacral trunk compression. The risk of permanent weakness with recurrent maternal obstetric palsies is unknown but necessitates recognition of underlying cephalopelvic disproportion and assessment of severity of the first neuropathy.

II. Myasthenia gravis. Myasthenia may improve, stabilize, or worsen in about equal proportions during pregnancy, but there is frequent immediate postpartum exacerbation. Pregnancy-associated exacerbation is less frequent after thymectomy. Myasthenia may come to medical attention during pregnancy or the postpartum period. Magnesium sulfate, scopolamine, and large amounts of procaine are contraindicated. Care must be taken in the use of anesthesia and sedative drugs. Newborns should be observed carefully for 72 hours for neonatal myasthenia caused by passive transfer of the acetylcholine receptor antibody from the maternal circulation. There is no contraindication to breast feeding because of anticholinesterase drugs or prednisone.

III. Myotonic dystrophy. Disability remains the same or worsens during pregnancy, especially during the third trimester. Regional anesthesia is preferred. Depolarizing muscle relaxants are contraindicated. Polyhydramnios suggests fetal myotonia.

IV. Movement disorders.
  A. *Chorea gravidarum:* Occurs in <1 per 100,000 pregnancies. Most chorea occurs during the first trimester and dramatically disappears after childbirth. It may recur with subsequent pregnancies. Approximately one third of patients have had Sydenham's chorea in the past. Differential diagnosis includes acute rheumatic fever, Wilson's disease, lupus erythematosus, polycythemia, hyperthyroidism, and idiopathic hypoparathyroidism.
  B. *Wilson's disease:* The infants are healthy, although penicillamine may be hazardous to the fetus. Pyridoxine therapy, 50 to 100 mg per day, is recommended, and a reduction in penicillamine dosage to 250 mg per day for the last 6 weeks of pregnancy is recommended if cesarean section is to be performed.

V. Multiple sclerosis (MS). Gestation, labor, and delivery may be normal in MS. Relapses may or may not be more frequent. Half of all pregnancy-associated relapses or first attacks occur during the first 3 postpartum months.

VI. Cerebrovascular disease.
  A. Subarachnoid hemorrhage: Incidence during pregnancy is estimated to range from 1 to 5 per 10,000 pregnancies. Cerebral arteriovenous malformations (AVMs) and aneurysms are the most common causes. Other causes include placental abruption, DIC, anticoagulants, endocarditis and mycotic aneurysm, metastatic choriocarcinoma, eclampsia, postpartum cerebral phlebothrombosis, and spinal cord AVMs. AVMs tend to bleed during the second trimester and during childbirth. Aneurysms commonly rupture during the third trimester; the greatest risk of rebleeding occurs in the first

few weeks after initial hemorrhage or in the postpartum period. The risk that an aneurysm will bleed increases with each trimester. The decision to operate should be based on the same criteria used in nonpregnant patients. The natural history of both AVMs and aneurysms shows that both can rebleed during childbirth, with fatal results. Hyperventilation, hypothermia, and steroids have been safely used during pregnancy, but mannitol should be restricted. An untreated aneurysm is a relative contraindication to future pregnancies.

B. *Cerebral ischemia:* Overall risk is 1 in every 3000 pregnancies, making cerebral ischemia one of the most common causes of stroke in young adults. The causes of stroke include arterial occlusion (60% to 80%) and cerebral venous thrombosis (20% to 40%). Mortality rate for cerebral venous thrombosis is around 30%, and residual disability varies with the extent and site of original insult. The assessment of the pregnant patient with transient ischemic attacks or stroke is the same as that for a young person with stroke.

C. *Sheehan's syndrome:* Postpartum hypopituitarism resulting from pituitary infarction (usually the anterior pituitary) during severe shock at the time of delivery. Failure to lactate is followed by amenorrhea, hypothyroidism, and hypoadrenocorticism.

D. *Carotid–cavernous sinus fistula* may develop during the second half of pregnancy.

E. *Reversible segmental cerebral vasoconstriction* is a rare syndrome that becomes evident as headache and focal deficits.

VII. Tumors. Excluding pituitary tumors, intracranial (primary) tumors do not have an increased incidence during pregnancy. Most primary brain tumors enlarge during pregnancy and shrink again in the postpartum period. This condition appears to result from the intrapartum increase in intravascular volume or tumor hormone dependence. Therefore symptoms or signs may be more apparent during the second half of pregnancy. Although slow-growing tumors can be resected in the postpartum period, malignant gliomas and many posterior fossa tumors require prompt surgery. Choriocarcinomas frequently metastasize to the brain.

VIII. Headache.

A. *Pseudotumor cerebri* has the same incidence during pregnancy as in the nonpregnant, age-matched population. Symptoms commonly begin in the first half of pregnancy.

B. *Muscle contraction or tension headache* is the most common.

C. *Migraines* may first become evident during pregnancy, usually during the first trimester. Approximately 75% of migraineurs improve or are free of headaches during pregnancy, especially during the second and third trimester; in the remainder of patients the condition fails to improve or worsens. Treatment is limited to acetaminophen therapy and avoidance of precipitants during pregnancy. Low-dose narcotics may be used with caution. Preventive therapy should be avoided. Biofeedback is a safe adjunctive therapy.

IX. Epilepsy. The rate of spontaneous abortions is comparable to that for the general population. It is unclear whether obstetric complications (pre-eclampsia, placental abruption, and premature labor) are increased in pregnant women with epilepsy. Perinatal mortality rate is increased 1.2-fold to threefold. These patients may have a normal vaginal delivery but have an increased rate of prolonged labor and bleeding at delivery. A convulsive seizure occurs during labor in 1% to 2% of women with epilepsy and within 24 hours postpartum in another 1% to 2%. The probability of a seizure during labor and the first postpartum day is nine times greater than the average probability of a seizure during pregnancy. It is advisable to give folate supplementation before conception and to administer monotherapy that is adjusted to the lowest effective level to avoid unnecessary fetal exposure. Total antiepileptic drug (AED) concentration declines as pregnancy progresses because of dynamic changes in plasma protein binding. Therefore it is recommended to measure free AED concentration and make appropriate dose adjustments on the basis of patient clinical condition, seizure frequency, and free AED concentration. If AED dosages are increased during pregnancy, they must be returned to prepregnancy levels during the initial weeks of puerperium to avoid toxic effects as a rebound increase in AED levels occurs. Drug levels should be checked periodically for at least the first 2 months after delivery.

More than 90% of women with epilepsy who receive AEDs deliver normal children free of birth defects. Both prospective and retrospective studies have identified unequivocal risks for major malformations and minor anomalies in a small but significant percentage of fetuses (6% to 8%) exposed in utero to AEDs (phenytoin, carbamazepine, valproate, and phenobarbital). Risks to the fetus are probably higher when AEDs are used in combination and when there is a family history of birth defects.

X. Eclampsia. Onset of hypertension, proteinuria, edema, oliguria, multi-organ failure, and seizures occurring after 20 weeks of gestation, usually in a young primigravida. Eclampsia is also associated with chronic hypertension and renal disease. Maternal mortality rates range from 0% to 14%. The use of magnesium for seizure control in eclampsia is controversial, but diazepam or phenytoin are also effective. Control of hypertension and fluid management are required. Delivery of the fetus and placenta is the definitive treatment for eclampsia occurring prepartum or intrapartum.

REF: Delgado-Escueta AV, Janz D: *Neurology* 42(suppl 5):8-11, 1992.
Donaldson JO: *Neurology of pregnancy*, ed 2, Philadelphia, 1989, WB Saunders.
Fox MW, Harms RW, Davis DH: *Mayo Clin Proc* 65:1595-1618, 1990.
Goldstein PJ, Stern BJ: *Neurological disorders of pregnancy*, ed 2, (revised), Mount Kisco, 1992, Futura.
Hiilesmaa VK: *Neurology* 42(suppl 5):149-160, 1992.

PRIMIDONE   (see Epilepsy)

PROGRESSIVE MULTIFOCAL LEUKOENCEPHALOPATHY   (see AIDS)

PROGRESSIVE SUPRANUCLEAR PALSY   (see Parkinsonism)

PSEUDOBULBAR PALSY

Most lower brainstem nuclei are bilaterally innervated. Unilateral involvement of supranuclear pathways, therefore, may not produce symptoms. Bilateral involvement of corticobulbar fibers and frontal efferents subserving emotional expression, which pass through the genu of the internal capsule and the medial cerebral peduncles, results in pseudobulbar palsy. This should be distinguished from nuclear involvement (see Bulbar Palsy). In pseudobulbar palsy decreased voluntary movement and spastic hyperreflexia of the involved muscles are present. Thus gag and jaw jerk reflexes may be hyperactive, even though the patient is unable to swallow or chew. Frequently there is a spontaneous release of emotional responses, such as crying or laughing with little or no provocation. Although a variety of lesions (demyelinating disease or motor neuron disease) can interrupt the corticobulbar and anterior frontopontomedullary fibers, infarction is most common. Dementia is frequently present in patients with pseudobulbar palsy, except those with motor neuron disease.

Frontal release signs (grasp, palmomental, suck, snout, rooting, and glabellar reflexes) may be prominent. These should be interpreted with caution, since many normal elderly persons exhibit palmomental and snout reflexes.

A syndrome similar to pseudobulbar palsy may occur with bilateral involvement of the opercular cortex, producing the anterior operculum syndrome *(Foix-Chavany-Marie syndrome)*. It differs from classic pseudobulbar palsy in that emotional symptoms are rare, and there is loss of voluntary control of facial, pharyngeal, lingual, masticatory, or ocular muscles with retention of reflexive and automatic movements in these muscle groups.

Successful treatment of pseudobulbar palsy has been reported with regimens of amitriptyline 50 to 75 mg per day, levodopa 0.6 to 1.5 g per day, and amantadine 100 mg per day.

PSEUDOMOTOR CEREBRI

Also called idiopathic intracranial hypertension, diagnosis of pseudotumor cerebri (PTC) is based on the following modified Dandy criteria for diagnosis:

1. Signs and symptoms of increased intracranial pressure.
2. Absence of localizing findings on neurologic examination.
3. Absence of deformity, displacement, or obstruction of the ventricular system and otherwise normal neurodiagnostic studies other than increased CSF pressure.
4. Awake and alert patient.
5. No other cause of increased intracranial pressure is present.

More than 90% of patients with PTC are obese, and more than 90% are women. Mean age at diagnosis is about 30 years. Symptoms of PTC include headache (94%), transient visual obscuration (68%), pulsatile intracranial noises (58%), photopsias (54%), retrobulbar pain (44%), diplopia (38%), vision loss (30%), and pain on eye movement (22%). Signs are mainly visual and include optic disc edema, cranial nerve VI palsies (10% to 20%), contrast sensitivity deficit (50% to 70%), color vision loss (20%), and visual field loss (in one study, present at initial visit in at least one eye in 96% of patients with Goldmann perimetry and in 92% with automated perimetry; 25% of this visual loss is mild and unlikely to be noticed by the patient). Blind-spot enlargement is always present with papilledema. Neuroimaging studies show normal morphologic characteristics of brain in patients with PTC.

The cause of PTC is unknown. Many disorders have been associated with PTC, including hypertension, endocrinopathies, vitamin A intoxication, pregnancy, and recent use of medications such as tetracycline, indomethacin, nalidixic acid, oral contraceptives, lithium, and corticosteroids. Systemic disorders linked with PTC include systemic lupus erythematosus, hyperthyroidism, iron deficiency, and venous sinus thrombosis.

General principles of management include close follow-up to detect progressive visual field loss and to stress the importance of weight loss. Regular ophthalmologic follow-up examinations of visual fields, stereophotographs of the optic discs, and visual acuity and contrast sensitivity testing are essential. Initial treatment is often with acetazolamide, which is generally well tolerated, but side effects include metabolic alkalosis, parasthesias of the extremities, liver dysfunction, and allergic reactions. Furosemide therapy has also been used. Repeated lumbar puncture, used in the past, is not recommended. Remission in some cases may occur after lumbar puncture. Therapy with corticosteroids provides symptomatic relief but increases weight and is not often useful for prolonged treatment. An algorithm for treatment based on the presence of visual loss follows.

PERIMETRY
No Visual Loss

1. Weight loss.
2. Symptomatic headache treatment (carbonic anhydrase inhibitor or loop diuretic).

Visual Loss

1. Weight loss.
2. Headache treatment.

If progression:

3. Optic nerve sheath fenestration.
4. As last resort, consider lumbar-peritoneal shunting.

REF: Giuseffi V et al: *Neurology* 41:239–244, 1991.

Wall M: *Neurol Clin* 9(1):73–95, 1991.

Wall M, George D: *Brain* 114:115–180, 1991.

PTOSIS
DEFICIENCY OF LEVATOR TONUS

I. Congenital ptosis.
  A. Isolated.
  B. With double elevator palsy.
  C. Anomalous synkinesis (including Gunn jaw winking).
  D. Lid or orbital tumor (hemangioma, dermoid).
  E. Neurofibromatosis.
  F. Blepharophimosis syndromes.
  G. First branchial arch syndromes (Hallerman-Streiff, Treacher Collins).
  H. Neonatal myasthenia.
II. Ptosis resulting from myopathy.
  A. Myasthenia gravis—ptosis may be variable and asymmetric. May see Cogan's lid twitch sign. Improves with edrophonium.
  B. Myopathy restricted to levator palpebrae superioris or including external ophthalmoplegia.
  C. Oculopharyngeal muscular dystrophy.
  D. Myotonic dystrophy.
  E. Polymyositis.
  F. Aplastic levator muscle.
  G. Dysthyroidism.
  H. Chronic progressive external ophthalmoplegia.
  I. Topical corticosteroid eye drops.
  J. Levator dehiscence-disinsertion syndrome. Resulting from aging, inflammation, surgery, trauma, or ocular allergy.
III. Ptosis resulting from sympathetic denervation (see Horner's Syndrome).
IV. Ptosis resulting from third-nerve lesions.
  A. Nuclear lesions involving the levator subnucleus produce severe bilateral ptosis, medial rectus weakness, skew deviation if the IV nerve is involved, or upgaze paresis and pupillary dilatation if entire third-nerve nucleus is involved.
  B. Peripheral third-nerve lesions produce unilateral ptosis with mydriasis, and ophthalmoplegia. Isolated ptosis is rare.
V. Pseudoptosis.
  A. Trachoma.

B. Ptosis adiposis.
C. Blepharochalasis.
D. Plexiform neuroma.
E. Amyloid infiltration.
F. Inflammation resulting from allergy, chalazion, blepharitis, conjunctivitis.
G. Hemangioma.
H. Duane's retraction syndrome.
I. Microphthalmos phthisis bulbi.
J. Enopthalmos.
K. Pathologic lid retraction on opposite side.
L. Chronic Bell's palsy.
M. Hypertropia.
N. Decreased mental status.
O. Hysterical.

REF: Glaser JS: *Neuro-ophthalmology*, Philadelphia, 1990, Lippincott.

PUPIL

Pupils are examined in both light and darkness, with attention to size, shape, and reactivity to a bright light.

Bilateral dilation (mydriasis) may be produced by the following:

1. Drugs (see Table 55).
2. Emotional state (startle, fear, pain).
3. Thyrotoxicosis.
4. Ciliospinal reflex.
5. Bilateral blindness resulting from severe visual system involvement anterior to the optic chiasm.
6. Parinaud's syndrome.
7. Seizures.
8. During rostral-caudal deterioration caused by supratentorial mass lesions.

Bilateral constriction (miosis) may be produced by the following:

1. Near triad (accommodation, convergence, miosis).
2. Old age.
3. Drugs (Table 55).
4. Pontine lesions.
5. Argyll Robertson pupils.

TABLE 55
Drug Effects on the Pupils

Constriction (Miosis)	Dilation (Mydriasis)
Systemic	
Narcotics	Anticholinergics
Morphine and opium alkaloids	Atropine
	Belladonna
Meperidine and congeners	Scopolamine
Methadone and congeners	Propantheline
Propoxyphene	Jimsonweed
Barbiturates	Nightshade
Diphenoxylate	Tricyclic antidepressants
Chloral hydrate	Trihexyphenidyl
Phenoxybenzamine	Benztropine
Dibenzyline	Antihistamines
Phentolamine	Diphenydramine
Tolazoline	Chlorpheniramine
Guanethidine	Phenothiazines
Bretylium	Glutethimide
Reserpine	Amphetamines
MAO inhibitors	Cocaine
Alpha-methyldopa	Ephedrine
Bethanidine	Epinephrine
Thymoxamine	Norepinephrine
Indoramin	Ethanol
Meprobamate	Botulinum toxin
Cholinergics	Snake venom
Edrophonium	Barracuda poisoning
Neostigmine	Tyramine
Pyridostigmine	Hemicholinium
Physostigmine	Hypermagnesemia
Cholinesterase inhibitor pesticides	Thiopental
	Lysergic acid diethylamide
Phencyclidine	Fenfluramine (patients receiving reserpine)
Thallium	
Lidocaine and related agents (extradural thoracic anesthesia)	
Marijuana	
Phenothiazines	

Continued.

TABLE 55—cont'd
Drug Effects on the Pupils

Constriction (Miosis)	Dilation (Mydriasis)
Local	
Miotics	Mydriatics and cycloplegics
Pilocarpine	Phenylephrine
Carbachol	Hydroxyamphetamine
Methacholine	Epinephrine
Physostigmine	Cocaine
Neostigmine	Eucatropine
Isoflurophate	Atropine
Echothiophate	Homatropine
Demecarium	Scopolamine
Aceclidine	Cyclopentolate
	Tropicamide
	Oxyphenonium

Adapted from Thurston SE, Leigh RJ. In Henning RJ, Jackson DL, eds: *Handbook of critical care neurology and neurosurgery*, New York, 1985, Praeger.

Anisocoria, or unequal pupil size, can be an important localizing sign. A difference of <1 mm exists in approximately 20% of the normal population; >1 mm, in as much as 5%. The asymmetry remains constant in light and dark. Drugs and toxins, including eye drops, may cause constriction or dilation of pupils (Table 55), which is usually symmetric unless agents are applied locally in one eye. Causes of significant anisocoria may be determined on clinical and pharmacologic bases using Table 56.

Causes of episodic anisocoria include the following:

1. Parasympathetic paresis (incipient uncal herniation, seizure, migraine).
2. Parasympathetic hyperactivity (cyclic oculomotor paresis).
3. Sympathetic paresis (cluster headache [paratrigeminal neuralgia]).
4. Sympathetic hyperactivity (Claude-Bernard syndrome following neck trauma).
5. Sympathetic dysfunction with alternating anisocoria (cervical spinal cord lesions).
6. Benign unilateral pupillary dilation (involved pupil has normal light and near responses).

TABLE 56
Characteristics of Pupils Encountered in Neuro-ophthalmology

	General Characteristics	Responses to Light and Near Stimuli	Room Condition in Which Anisocoria is Greater	Response to Mydriatics	Response to Miotics	Response to Pharmacologic Agents
Essential anisocoria	Round, regular	Both brisk	No change	Dilates	Constricts	Normal and rarely needed
Horner's syndrome	Small, round, unilateral	Both brisk	Darkness	Dilates	Constricts	Cocaine 4%, poor dilation; paredrine 1%, no dilation if third-order neuron damage
Tonic pupil syndrome (Holmes-Adie syndrome)	Usually larger* in bright light; sector pupil palsy, vermiform movement; unilateral or, less often, bilateral	Absent to light, tonic to near; tonic redilation	Light	Dilates	Constricts	Pilocarpine 0.1% or 0.125% constricts; mecholyl 2.5% constricts

Argyll Robertson pupils	Small, irregular, bilateral	Poor to light, better to near	No change	Poor	Constricts	
Midbrain pupils	Mid-dilated; may be oval; bilateral	Poor to light, better to near (or fixed to both)	No change	Dilates	Constricts	
Pharmacologically dilated pupils	Very large,† round, unilateral	Fixed‡	Light		No‡	Pilocarpine 1% does not constrict
Oculomotor palsy (nonvascular)	Mid-dilated (6–7 mm), unilateral (rarely bilateral)	Fixed	Light	Dilates	Constricts	

From Glaser JS: *Neuro-ophthalmology,* Philadelphia, 1989, Lippincott.

*Tonic pupil may appear smaller following prolonged near-effort or in dim illumination; affected pupil is initially large, but with passing time gradually becomes smaller.

†Atropinized pupils have diameters of 8 mm to 9 mm. No tonic, midbrain, or oculomotor palsy pupil ever is this large.

‡Pupils may be weakly reactive, depending on interim after instillation.

Afferent pupillary defects (Figure 39), (Marcus-Gunn pupil), resulting from a lesion of the optic nerve. Resting pupil sizes are normal.
Both direct and consensual pupillary responses are decreased with bright
illumination of the involved side, whereas both responses are normal
with illumination of the normal side. When alternately stimulating
each eye ("swinging flashlight test"), both pupils dilate with stimulation

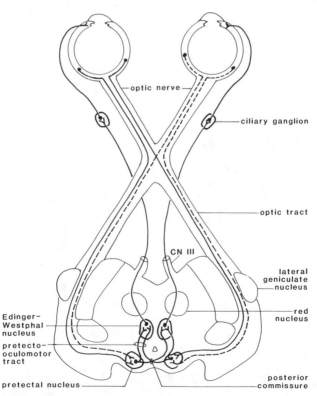

FIGURE 39
Pupillary light reflex pathways.

on the abnormal side, and both constrict with stimulation on the normal side.

The *near reflex* should be tested whenever pupils react poorly to light. Have the patient fixate a distant target, then quickly fixate his own fingertip held immediately in front of his nose. Light-near dissociation may occur in the following:

1. Severe anterior visual system dysfunction (such as severe glaucoma, bilateral optic neuropathy)
2. Neurosyphilis (Argyll Robertson pupil)—associated with miosis, irregular pupils, poor dilation, and usually, relatively normal vision.
3. Adie's tonic pupil.
4. Rostral dorsal midbrain (Parinaud's syndrome).
5. Aberrant III nerve regeneration.
6. Diabetes (out of proportion to any retinopathy).
7. Amyloidosis.
8. Myotonic dystrophy.

REF: Loewenfeld IE: *The pupil: anatomy, physiology and clinical applications, vol 1*, Ames, Ia, 1993, Iowa State University.

PYRIDOXINE DEFICIENCY   (see Epilepsy, Nutritional Deficiency Syndromes)

RABIES   (see Encephalitis)

RACHISCHISIS   (see Developmental Malformations)

RADIAL NERVE   (see Peripheral Nerve)

RADIATION INJURY

Injury to the nervous system occurs either as a result of treatment of CNS tumors or when nervous tissue falls into the field of treatment of another organ system. The five major manifestations of radiation injury are outlined as follows.

I. Cerebral injury.
   A. *Acute encephalopathy* occurs during the first few days of radiotherapy with headache, fever, nausea, depressed sensorium, and worsening of previous focal deficits. It is more frequent and severe in patients with large brain masses or those receiving

daily dose fractions greater than 300 cGy of whole-brain ir-radiation. It is probably caused by increases in pre-existing cerebral edema and responds well to increased corticosteroid dose. It may be prevented by use of corticosteroid 24 to 72 hours before radiotherapy.

B. *Early delayed encephalopathy* occurs 1 to 4 months after ir-radiation, becomes evident as headache, somnolence, nausea, irritability, fever, and transient papilledema, and usually re-solves after several weeks. It occurs in 40% to 60% of pediatric patients with leukemia who are receiving 1800 to 2400 cGy of prophylactic whole brain irradiation. Corticosteroids may be beneficial. This syndrome may be due to damaged myelin and glia.

C. *Focal cerebral necrosis* may develop several months to 10 years after focal or whole brain irradiation and becomes evident as a subacutely evolving mass lesion. Frequency is 3% to 5% after receiving 5000 cGy of radiation. "Tolerable" dose esti-mates vary (up to 6500 to 7000 cGy), but above the critical exposure level the frequency increases markedly. Peritumoral edema may predispose to injury, and corticosteroids may be protective. CT or MRI show edema and a patchy or ring-enhancing mass lesion. PET scanning may help differentiate cerebral necrosis from tumor recurrence. Corticosteroids fre-quently cause improvement, albeit temporary. Radiation ne-crosis occurs around the tumor and primarily involves the white matter, mostly sparing of cortex and deep gray structures, with demyelination, loss of oligodendrocytes, axonal loss and swelling, calcification, fibrillary gliosis, and mononuclear perivascular infiltrate with extensive vascular injury.

D. *Diffuse cerebral injury*, the most frequent (2% to 19%) delayed effect of radiation therapy, occurs in adults with primary brain tumors receiving 4000 to 6000 cGy of whole brain irradiation and becomes evident as moderate to severe cortical dysfunc-tion, progressive dementia, and gait disturbance. On patho-logic study cerebral atrophy, diffuse demyelination, and spon-giform changes with sparing of axons and blood vessels are present.

E. *Leukoencephalopathy* occurs 4 to 24 months after CNS irra-diation, primarily in children who have received radiation therapy and chemotherapy (especially methotrexate). Initial signs include memory, attentional, and visuospatial difficulties (especially in children younger than 4 or 5 years of age); ataxia; and focal motor deficits. CT or MRI shows enlarged ventricles, widened sulci, areas of calcification (especially basal ganglia), and areas of decreased density or signal. Pathologic study shows multifocal white matter destruction, especially in the centrum semiovale and periventricular white matter, dystrophic calcification of the lenticular nuclei, and mineralizing microangiopathy.

II. Spinal cord injury.

A. *Transient myelopathy*, the most common radiation-induced spinal injury, usually occurs 1 to 30 months after completion of radiotherapy, with peak onset at 4 to 6 months. There is a positive correlation with radiation dose greater than 3500 to 4400 cGy. Lhermitte's sign (paresthesias radiating down the spine and limbs, precipitated by neck flexion), is often present. Myelopathic signs are usually absent. CT, MRI, and myelography results are normal. The syndrome resolves gradually over 1 to 9 months without risk of delayed, severe radiation myelopathy.

Delayed progressive myelopathy has a peak time of onset of 9 to 18 months after radiotherapy and a reported frequency of 1% to 2%. Risk is mostly correlated with the dose and dose schedule; risk is less than 5% with total doses of 4500 cGy in daily fractions of 180 cGy. Delayed progressive myelopathy usually begins with hypoesthesias or dysesthesias in lower extremities, then weakness and sphincter dysfunction. The level of dysfunction ascends up to the area irradiated. Symptoms progress over weeks to months, with paraplegia or quadriplegia in about 50% of those affected by this syndrome. Results of imaging studies are usually normal but may show focal or diffuse fusiform spinal cord enlargement. CSF is usually normal but may show increased levels of protein or white blood cells. The clinical picture may stabilize spontaneously or improve temporarily with dexamethasone therapy. Pathologic study shows a coalescing foci of demyelination and axonal degeneration more severe in white than in gray matter, especially in the posterior columns and superficial lateral tracts.

C. *Motor neuron syndrome.* Beginning 4 to 14 months after radiotherapy, this rare syndrome becomes evident as subacute, diffuse leg weakness, atrophy, fasciculations, depressed deep tendon reflexes, and flexor planter responses without sensory or sphincter involvement. Symptoms gradually progress over several months, then stabilize without improvement. Results of EMG show diffuse denervation. CSF may be normal or have slight increase in protein level. This syndrome may result from damage to lumbosacral anterior horn cells, motor axons, or nerve roots.

III. Peripheral nerve. Radiation plexopathy of the brachial or lumbosacral plexuses must be distinguished from recurrent tumor. Radiation plexopathies tend to have less pain, more weakness, and myokymia on EMG. Contrast-enhanced CT or MRI helps differentiate these conditions.

IV. Cerebrovascular disease. Extracranial carotid disease, which comes to medical attention with transient ischemic attacks or strokes, may develop 6 months to many years (median, 19 years) after radiation therapy. Occlusive disease of the intracranial arteries follows irradiation of optic gliomas, pituitary, or suprasellar tumors (2 to 20 years later; median, 5 years later). The most frequent finding on arteriography is narrowing or occlusion of the supraclinoid internal carotid artery, and two thirds of patients may show a "moyamoya" pattern.

V. Radiation-induced tumors. In order of decreasing frequency, meningiomas, sarcomas, and gliomas may occur after radiation therapy. Meningiomas have a latency of 15 to 50 years after irradiation, and gliomas may develop around 10 years after irradiation. Diagnosis of a radiation-induced malignancy depends on the following:

1. The second tumor should occur within the field of radiation.
2. There should be a significant delay between end of irradiation and appearance of the secondary tumor.
3. The primary and secondary tumors must have different histologic features.
4. There should be no family history of neurocutaneous syndromes.

REF: Dropcho EJ: *Neurol Clin* 9(4):969–988, 1991.

Duffner PK, Cohen ME: *Neurol Clin* 9(2):479–495, 1991.

Gutin PH, Leibel SA, Sheline GE, eds: *Radiation injury to the nervous system*, New York, 1991, Raven.

RADICULOPATHY (see also Dermatomes, Myotomes)

Radiculopathy is usually manifested by radiating pain, weakness, loss of deep tendon reflexes, and sensory changes in a segmental distribution. Neck or lower back pain and stiffness are common in cervical and lumbar radiculopathies. The symptoms are aggravated by sneezing, coughing, and straining with defecation or by neck or trunk movement. Bed rest usually offers relief. On examination straight leg raising sign may be present in cases of lumbar radiculopathy. Crossed straight leg raising usually indicates a larger lesion. An isolated root lesion may result in a smaller area of sensory disturbance than expected because of dermatomal overlap. Hyporeflexia is restricted to the involved root level. Weaknesses may occur in the appropriate myotomal distribution and may indicate a larger lesion with greater anterior root involvement. Central lumbar lesions may result in a cauda equina syndrome.

Diagnostic studies should include plain radiographs with oblique views. Nerve conduction studies and EMG may identify evidence of denervation in a root distribution and exclude more peripheral lesions. The use of myelogram followed by CT is being supplanted in many centers by MRI.

Although herniated intervertebral disk material is the most common cause of radiculopathy, other mass lesions and structural abnormalities should be excluded. Central disk herniation is relatively uncommon as a cause of radiculopathy. Differential diagnosis includes tumors, epidural abscess, rheumatoid spondylosis, brachial or lumbar plexopathy, and peripheral neuropathy.

Treatment of disk disease should begin conservatively with bed rest, traction, and nonsteroidal anti-inflammatory agents. Surgical decompression is indicated when symptoms are unresponsive to medical therapy, when there is progressive weakness, or when central herniation results in myelopathy or a cauda equina syndrome.

COMMON CERVICAL ROOT SYNDROMES

1. C5 or C6 radiculopathy (C4-5 or C5-6 disk space, respectively): Pain and sensory loss in shoulder, upper arm, radial and anterior aspect of forearm, and first 1½ digits. Hyporeflexia in biceps and brachioradialis. Weakness in clavicular head of pectoralis, supraspinatus, infraspinatus, deltoid, biceps, and brachioradialis.
2. C7 radiculopathy (C6-7 disk space, most common level for disk herniation): Pain and sensory loss in posterior arm and third and fourth digits. Hyporeflexia in triceps. Weakness in triceps and wrist extensors.
3. C8 radiculopathy (C7-T1 disk space): Pain and sensory loss in medial forearm and hand and in fifth digit. Hyporeflexia in finger flexors. Weakness in intrinsic hand muscles. Ipsilateral Horner's syndrome.

COMMON LUMBAR ROOT SYNDROMES

1. L4 radiculopathy (L3-4 disk space): Pain and sensory loss in hip and anterolateral thigh (pain), knee, anteromedial leg, medial foot, and possibly, great toe. Hyporeflexia-quadriceps (patellar). Weakness in quadriceps, anterior tibialis, and sartorius.
2. L5 radiculopathy (L4-5 disk space): Pain and sensory loss in hip and lateral thigh (mainly pain), anterolateral leg, dorsum of foot, and medial toes (including great toe). Hyporeflexia, possibly patellar. Weakness in peroneus, toe extensors, anterior tibialis, and gluteus medius and minimus.
3. S1 radiculopathy (L5-S1 disk space): Pain and sensory loss in buttock and posterior thigh (mainly pain), posterolateral leg, lateral foot, lateral toes, and heel. Hyporeflexia in ankle (Achilles). Weakness in hamstrings, gluteus maximus, and plantar flexors of foot and toes. S1-5 radiculopathies (see Cauda Equina).

REF: Brazis PW, Masdeu JC, Biller J: *Localization in clinical neurology*, ed 2, Boston, 1990, Little Brown.

RAMSAY-HUNT *(see Facial Nerve, Zoster)*

READING DISORDERS *(see Alexia)*

REFLEXES *(see also Myotomes)*

Evaluate latency of response, degree of activity, and duration of the contraction. Reflexes should be both observed and palpated. Compare right and left sides. In general, reflexes are not pathologic if they are symmetric unless they are absent or 4+ (see Table 57).

TABLE 57
Grading of Muscle Stretch Reflexes

0	Absent, abnormal
1+	Diminished, may or may not be abnormal
2+	Normal
3+	Increased, may or may not be abnormal
4+	Markedly increased, abnormal. May be associated with clonus

Hyporeflexia results from dysfunction of any part of the reflex arc. Conditions include neuropathy, radiculopathy, tabes dorsalis, syringomyelia, intramedullary tumors, and spinal motor neuron dysfunction. Bilateral hyporeflexia is the hallmark of neuropathies. Isolated, unilateral absent reflexes suggest radiculopathy. Hyporeflexia may occur in late stages of primary muscle diseases because of loss of muscle mass. Areflexia with rapidly progressive weakness and only mild sensory loss is the hallmark of Guillain-Barré syndrome. Hyporeflexia is seen transiently in acute upper motor neuron lesions such as cerebral infarction or spinal cord compression (spinal shock). Prolongation of both the contraction and relaxation times ("hung-up" reflex) is seen with hypothyroidism. This prolongation is most evident in the knee jerks. Areflexia may be a component of Adie's syndrome (see Pupil) (see also Hypotonic Infant).

Hyperreflexia usually results from an upper motor neuron lesion with loss of corticospinal inhibition. The extrapyramidal system may also play a role. Involvement may occur anywhere from the cortical Betz cell to just proximal to the spinal cord motor neuron. Unilateral hyperreflexia results from a unilateral lesion anywhere along the corticospinal tract, most commonly in the cerebral hemispheres or brainstem. Bilateral hyperreflexia occurs more commonly with myelopathy but also occurs with bilateral cerebral hemisphere or brainstem involvement. Symmetric, 3+ reflexes in the absence of clonus, Babinski, Tromner's, or Hoffmann's signs, or weakness and with a normal result of neurologic examination is usually benign. Reflexes are variable (usually normal) with extrapyramidal system dysfunction. Reflexes are normal, slightly decreased, or pendular with cerebellar tract dysfunction (see also Rigidity, Spasticity).

"*Pathologic reflexes*" (pyramidal tract reflexes) indicate upper motor neuron dysfunction. The extensor plantar response (Babinski's sign) consists of dorsiflexion of the great toe and fanning of the remaining toes on stimulating the plantar surface of the foot. Hoffmann and Tromner signs are elicited by "flicking" the index or middle finger down or up, respectively, producing flexion of the thumb; they may be normal if present bilaterally, especially if reflexes are 3+ and symmetric. Ankle clonus is the continuing rapid flexion and extension of the foot elicited by forcibly and quickly dorsiflexing the foot. Pyramidal tract reflexes are normally present in infants (see Child Neurology).

Segmental muscle stretch and cutaneous reflexes are listed in Table 58.

REFLEX SYMPATHETIC DYSTROPHY *(see Pain)*

TABLE 58

Segmental Muscle Stretch and Cutaneous Reflexes

Reflex	Level	Nerve
Muscle Stretch ("Deep Tendon") Reflexes		
Jaw (masseter and temporal muscle)	CNV	Mandibular branch
Biceps	C5, 6	Musculocutaneous
Brachioradialis	C5, 6	Radial
Pectoral major	C5, 6, 7	Lateral pectoral
Triceps	C6, *7*, 8	Radial
Finger flexors	C*8*	Medial (ulnar)
Adductor	L2, *3*, 4	Obturator
Quadriceps (patellar, knee jerks)	L2, *3*, 4	Femoral
Internal hamstring	L4, *5*, S1	Sciatic
External hamstring	L5, S*1*	Sciatic
Gastrocnemius-soleus (Achilles, ankle jerks)	L5, S*1, 2*	Tibial
Cutaneous ("Superficial") Reflexes		
Corneal	Pons	CN V (afferent), VII (efferent)
Pharyngeal Gag reflex	Medulla	CN IX (afferent), X (efferent)
Upper abdominal	T6-9	
Middle abdominal	T9-11	
Lower abdominal	T11-L1	
Cremasteric	L1, 2	Femoral (afferent), genitofemoral (efferent)
Plantar	L5, S1, 2	Tibial
Anal	S3, 4, 5	Pudendal
Bulbocavernosus	S3, 4	Pudendal, pelvic autonomics

REFSUM'S DISEASE *(see Neuropathy)*

RENAL DISEASE *(see Dialysis, Uremia)*

RESPIRATION *(see Coma, Herniation, Hyperventilation)*

RESPIRATORY ACIDOSIS *(see Electrolyte Disorders)*

RESPIRATORY ALKALOSIS *(see Electrolyte Disorders)*

RESTLESS LEGS SYNDROME *(EKBOM SYNDROME)*

Restless legs syndrome is characterized by ill-defined, deep, "crawling" paresthesias in the lower legs, thighs, and occasionally, the arms; it is usually bilateral and occurs especially while at rest or during drowsiness, resulting in insomnia. There is a strong impulse to move or walk, to avoid the sensations. It is usually intermittent and lasts from minutes to hours. There is frequently an overlap between the restless legs syndrome and periodic movements of sleep (nocturnal myoclonic movements consisting of discrete, brief, repetitive flexion at the hips, knees, and thighs during light sleep). There may be a familial predisposition. Some similarities exist between this syndrome and growing pains in children.

A variety of conditions have been described in association with restless legs syndrome, including the following.

Uremia.	Chronic obstructive pulmonary disease.
Pregnancy.	Carcinoma.
Iron deficiency anemia.	Diabetes.
Exposure to cold.	Acute intermittent porphyria.
Parkinson's disease.	Amyloidosis.
Vitamin deficiencies.	Caffeine.
Hyperlipidemia.	Barbiturate withdrawal.
Prochlorperazine.	

Treatment involves correcting the underlying condition. Diazepam, clonazepam, baclofen, dopamine agonists (levodopa and bromocriptine), carbamazepine, propoxyphene, and amitriptyline have been used with varying success.

REF: Ekbom KA: *Neurology* 10:388, 1960.

Mahowald MW, Ettinger MG: *J Clin Neurophysiol* 7:119–143, 1990.

Walters AS, Hening WA, Chokroverty S: *Mov Disord* 6:105–110, 1991.

RETINA AND UVEAL TRACT   *(see also Uveitis)*

I. Systemic and neurologic disorders associated with retinal pigmentary degeneration.
   A. Typical retinitis pigmentosa changes include early-onset nyctalopia, progressive visual loss, bone spicules, narrowing of retinal arterioles, and electroretinogram (ERG) changes. They may be associated with the following:
      1. Myotonic dystrophy (rarely).
      2. Leber's congenital amaurosis.
      3. Senear-Loken disease (Leber's + juvenile nephronophthisis).
      4. Friedreich's ataxia (may also rarely be associated with optic atrophy and deafness).
      5. Spielmeyer-Vogt disease.
      6. Neonatal and childhood adrenoleukodystrophy.
      7. Usher's syndrome (vestibulocochlear dysfunction, mutism).
      8. Pelizaeus-Merzbacher disease (mental retardation, ataxia).
      9. Hallgren's disease (mental retardation, ataxia, deafness).
   B. Atypical central and peripheral retinal pigmentary changes with variable degrees of visual impairment. The presumed mechanism in storage diseases is disruption of pigment epithelial function by accumulated metabolic material with secondary retinal receptor degeneration. Primary rod cone dystrophy may exist in the first four of the following syndromes.
      1. Laurence-Moon-Biedl (hypogenitalism, mental retardation, polydactyly).
      2. Biemond (hypogenitalism, mental retardation, iris coloboma).
      3. Alström (hypogenitalism, deafness, diabetes mellitus).
      4. Bassen-Kornzweig (abetalipoproteinemia, ataxia, acanthocytosis).
      5. Refsum's disease (polyneuropathy, ataxia).

      6. Sjögren-Larsson syndrome (ichthyosis, spastic paresis, mental retardation).

      7. Amalric-Dialinos syndrome (deafness).

      8. Cockayne's syndrome (dwarfism, neuropathy, deafness).

      9. Hallervorden-Spatz syndrome (neuropathy, basal ganglia degeneration).

     10. Alport's syndrome (nephritis, hearing loss).

     11. Hurler's (mucopolysaccharidosis [MPS] I), Hunter's (MPS II), Sanfilippo's (MPS III), and Scheie's disease (MPS V).

C. Postinflammatory.

    1. Congenital and acquired syphilis.

    2. Congenital rubella (German measles)—"salt and pepper fundus."

    3. Congenital rubeola (measles).

D. Avitaminoses and vitamin metabolism disorders.

    1. Pellagra.

    2. Vitamin B_{12} metabolism disorder associated with aminoaciduria.

E. Toxic.

    1. Chlorpromazine.

    2. Thioridazine.

    3. Indomethacin.

II. Hereditary cerebromacular dystrophies.

A. With cherry red spot of the macula.

    1. Sphingolipidoses—Tay-Sachs, Niemann-Pick, Gaucher's, metachromatic leukodystrophy (infantile form), Sandhoff's.

    2. Mucolipidoses—GM_1 gangliosidosis, Farber's syndrome.

    3. Mucolipidosis I.

    4. Mucopolysaccharidoses—Hurler's (MPS I), MPS VII.

    5. Goldberg's disease.

B. Without cherry red spot.

    1. Ceroid lipofuscinoses—Jansky-Bielschowsky disease.

    2. Batten-Mayou, Spielmeyer-Vogt disease.

    3. Kufs-Hallervorden.

III. CNS vasculitides.

All vasculitides may involve the retinal circulation with variable manifestations (arterial occlusive retinopathy, hemorrhages, retinal infiltrates, and the like).

IV. Phakomatoses.

A. Vascular malformations of the choroid or retina and the CNS.

    1. Von Hippel-Lindau syndrome (retinal angiomas and cerebellar hemangioblastomas).

    2. Sturge-Weber syndrome (choroidal hemangioma, parieto-occipital arteriovenous malformations [AVMs]).
    3. Wyburn-Mason syndrome (AVMs in the retina and brainstem).
    4. Retinal cavernous hemangioma (unclassified phakomatosis, rarely associated with intracranial AVMs).
  B. Retinal and intracranial tumors.
    1. Tuberous sclerosis.
    2. Neurofibromatosis.
V. Dystrophies of the uvea.
  A. Angioid streaks (ruptures of Bruch's membrane) occur in the following diseases, which may be associated with neurologic dysfunction.
    1. Francois dyscephalic syndrome.
    2. Paget's disease.
    3. Acromegaly.
    4. Sickle cell anemia.
  B. Gillespie's syndrome (aniridia, ataxia, psychomotor retardation).
VI. Retinovitreal syndromes and vitreal involvement.
  A. Wagner's vitreoretinopathy (rarely associated with encephaloceles).
  B. Dominant familial amyloidosis (diffuse vitreous opacification).

RETINAL ISCHEMIA   *(see Amaurosis Fugax)*

RETINITIS PIGMENTOSA   *(see Retina and Uveal Tract)*

RHABDOMYOLYSIS   *(see Myoglobinuria)*

RHEUMATOID ARTHRITIS

Neurologic complications usually occur in patients with moderate to severely affected rheumatoid arthritis (RA) and consist of neuropathy, myopathy, myelopathy, and involvement of the brain and meninges.

Peripheral neuropathy is the most frequent complication of RA and includes the following main types: (1) entrapment, (2) distal sensory polyneuropathy, and (3) mononeuritis multiplex (sensorimotor). *Entrapment neuropathies*, the most common complication, result from inflammation around the joints, causing nerve compression. Carpal tunnel syndrome is the most common. Other nerves involved include ulnar (at wrist or elbow), posterior interosseous (at elbow), posterior tibial (at popliteal fossa or tarsal tunnel), peroneal (at popliteal fossa), and medial and lateral plantar. Distal sensory neuropathy is also common and may be asymptomatic or can cause dysesthesias. All sensory modalities are affected, vibratory often the most. Segmental demyelination is the presumed cause. *Mononeuritis multiplex* is usually of sudden onset as a result of ischemic injury causing both demyelination and axonal loss. Mononeuritis multiplex may be severe and may result in quadriparesis. Autonomic dysfunction can also occur.

Myelopathy resulting from subluxation of the cervical spine is frequently observed in severe RA. Atlantoaxial subluxation, separation of the anterior arch of the atlas from the dens by more than 3 mm, is most frequent. Lateral cervical spine radiographic films during flexion and extension are usually sufficient for diagnosis. The patient, not the technician, should flex and extend the neck. MRI, CT, myelography, and vertebral angiography may be needed in selected cases. Vertical upward subluxation of the odontoid process resulting from lack of lateral support of the atlas usually occurs on the background of atlantoaxial subluxation. Sensory loss in the trigeminal and C2 distributions, nystagmus, and pyramidal tract signs can result. Basilar invagination, the penetration of the odontoid through the foramen magnum with compression of ventral medulla, is occasionally seen (see Craniocervical Junction).

Complications affecting muscle include disuse atrophy, focal myositis (usually adjacent to actively involved joints), disseminated nodular myositis (nonnecrotizing lymphocytic and plasma cell perivascular infiltrates), corticosteroid myopathy, polymyositis (rare, more malignant course), and ischemia resulting from vasculitis.

CNS complications of RA include vasculitis (systemic vasculitis or isolated CNS angiitis); cranial neuropathies; infarction, hemorrhage, and encephalopathy; dural nodules (often asymptomatic); rheumatoid pachymeningitis (seizures and encephalopathy); and hyperviscosity syndrome (rare). Neurologic symptoms may also be caused by drugs used to treat RA, such as gold (myokymia), steroids (myopathy), and penicillamine (myasthenia).

REF: Brick JE, Brick JF: *Neurol Clin* 7(3):629-639, 1989.

RIGIDITY

Rigidity is a form of increased muscle tone that is present throughout the range of motion of a limb (compare Spasticity). When released, the rigid limb does not spring back to its original position. Rigidity is not associated with increased reflexes. EMG reveals persistent motor unit activity during apparent relaxation.

Forms of rigidity include the following:

1. Cogwheel rigidity: An increased resistance to stretch interrupted by rhythmic yielding (that is, variable resistance) seen in extrapyramidal disease.
2. Lead-pipe rigidity: Constant resistance to movement of a limb, which may maintain its position at the end of the displacement; may also be seen in catatonia.
3. Gegenhalten or paratonia: Refers to increasing tone equal in response to increasing effort to move a limb passively throughout its range of motion (that is, velocity and load-dependent resistance); seen in bilateral frontal lobe or mesial basal temporal lobe disease, encephalopathies, and dementias.

The following are not true rigidity:

1. Voluntary rigidity: Agonist-antagonist cocontraction associated with heightened emotional states.
2. Involuntary rigidity: For example, an acute condition in the abdomen.
3. Hysterical rigidity.
4. Reflex rigidity: Spasms in response to pain or cold.
5. Decorticate and decerebrate posturing are imprecise terms. Decorticate posturing is a slow, stereotyped flexion of arm, wrist, and fingers with adduction at the shoulder and leg extension with plantar flexion of the foot. It occurs with supratentorial processes compressing the diencephalon. Decerebrate posturing is pronation of the arm with adduction and internal rotation of the leg, along with plantar flexion of the foot. It occurs with more caudal compression of the midbrain and rostral pons. Extension in the arms with flexion or flaccidity in the legs is associated with lesions of the pontine tegmentum (see also Herniation).

RILEY-DAY SYNDROME *(see Autonomic Dysfunction, Neuropathy)*

RINNE TEST *(see Hearing)*

ROMBERG SIGN

A test comparing the stability of a person standing with both feet together and eyes open with that with eyes closed. A normal response is a slight increase in sway. A marked increase in sway indicates proprioceptive sensory loss. Increased sway may also indicate cerebellar ataxia, vestibulopathy, frontal lobe impairment, or other motor impairment. Patients with cerebellar or vestibular dysfunction tend to fall toward the side of the lesion.

ROUSSY-LÉVY SYNDROME   (see Neuropathy)

SACRAL PLEXUS   (see Lumbosacral Plexus)

SARCOIDOSIS

Sarcoidosis is a multisystem disorder of unknown etiology characterized by noncaseating granulomas in affected tissues. The disease may affect any organ, and the nervous system is affected in 5% of cases of sarcoidosis. Generally it affects young adults and is more common in blacks. It usually begins with bilateral hilar adenopathy, pulmonary infiltrate, uveitis, or skin lesion. Hypercalcemia and hypercalciuria are common.

MANIFESTATIONS OF NEUROSARCOIDOSIS

1. Muscle: Slowly progressive myopathy with proximal weakness.
2. Peripheral nerve: Mononeuritis multiplex, polyneuropathy, Guillain-Barré syndrome, polyradiculopathy.
3. Cranial nerves: Peripheral facial nerve palsy of one or both sides is common. Other cranial nerves can be affected, but ophthalmoplegia is rare. A paralyzed pupil is an occasional finding.
4. Spinal cord: May be compressed by an extramedullary or intramedullary granuloma. Spinal block may occur.
5. Intracranial: Most common presentations relate to basilar meningitis with involvement of neighboring structures (cranial nerves, hypothalamus, pituitary), obstruction of CSF pathways, and hydrocephalus. Mass lesions are often found in the hypothalamic region. Infrequently neurosarcoidosis comes to medical attention as a mass lesion mistaken for a meningioma before surgery.
6. Opportunistic infections occur because of defective immune

system or as treatment complication and may include tuberculous meningitis, progressive multifocal leukoencephalopathy, nocardiosis, herpes simplex encephalitis, and cryptococcal meningitis.

DIAGNOSTIC TESTS

Definitive diagnosis is based on biopsy demonstration of typical granulomas. CT and MRI are helpful in localizing CNS lesion. Gallium scan helps in detecting systemic involvement and is more sensitive than chest x-ray. CSF examination may show increased protein level, pleocytosis, and low glucose level. Oligoclonal bands and high IgG index may occur. Angiotensin-converting enzyme has 56% to 86% sensitivity in serum and is not specific. Its level in CSF is presumed to reflect disease activity.

TREATMENT AND PROGNOSIS

A regimen of prednisone, 40 to 80 mg daily, is the mainstay of treatment. If treatment fails or if corticosteroids cannot be tapered, cytotoxic agents may be added. Most patients respond to treatment but one third relapse when treatment is discontinued. Prognosis is usually better when disease is limited to peripheral nerve. Effective response to radiotherapy for intracranial sarcoidosis has been reported.

REF: Scott TF: *Neurology* 43:8–12, 1993.

SCHILDER'S DISEASE   *(see Demyelinating Diseases)*

SCHIZENCEPHALY   *(see Developmental Malformations)*

SCHWANNOMA   *(see Tumor, Hearing)*

SCIATIC NERVE   *(see Radiculopathy, Peripheral Nerve)*

SEPSIS

Sepsis is the constellation of active infection and changes in respiratory rate, pulse, and temperature. Neurologic complications most frequently include obtundation (up to 70%) and less commonly include paratonic rigidity, seizures, and asterixis. It is important to distinguish septic encephalopathy from disorders producing primary neurologic disease (for example, meningitis, stroke, and brain abscess), metabolic encephalopathies (such as hypoxia, hypoglycemia and hyperglycemia, thyrotoxicosis, adrenal failure, and Reye's syndrome), drug reactions, some hematologic conditions (such as hyperviscosity syndromes, leukemia, and sickle cell crises), and other disorders of thermoregulation.

Neuromuscular complications of sepsis include critical illness polyneuropathy, a pure axonal sensorimotor polyneuropathy that becomes evident as respiratory failure, distal weakness, and reduced reflexes with relative sparing of cranial musculature. Other syndromes include disuse atrophy and myositis. These conditions must be distinguished from Guillain-Barré syndrome, nutritional deficiency neuropathies, paraneoplastic syndromes, and neuromuscular blockade resulting from some antibiotics (for example, aminoglycosides).

REF: Bolton CF, Young GB, Zochodne DW: Ann Neurol 33:94–100, 1993.

SEXUAL FUNCTION   *(see Autonomic Dysfunction, Impotence)*

SHINGLES   *(see Zoster)*

SHUNTS   *(see also Hydrocephalus, Macrocephaly)*

Ventriculoperitoneal (VP) shunts are favored in infants and growing children because extra tubing can be left in the peritoneal cavity, allowing for growth and extending the time between shunt revisions. Ventriculojugular (VJ) shunts may be used after major growth is completed; complications (thrombi, endocarditis, septic or tubing emboli, and arrhythmias) are more frequent and serious than with VP shunts. Lumboperitoneal (LP) shunts are useful in communicating (especially "normal pressure") hydrocephalus. External ventriculostomy is useful immediately after cranial surgical procedures, when CSF protein level is very high or when there is debris in the CSF.

Mechanical malfunction can be due to disconnection, breakage, or obstruction (ventricular catheter plugged with glia or choroid plexus; valve plugged with high-protein CSF or debris; distal catheter plugged with thrombus (VJ) or omentum (VP). Classic symptoms of shunt dysfunction in older children and adults are headache, lethargy, nausea, and vomiting. Gradual shunt malfunction may come to medical attention as impaired school performance, irritability, or personality change. Infants may have irritability, poor feeding, vomiting, and an abnormally shrill cry. Children with repeated episodes of shunt malfunction generally come to medical attention in a similar manner with each episode.

Begin the evaluation by pumping the valve. Difficulty compressing the valve ("pumps hard") suggests distal obstruction; slow refill suggests proximal obstruction or slit ventricles. Even if the shunt pumps, it may not be working properly. Palpate the shunt tubing for any interruption. Obtain a shunt series (plain x-rays of the entire shunt system; reservoirs and pumps may be radiolucent) to look for interruption and a non-contrasted head CT scan to assess ventricular size (old films are invaluable for comparing ventricular size). Tap the shunt (Huber needle only) for CSF pressure (if obstructed proximal to reservoir, measured pressure will not be elevated) and CSF examination.

A shunt tap is not always necessary when a fever develops in a child with a shunt. Upper respiratory infection, otitis media, pharyngitis, urinary tract infection, and gastroenteritis are frequent causes of febrile illness in any child, including those with shunts. A tap should be performed if the child is lethargic, unusually irritable, photophobic, or has neck stiffness. A shunt tap should also be considered if there is a history of similar presentation with a previous shunt infection or if there is unexplained fever or leukocytosis. Although intrathecal antibiotics may be successful, removal of an infected shunt is usually necessary for effective treatment.

CNS complications of shunts include meningitis, seizures, hematomas, and hygromas. Asymptomatic bilateral subdural effusions are common and require no treatment. Peritoneal complications include ascites and cyst formation, perforation of viscus or abdominal wall, infection with obstruction of the distal end of the catheter, and peritoneal metastases from CNS tumors (for example, medulloblastoma). Other complications include soft-tissue infection along the shunt tract and pressure necrosis of the skin.

Figure 40 shows the major components of typical shunt systems.

REF: Wilkins RH, Rengachary SS: *Neurosurgery update II*, New York, 1991, McGraw-Hill.

Youmans JR: *Neurological surgery*, ed 3, Philadelphia, 1990, WB Saunders.

SHY-DRAGER SYNDROME   *(see Autonomic Dysfunction, Parkinsonism)*

SICKLE CELL DISEASE

Sickle cell anemia is due to a genetic defect in hemoglobin in which valine is substituted for glutamic acid at position six of the beta-

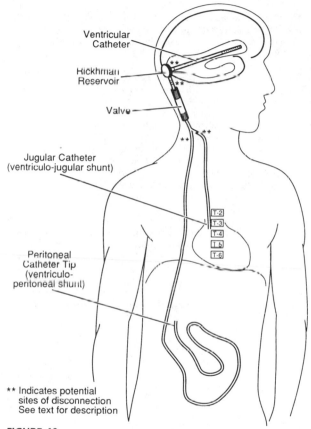

Ventricular
Catheter

Hickhman
Reservoir

Valve

Jugular Catheter
(ventriculo-jugular shunt)

T-2
T-3
T-4
T-5
T-6

Peritoneal
Catheter Tip
(ventriculo-
peritoneal shunt)

** Indicates potential
   sites of disconnection
   See text for description

FIGURE 40
Typical shunt system (many variations exist).

hemoglobin chain, creating hemoglobin S (Hb S). This leads to red cells that are rigid and easily damaged and results in a hemolytic anemia. Sickle cell trait is unlikely to produce neurologic manifestations.

Neurologic manifestations are seen in one third of patients with sickle cell disease (SS) and may be the presenting sign. The frequency of neurologic manifestations is proportional to the propensity for sickling: 6% to 35% in SS, 6% to 24% in SC disease, and 0% to 6% in sickle trait (AS).

Stroke, including thrombosis and hemorrhage, occurs in 13% to 17% of patients. About 75% have ischemia; the remainder have hemorrhage. Venous thrombosis may occur rarely. Cerebral infarcts occur at a mean age of 7 years; recurrence rates are as high as 67%, with a mean interstroke interval of 28 months. 80% of recurrences occur within 36 months of the initial infarct. Intracranial hemorrhage occurs in 3% of sickle cell patients at a mean age of 25 years. Hemorrhages are more often subarachnoid in children and intraparenchymal in adults. They may occur in association with aneurysms, rupture of dilated vessels, hemorrhage into infarcted tissue, or "moyamoya." Angiography may precipitate sickling but may be safely performed after abnormal hemoglobin is reduced to less than 20% by transfusions.

Patients with SS disease have a higher stroke rate than patients with SC disease. The level of fetal hemoglobin (Hb F) correlates inversely with stroke incidence. Three intrinsic mechanisms contribute to ischemia in sickle cell disease. (1) There may be large vessel endothelial injury because of the sickled cells, resulting in endothelial hyperplasia and vessel occlusion. Particularly common are middle cerebral artery infarcts and watershed infarcts. (2) There may be sludging of sickled cells during a sickle crises, with resultant ischemia in small vessels. (3) The chronic anemia leads to chronically increased cerebral perfusion and vasodilation and lack of cerebral autoregulatory reserve in meeting regional cerebral metabolic demands. These abnormal, dilated vessels may also rupture, with resultant hemorrhage.

Recurrence of stroke may be prevented by exchange transfusion to keep the percentage of sickle cells below 20%. Transfusions are typically repeated for approximately 2 years after a stroke (peak time for recurrences).

Acute or chronic *encephalopathy* may occur and possibly represents a manifestation of cerebrovascular disease.

Seizures occur in 8% to 12% of patients and are usually generalized tonic-clonic. In SS disease, they can occur in the absence of recognized cerebrovascular involvement or intercurrent illness, although there may be precipitating factors such as medications, surgery, or anesthesia. In SC disease intercurrent illness is frequently responsible.

CNS infections with encapsulated organisms (such as *Streptococcus pneumoniae* occur in patients with SS disease as a result of decreased phagocytic ability of the reticuloendothelial system (autosplenectomy).

Pain during sickle crisis is often severe and localizes to the affected organ. It is commonly treated with opiate analgesics. Idiopathic headache is common and may be related to increased cerebral blood flow.

Myelopathy resulting from vertebral body infarction, extramedullary hematopoiesis, and spinal cord infarction has been reported.

Visual disturbances are much more frequent in SC than in SS disease. About one third of patients with SC disease first seek medical attention for visual impairment. Visual complications include vitreous, retinal, and subretinal hemorrhages; central retinal artery and vein occlusions; retinitis proliferans; and other retinal vascular changes.

REF: Pavlakis SG, Prohovnik I, Piomelli S, DeVivo DC: *Adv Pediatr* 36:247–276, 1989.

SIMULTANAGNOSIA *(see Agnosia)*

SINGLE PHOTON EMISSION COMPUTED TOMOGRAPHY *(see PET AND SPECT)*

SLEEP DISORDERS
ABRIDGED CLASSIFICATION OF SLEEP DISORDERS

I. Disorders of initiating and maintaining sleep (insomnias).
    A. Associated with psychiatric disorders such as personality disorders, affective disorders, or psychoses.
    B. Associated with abuse of or withdrawal from drugs or alcohol.
    C. Sleep apnea syndromes.
    D. Alveolar hypoventilation, including Ondine's curse.
    E. Sleep-related myoclonus.
    F. Restless legs syndrome.
    G. Neurologic and medical disorders that interfere with sleep.
    H. "Pseudoinsomnia" (subjective symptoms without laboratory evidence of a sleep disturbance).
    I. Normal short sleeper.
    J. Rapid eye movement (REM) interruptions and other polysomnographic abnormalities.
II. Disorders of excessive somnolence.
    A through G, as listed above, are also associated with excessive somnolence.
    H. Narcolepsy.
    I. Idiopathic CNS hypersomnolence.
    J. Klein-Levin syndrome.
    K. Insufficient sleep.
    L. Normal long sleeper.

III. Disorders of the sleep-wake cycle.
    A.   Jet lag.
    B.   Shift work.
IV. Parasomnias.
    A.   Sleepwalking (somnambulism).
    B.   Sleep terror (pavor nocturnus).
    C.   REM behavior disorder.
    D.   Others.

Insomnia is the most common sleep disorder. Associated medical or psychiatric conditions should be treated. General management of insomnia includes optimizing the patient's "sleep hygiene" as follows: Wake and retire at the same time each day (including weekends); use the bed only for sleep and sex; leave the bed if not asleep within 10 minutes of retiring; avoid heavy exercise or large meals just before bedtime; avoid daytime napping; make sure the bedroom is not too warm or cold; exercise regularly; and discontinue use of alcohol, caffeine, cigarettes, and psychoactive drugs. Other treatments include biofeedback and sleep restriction therapy. Short-acting benzodiazepines may offer temporary adjunctive benefit, but their long-term use is not recommended. Other sedatives, including chloral hydrate, zolpidem, and diphenhydramine, may be used judiciously.

REF: Gillin JC, Byerley WF: *N Engl J Med* 322:239–248, 1990.

Sleep apnea syndrome is characterized by daytime somnolence and nighttime, or sleep-related, apnea resulting from either upper airway obstruction or central causes, or both. The typical patient is obese and snores loudly. Recurrent hypoxemia, hypercapnia, heart failure, arrhythmia, and sudden death may result. Diagnosis is made by polysomnography, including EEG, nasal and oral airflow recording, chest and abdominal respiratory movement, ECG, and pulse oximetry. Treatment consists of weight reduction, lateral sleep position, avoidance of sedatives or alcohol, and nasal continuous positive airway pressure (CPAP). Some patients may benefit from surgical correction of upper airway obstruction.

REF: Kaplan J, Staats BA: *Mayo Clin Proc* 65:1087–1094, 1990.

Narcolepsy is a disorder of excessive daytime somnolence characterized on clinical study by sleep attacks, cataplexy (sudden weakness or loss of tone elicited by emotional stimuli), hypnagogic hallucinations, and sleep paralysis. Polysomnographic confirmation includes absence of sleep apnea and daytime mean sleep latency of less than 5 minutes accompanied by REM sleep in at least two of five daytime naps on the multiple sleep latency test (MSLT). Ninety-eight percent of patients have HLA-DR2 and HLA-DQwl antigens. Treatment consists of a regimen of stimulants (such as methylphenidate, 10 to 60 mg daily, or dextroamphetamine, 5 to 50 mg daily) for sleepiness, tricyclic antidepressants (such as protriptyline, 15 to 40 mg daily) for cataplexy and sleep paralysis, and regular, brief daytime naps. Tolerance to stimulants may develop and is sometimes relieved by a "drug holiday." Abuse potential is high for stimulants. Monoamine oxidase (MAO) inhibitors are also useful but should not be used with tricyclics. Selegiline, a selective MAO-B inhibitor, improves daytime alertness and may have fewer side effects than amphetamines.

REF: Aldrich MS: N Engl J Med 323:389–394, 1990.

Sleep terrors (pavor nocturnus) typically occur in the first third of sleep. Patients often arouse with a blood-curdling cry and cannot explain what is frightening them. In contrast to common nightmares, with sleep terrors the patient is amnestic for them the next morning. Sleep terrors occur almost exclusively in children and disappear by adolescence. Treatment usually consists of reassuring the parents; occasionally a regimen of benzodiazepines or imipramine is useful.

Restless legs syndrome (see Restless Legs Syndrome).

SMELL *(see Olfaction)*

SODIUM *(see Electrolyte Disorders)*

SPASMODIC TORTICOLLIS *(see Dystonia)*

SPASTICITY

Spasticity is a velocity-dependent increase in muscle tone. It is one component of the upper motor neuron syndrome. Other components include flexor spasms, weakness, tonic flexor and extensor dystonia, increased stretch reflexes, extensor plantar response (Babinksi's sign), and loss of dexterity. It results from damage to various descending pathways. Isolated lesions of the pyramidal tract are not sufficient to produce spasticity or the complete syndrome.

Overall, no medication is particularly useful in relieving the disabling spasticity of cerebral lesions (tightly flexed and adducted upper extremities, extended and adducted lower extremities). Painful flexor spasms can be markedly reduced by administration of baclofen or diazepam. Dantrolene may be helpful but causes mild to moderate muscle weakness, sedation, and dizziness. Combinations may be more effective, with fewer side effects.

Baclofen is a gamma aminobutyric acid (GABA) agonist and also interferes with the release of excitatory transmitters. Starting dosage is 5 mg three times a day (tid), increased by 5 mg every three days to a maximum dosage of 80 to 120 mg per day in divided doses. Adverse effects are mood changes, hallucinations, gastrointestinal symptoms, hypotension, changes in accommodation and ocular motor function, and deterioration in seizure control. Care should be used if renal disease is present; avoid abrupt withdrawal of the drug. Continuous infusion of intrathecal baclofen by means of an implanted infusion pump at a rate of 15 to 450 μg per day is useful in spasticity caused by spinal cord lesions or demyelinating disease and may be useful in spasticity of cerebral origin in cerebral palsy.

Diazepam facilitates GABA-mediated presynaptic and postsynaptic inhibition. Starting dosage is 2 mg twice daily, increased slowly to a maximum dosage of 60 mg per day in divided doses.

Dantrolene sodium interferes with excitation-contraction coupling by decreasing the release of calcium at the sarcoplasmic reticulum. Starting dosage is 25 mg every day, increased by 25 mg every three to four days to a maximum dosage of 100 mg qid. Side effects are hepatotoxicity (follow liver enzymes) and diarrhea. A regimen of clonidine, 0.2 to 1 mg per day in divided doses, has also been useful, but orthostatic hypotension may limit its use. Clonidine binds to $\alpha 2$ adrenoreceptor sites, decreasing sympathetic outflow along with subsequently inhibiting afferent inputs into the spinal reflex arc.

A regimen of chlorpromazine (25 to 75 mg per day) causes alpha adrenergic blockade and has been used to reduce spasticity, but sedation and fear or tardive dyskinesia have limited its use.

Phenytoin (100 to 400 mg per day) and carbamezepine (600 to 1200 mg per day) act on the Ia afferent muscle spindle to reduce spontaneous and stretch-evoked discharges.

Surgical intervention with selective posterior rhizotomy has been used in patients with cerebral palsy and severe spasticity. Longitudinal myelotomy has been used to control severe flexor spasms. Spinal cord and cerebellar stimulation act by stimulating inhibitory pathways. Botulinum toxin may also be useful in the treatment of spasticity.

REF: Alonso PJ, Mancall EL: *Semin Neurol* 2(3):215–218, 1991.

National Institutes of Health: *Conn Med* 55:471-477, 1991.

Young RR, Wiegner AW: *Clin Orthop* 219:50, 1987.

SPECT   *(see PET AND SPECT)*

SPEECH DISORDERS   *(see Aphasia, Dysarthria)*

SPHINCTER   *(see Bladder)*

SPINA BIFIDA   *(see Developmental Malformations)*

SPINAL ARTERY   *(see Spinal Cord)*

SPINAL CORD   *(see also Bladder, Cauda Equina, Craniocervical Junction, Radiculopathy)*

Relation of the spinal cord segments and roots to the vertebral column is depicted in Figure 41. Cross-sectional anatomy of the cervical cord is shown in Figure 42.

SPINAL CORD SYNDROMES

An acute *spinal cord* lesion causes "spinal shock," which becomes evident as paralysis, areflexia, anesthesia and bowel or bladder dysfunction below the level of the lesion. Spinal shock may last weeks and may evolve into spasticity, exaggerated tendon and withdrawal reflexes, and Babinski's signs.

Anterior cord syndrome is characterized by paresis and impaired pain perception; proprioception is preserved below the lesion. The syndrome is usually caused by spinal cord compression or anterior spinal artery occlusion. Posterior cord syndrome consists of pain and parathesias out of proportion to motor impairment that are referable to the affected segments; the syndrome is commonly associated with demyelinating lesions. Central cord syndrome, often seen with hyperextension injuries in the neck, results in patchy sensory loss, urinary retention, and weakness disproportionately affecting the legs.

Spinal cord hemisection produces the Brown-Sequard syndrome, consisting of (1) ipsilateral spastic paresis; (2) ipsilateral loss of touch and vibratory and joint position sense; and (3) contralateral loss of pain and temperature sensation below the level of the lesion.

CAUSES OF MYELOPATHY

Congenital or developmental: Spinal dysraphism (see Developmental Malformations), craniocervical junction abnormalities, syrin-

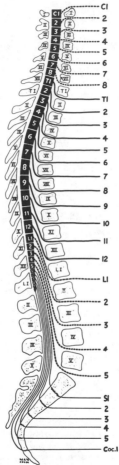

FIGURE 41
Relation of spinal segments and roots to the vertebral column. (From Haymaker W, Woodhall B: *Peripheral nerve injuries: Principles of diagnosis,* Philadelphia, 1953, WB Saunders.)

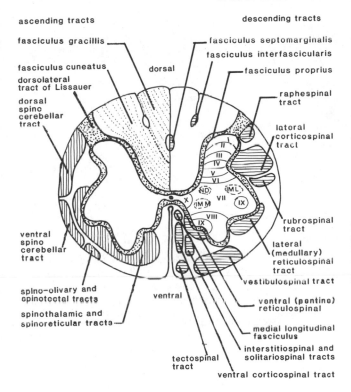

ascending tracts

fasciculus gracillis

fasciculus cuneatus

dorsolateral
tract of Lissauer

dorsal
spino
cerebellar
tract

dorsal

descending tracts

fasciculus septomarginalis

fasciculus interfascicularis

fasciculus proprius

raphespinal
tract

lateral
corticospinal
tract

ventral
spino
cerebellar
tract

rubrospinal
tract

lateral
(medullary)
reticulospinal
tract

vestibulospinal tract

spino-olivary and
spinotectal tracts

ventral

spinothalamic and
spinoreticular tracts

ventral (pontine)
reticulospinal

medial longitudinal
fasciculus

interstitiospinal and
solitariospinal tracts

tectospinal
tract

ventral corticospinal tract

FIGURE 42
Cervical spinal cord (cross section). Gray matter columns: *I-X,* Rexed's lami-
nae; *IML,* interomediolateral column; *ND,* nucleus dorsalis (Clarke's column);
PM, posteromedial column.

gomyelia, congenital cervical spinal stenosis, tethered-cord syndromes,
diastatomyelia.

Degenerative (see Degenerative Joint Disease on p. 390): Spondylosis, motor neuron disease, spinocerebellar degeneration, hereditary
spastic paraplegia.

Demyelinating: Multiple sclerosis, neuromyelitis optica (Devic's
disease).

Infectious: Poliomyelitis, herpes zoster, rabies, viral encephalomyelitis, bacterial meningitis, epidural or subdural abscess, syphilis, tuberculosis, typhus, spotted fever, fungal infections, trichinosis, schistosomiasis, HTLV-1, human immunodeficiency virus (HIV), cytomegalovirus.

Inflammatory or immune response: Postinfectious, postvaccination, arachnoiditis, sarcoidosis, lupus erythematosus.

Metabolic or nutritional: Pernicious anemia (B_{12} deficiency), pellagra, chronic liver disease.

Neoplastic: Extramedullary or intramedullary tumors (see Tumors), meningeal carcinomatosis, paraneoplastic.

Toxic: Ethanol (direct effect and through hepatic cirrhosis and portocaval shunting), arsenic, cyanide, lathyrism, clioquinol, intrathecal contrast or chemotherapeutic agents.

Traumatic (see below): Vertebral subluxation or fracture, transection, contusion, concussion, hemorrhage, birth injury (particularly breech delivery), electrical injury.

Vascular (see below): Arterial and venous infarction, hemorrhage (epidural, subdural, intraparenchymal), vasculitides, vascular malformations, aneurysms, effects of radiation therapy (see Radiation).

DEGENERATIVE JOINT DISEASE

Degenerative joint disease of the spine occurs as a result of changes in the intervertebral disks (spondylosis) with aging. Spondylosis leads to osteophyte formation, meningeal fibrosis, and disk herniation.

Spondylosis in the cervical spine can cause progressive myelopathy, radiculopathy, or both. Thoracic lesions become evident mainly as paraparesis. Lumbar lesions cause radiculopathies, neurogenic claudication, or acute back pain syndromes. Neurogenic claudication, like vascular claudication, causes exertional pain, but it differs from vascular claudication as follows: (1) the pain may be felt in buttock or thigh with prolonged standing or walking; (2) the pulses are normal; (3) reflexes may be decreased while at peak pain; and (4) the pain is relieved with waist flexion or rest but generally takes several minutes or more to resolve.

Syringomyelia describes a condition in which there is an abnormal cavity or cyst in the spinal cord. Syrinxes are usually cervical but may extend rostrally (syringobulbia) or caudally. They are frequently associated with developmental malformations of the craniocervical junction (Arnold-Chiari malformations, platybasia, myelomeningocele, kyphoscoliosis, intramedullary tumors, vascular malformations or trauma. Hand numbness is the usual initial complaint with cervical syrinxes. Loss of pain and temperature sensation in a capelike (suspended) distribution with sparing of vibratory and joint position sense (dissociated sensory loss) is due to destruction of crossing pain fibers at the lesion level. Segmental weakness, atrophy, fasciculations, spasticity, incontinence, and hyperreflexia occur frequently. The course is usually slowly progressive; a sudden decline may indicate development of hematomyelia or progression of an underlying condition. Management includes cyst drainage and scrupulous hand care to prevent painless cuts and wound infections.

TRAUMA

Initial management of spinal cord trauma should include maintenance of airway, breathing, and circulation; immobilization (spine board, collars); bladder catheterization; nasogastric intubation; administration of high-dose IV corticosteroids; and serial neurologic examinations. Radiographic studies are directed to the area of interest but generally include cross-table lateral and AP cervical views (all seven cervical vertebrae must be seen) and films of the thoracic and lumbar spine. An open-mouth odontoid film may be obtained in conscious patients. CT is sensitive for identification of fractures. Myelography or MRI can identify acute compressive lesions such as hematomas.

VASCULAR SYNDROMES

Anterior spinal artery infarctions typically affect the midthoracic region, causing severe local, radicular, and deep pain; paraparesis; sphincter disturbance; and dissociated distal sensory loss (pain and temperature sensation more affected than vibration, touch, and joint position sense). Sacral sensation may remain intact. Causes include systemic hypotension, aortic dissection, vasculitis, embolism, sickle cell disease, and extrinsic arterial compression by tumor, bone, or disk material. Posterior spinal artery infarction is less common and produces pain, loss of proprioception, and variable involvement of corticospinal and spinocerebellar tracts.

Spinal subdural and epidural hemorrhage most commonly occurs after trauma, lumbar puncture, or spinal or epidural anesthesia. Other causes include anticoagulant use, blood dyscrasias, thrombocytopenia, neoplasm, and vascular malformation. The initial symptom is severe back pain at the level of the bleed. Myelopathy or cauda equina syndrome with symptoms dependent on lesion level develop over hours to days. MRI is especially useful in determining lesion location. Laminectomy with clot evacuation should be performed as soon as possible, since prognosis for recovery is better when surgery is performed early and the preoperative deficits are not severe.

Spinal subarachnoid hemorrhage most commonly results from aneurysm rupture but may occur with vascular malformations. Other causes include aortic coarctation, spinal artery rupture, mycotic aneurysms, polyarteritis nodosa, spinal tumors, lumbar puncture, blood dyscrasias, and anticoagulants. Severe back pain followed by signs of meningeal irritation are usually the first manifestations. Multiple radiculopathies and myelopathy may develop. Headache, cranial neuropathies, and obtundation are associated with diffusion of blood above the foramen magnum. Cerebrospinal fluid is bloody and intracranial pressure may be elevated; treatment is directed at the underlying cause.

Hematomyelia: Intramedullary spinal hemorrhage is rare but occurs after trauma, spinal arteriovenous malformation rupture, hemorrhage into tumor or syrinx, or venous infarction or with clotting or bleeding disorders. Emergency surgical decompression is often indicated.

Spinal cord compression and tumors are discussed in the Tumors section.

SPINOCEREBELLAR DEGENERATION

Spinocerebellar degeneration is a general term used to describe a heterogeneous group of inherited disorders in which ataxia may be prominent. The classification below (adapted from Harding and Deufel, 1993) is based on clinical, genetic, and pathologic findings.

Olivopontocerebellar atrophy is a pathologic diagnosis applied to diverse clinical entities. The course may include progressive ataxia, tremor, spasticity, involuntary movements, optic atrophy, and sensory abnormalities; it may be indistinguishable on clinical examination from the hereditary ataxias listed below.

CLASSIFICATION

	Decade of Onset
I. Disorders with known metabolic or other cause.	
A. Metabolic disorders.	
1. Progressive, unremitting ataxia.	
a. Abetalipoproteinemia (Bassen-Kornzweig).	1st–2nd
b. Hypobetalipoproteinemia.	2nd–4th
c. Hexosaminidase deficiency.	1st
d. Glutamate-dehydrogenase deficiency.	2nd–6th
e. Cholestanolosis.	3rd–6th
f. Mitochondrial myopathy.	1st–6th
2. Intermittent ataxia.	
a. Disorders of pyruvate and lactate metabolism.	1st

      b. Aminoacidurias (Hartnup disease and in-
         termittent branched chain ketoaciduria).   1st
      c. Urea cycle enzyme deficiencies (autoso-
         mal recessive and X-linked).   1st
  B. Disorders characterized by defective DNA repair.
    1. Ataxia telangiectasia (Louis-Bar syndrome).   1st
    2. Xeroderma pigmentosa   1st–2nd
    3. Cockayne's syndrome.   1st
II. Disorders of unknown etiology.
  A. Early onset cerebellar ataxia—before age 20 (all
    are autosomal recessive unless indicated).
    1. Friedreich's ataxia.   1st–2nd
    2. Early onset cerebellar ataxia with retained
       tendon reflexes.   1st–2nd
    3. With hypogonadism with or without deaf-
       ness; dementia.   1st–3rd
    4. With congenital deafness.   2nd–3rd
    5. With childhood deafness and mental retarda-
       tion.   1st
    6. With pigmentary retinal degeneration with or
       without mental retardation, dementia, or
       deafness.   1st
    7. With optic atrophy, mental retardation with
       or without deafness, or spasticity (Behr's syn-
       drome).   1st
    8. With cataracts and mental retardation (Mari-
       nesco-Sjögren's syndrome).   1st
    9. With myoclonus (Ramsay Hunt syndrome)
       (autosomal recessive or dominant).   1st–2nd
    10. X-linked recessive spinocerebellar ataxia.   1st–2nd
    11. With extrapyramidal features.   1st–3rd
  B. Late onset cerebellar ataxia—after age 20 (all are
    autosomal dominant).
    1. With optic atrophy, ophthalmoplegia, de-
       mentia, amyotrophy, and extrapyramidal fea-
       tures (includes Machado-Joseph disease).   3rd–5th
    2. With pigmentary retinal degeneration with or
       without opthalmoplegia and extrapyramidal
       features.   2nd–4th
    3. Pure cerebellar ataxia of late onset.   6th–7th
    4. With myoclonus and deafness.   2nd–5th

Friedreich's ataxia is the most common of the spinocerebellar degenerations of unknown etiology. Symptoms develop from 18 months

to 24 years of age and consist of progressive limb and truncal ataxia, dysarthria, and areflexia in the lower extremities. Pyramidal signs and loss of position and vibration sense evolve gradually. Kyphoscoliosis with restrictive lung function and cardiomyopathy with electrocardiographic abnormality are seen in more than two thirds of patients. Pes cavus, optic atrophy, distal amyotrophy, and horizontal nystagmus are less common. Sensory conduction is absent in lower extremities and slowed in upper extremities. Diabetes may be present. Ambulation is usually lost by 25 years of age, and death occurs in the fourth or fifth decade of life. Treatment is aimed at symptomatic management of diabetes, cardiomyopathy, and arrhythmias.

On pathologic study Friedreich's ataxia is characterized by a narrowed spinal cord with gliosis and cell loss in the posterior columns and corticospinal and spinocerebellar tracts. Clarke's column and dorsal root ganglia are depleted. Cranial nerve nuclei VIII, X, and XII are depleted, as may be dentate nuclei and superior cerebellar peduncles. Large, myelinated peripheral nerves are lost. Myocardial fibers are degenerated.

Early-onset cerebellar ataxia with retained reflexes is not uncommon and is often confused with Friedreich's ataxia. Reflexes are normal or brisk. Optic atrophy, cardiomyopathy, diabetes, and skeletal deformities are not seen. Life span is considerably longer than with Friedreich's ataxia.

The adult forms of spinocerebellar degeneration occur less frequently than does Friedreich's ataxia, and there may be several clinical manifestations within a kindred. The conditions tend to progress more rapidly in patients with early onset of symptoms than in those with late-onset ataxia.

REF: de Jong JMBV et al. In Vinken PJ, Bruyn GW, Klawans HL, eds: *Handbook of Clinical Neurology*, 60, Amsterdam, 1991, Elsevier.

Harding AE, Deufel T, eds: *Adv Neurology* 61, 1993.

Rosenberg R: *Neurology* 40:1329, 1990.

SPONDYLOSIS—CERVICAL   *(see Spinal Cord)*

STATUS EPILEPTICUS   *(see Epilepsy)*

STATUS MIGRAINOSUS   *(see Headache)*

STIFF-MAN SYNDROME   *(see Cramps)*

STOKES-ADAMS ATTACK   *(see Syncope)*

STRABISMUS   *(see Eye Muscles)*

STROKE   *(see Amaurosis Fugax, Hemorrhage, Ischemia, Spinal Cord)*

STUPOR   *(see Coma, Confusional State)*

STURGE-WEBER SYNDROME   *(see Neurocutaneous Syndromes)*

SUBACUTE COMBINED DEGENERATION   *(see Nutritional Deficiency Syndromes)*

SUBARACHNOID HEMORRHAGE   *(see Aneurysm, Hemorrhage)*

SUBDURAL HEMORRHAGE   *(see Hemorrhage)*

SYDENHAM'S CHOREA   *(see Chorea)*

SYMPATHETIC NERVOUS SYSTEM   *(see Autonomic Dysfunction)*

SYNCOPE   *(see also Autonomic Dysfunction, Dizziness)*

Syncope is the brief loss of consciousness and postural tone that results from decreased cerebral perfusion. Onset is usually gradual but may be rapid, with cardiac arrhythmias. If cerebral hypoperfusion persists, tonic-clonic jerks and urinary incontinence (convulsive syncope) may result. After the syncopal event some patients have muscular weakness, but confusion, headache, and drowsiness are uncommon.

Syncope is classified as follows according to the pathophysiologic mechanism involved, although all pathophysiologic mechanisms involve cerebral hypoperfusion.

  I. Orthostatic syncope usually occurs as patients are sitting or standing up and results in global cerebral hypoperfusion and syncope. Marked autonomic dysfunction, including diaphoresis, pallor, bradycardia, blurred vision, epigastric distress, and dilated pupils, usually precedes orthostatic syncope. Attaining recumbency may abort the syncopal spell and results in recovery.

II. *Vasovagal or vasodepressor syncope* usually occurs in young patients and is associated with little or no pathologic involvement. Fear, emotional distress, pain, prolonged fasting, stress, fatigue, and standing immobile while overheated are common precipitants. These events trigger increased ventricular systolic contraction via increased sympathetic release. This exaggerated inotropic response stimulates afferent unmyelinated C fibers located in the atria, ventricles, and pulmonary artery. These communicate with the dorsal vagal nucleus of the brainstem, which completes a vagal efferent arc that results in bradycardia, vasodilation, and subsequent hypotension.

III. *Impaired splanchnic and visceral vasoconstriction* is essentially a defective vasopressor response. Causes include medications (antihypertensive agents, tricyclic antidepressants, phenothiazines, levodopa, and lithium), autonomic neuropathy (diabetes, Guillain-Barré syndrome, uremia, amyloidosis, Riley-Day syndrome, porphyria, and following sympathectomy), central dysautonomias (see Autonomic Disorders), and prolonged confinement to bed.

IV. *Reflex hypotension* and other inappropriate vagal stimuli, including micturition syncope (mostly in men), defecation syncope, glossopharyngeal neuralgia, carotid sinus hypersensitivity, swallowing cold fluids, vagal irritation (such as esophageal diverticula, mediastinal masses, and gall bladder disease).

V. *Cardiac syncope* is usually unrelated to posture. It may be due to the following:
   A. Arrhythmias.
      1. *Stokes-Adams attack* is disturbance of consciousness associated with atrioventricular block. Electrocardiography shows independent P wave and QRS complexes.
      2. Sick sinus syndrome.
      3. Supraventricular tachycardias, including atrial fibrillation, atrial flutter, and Wolff-Parkinson-White syndrome.
      4. Long QT syndrome.
      5. Pacemaker failure.
      6. Ventricular fibrillation, ventricular tachycardia.
   B. Decreased cardiac output.
      1. Mechanical obstruction: left ventricular outflow obstruction.
      2. Pericardial effusion with cardiac tamponade.
      3. Myocardial infarction.

       4. Congestive heart failure.
       5. Tension pneumothorax.
       6. Superior or inferior vena cava obstruction.
       7. Congenital heart disease (tetralogy of Fallot)

  VI. Neurologic causes.
     A. Seizures (especially atonic seizures in children).
     B. Craniocervical junction lesions (may be induced by cough or sneeze).

 VII. Vascular causes.
     A. Vertebrobasilar insufficiency (diagnosis should be made only when other symptoms of brainstem ischemia are present).
     B. Subclavian steal syndrome.

VIII. Metabolic causes.
     A. Hypovolemia.
     B. Hypoglycemia (onset is usually gradual).
     C. Hyperventilation.
     D. Carbon monoxide toxicity.

  IX. Psychiatric.
     A. Panic disorder.
     B. Conversion reaction.
     C. Factitious syncope.

Medical evaluation of syncope depends on the clinical situation, and many of the tests have a low yield. The most useful tests are ECG, prolonged ambulatory monitoring (loop recorder or Holter monitor), echocardiogram, and tilt table testing. Complete blood cell count, serum chemistry studies, toxicology screens, and electrophysiologic studies are occasionally useful. Electroencephalography (EEG), carotid ultrasound, and CT scan have a low diagnostic yield in the presence of negative results of neurologic examination and history. If the history suggests seizure, EEG may be useful. Brain MRI with attention to the posterior fossa may be indicated when the history suggests vertebrobasilar insufficiency.

SYNDROME OF INAPPROPRIATE ANTIDIURETIC HORMONE (SIADH)

The syndrome of inappropriate antidiuretic hormone (SIADH) is due to antidiuretic hormone (ADH)–stimulated water conservation, which results in hyponatremia with inappropriately high urine osmolality and urine sodium excretion (>20 mEq/L). The diagnosis is made when the patient has euvolemia; normal adrenal, renal, and thyroid function; and is not taking medications that stimulate ADH release.

Manifestations are due to the hyponatremia and include mental status changes, behavioral changes, weakness, anorexia, nausea, vomiting, muscle cramps, and extrapyramidal signs. Seizures, coma, and death may occur.

Neurologic causes include stroke, subdural hematoma, subarachnoid hemorrhage, head trauma, intracranial surgery, tumors, basal skull fractures, infections, central pontine myelinolysis, vasculitis, Guillain-Barré syndrome, acute intermittent porphyria, and other neuropathies.

Therapy involves removing the underlying cause and restricting fluid intake. If hyponatremia is severe or the patient is symptomatic, correction to a serum sodium level of 125 mEq/L should be carried out by sodium repletion at a rate that increases serum sodium by 0.5 mEq per hour. Correction to normal sodium levels should then be slowly accomplished.

SYPHILIS

Neurosyphilis results from meningeal invasion by *Treponema pallidum*; parenchymal involvement occurs in later stages (that is general paresis and tabes dorsalis). Symptomatic neurosyphilis develops in only 4% to 9% of patients with syphilis who do not receive treatment. Clinical syndromes include the following:

1. *Asymptomatic neurosyphilis* refers to the presence of CSF abnormalities in the absence of neurologic signs and symptoms. The highest rate of abnormalities occurs early, 13 to 18 months after initial infection; the diagnosis is made on the basis of positive results of serum or CSF serologic tests and abnormal CSF, usually with mildly increased level of protein (40 to 200 mg/dl); normal glucose level; and a mild, lymphocytic pleocytosis (50 to 400 cells/mm³). The level of CSF gammaglobulins may be increased. Normal CSF 5 years after infection reduces the risk of CNS syphilis to 1%. Ten percent to 25% of patients with asymptomatic neurosyphilis who do not receive treatment become symptomatic. Lumbar puncture, therefore, should be performed in all patients in whom a diagnosis of syphilis is made beyond the primary stage or in whom the dating of primary infection cannot be established.
2. *Acute syphilitic meningitis* usually occurs within the initial 2 years of infection and becomes evident as headache, nuchal rigidity, confusion, and cranial nerve (CN) palsies (especially, CN II, III, VI, and VIII).

3. *Meningovascular syphilis* usually occurs within 4 to 7 years after initial infection and results from an endarteritis, most commonly of the middle cerebral artery. Meningovascular syphilis becomes evident as a focal CNS ischemia that evolves acutely or over days and is often associated with a prodrome (weeks to months) of headache, dizziness, and psychiatric disturbances.

4. *General paresis (meningoencephalitis)* usually occurs 15 to 20 years after initial infection as a result of spirochete invasion of the cortex. Dementia is the initial manifestation. Seizures may occur. Untreated, the condition is fatal within 4 years.

5. *Tabes dorsalis* occurs 20 to 25 years after infection and results from inflammation of the posterior roots and posterior columns. Classic presentation includes triads of symptoms (lightning pains, dysuria, and ataxia) and signs (Argyll-Robertson pupils, areflexia, and proprioceptive loss). Later involvement includes visceral crises, optic atrophy, ocular motor palsies, Charcot joints, and foot ulcers. Early treatment usually arrests the progression and may reverse some of the symptoms.

6. Less common manifestations include optic neuropathy, eighth-nerve neuropathy, spinal neurosyphilis (for example, meningomyelitis and meningovascular), and gumma (granulomatous mass lesions in brain or spinal cord).

7. Patients co-infected with human immunodeficiency virus (HIV) have a higher rate of early neurosyphilis (meningitis or meningovascular) and may be at an increased risk for neurologic relapse after treatment of primary and secondary syphilis with IM benzathine penicillin. This may indicate that the CNS is a "sheltered" site from which relapse may proceed.

Diagnosis depends on clinical findings, serum serology results, and CSF examination. Serum treponemal serologic tests (VDRL and RPR) become nonreactive with treatment and therefore can be used to assess therapeutic efficacy. However, their titers progressively decline, even during the course of untreated disease, becoming nonreactive in 25% of patients with late (neuro) syphilis. Serum treponemal tests (FTA-ABS, MHA-TP) are usually unaffected by treatment, their titers remaining elevated indefinitely. Therefore a nonreactive FTA-ABS result excludes neurosyphilis.

The CSF in neurosyphilis usually shows elevated protein level, normal glucose level, and lymphocytic pleocytosis (10 to 400 cells/mm^3). The CSF VDRL has very high specificity but low sensitivity (30% to 70%). Thus nonreactive CSF VDRL does not exclude neurosyphilis. The CSF FTA-ABS test has a high false-positive rate, and its role in diagnosis is unclear. As with all CSF serologic studies, a traumatic spinal fluid sample may also give misleading results.

Treatment of neurosyphilis consists of a regimen of aqueous penicillin G, 2 to 4 million units IV q4h for 10 to 14 days. An alternative treatment is penicillin G procaine 2 to 4 million units IM qd with probenecid 500 mg po qid for 10 to 14 days. In cases of penicillin allergy treatment options include penicillin desensitization followed by standard penicillin therapy; other regimens, such as tetracycline hydrochloride 500 mg PO qid for 30 days, erythromycin 500 mg PO qid for 30 days, or ceftriaxone 250 mg IM qd, are recommended for primary, secondary or latent syphilis but are of unproven value for tertiary neurosyphilis.

Follow-up CSF examination should be performed at 6 and 12 months. The CSF cell count is the earliest indicator of response and relapse and should normalize within 6 months. CSF protein level declines more slowly, taking as long as 2 years to normalize. CSF VDRL titers are the last to decline and may remain mildly elevated despite adequate treatment. Repeat treatment is indicated if the CSF pleocytosis persists after 6 months or is abnormal 2 years after treatment. Because CSF protein level and VDRL titers take much longer to normalize, treatment cannot be considered inadequate unless these values unequivocally increase.

REF: Hook EW, Marra CM: N Engl J Med 326:1060–1069, 1992.

Katz DA, Berger JR, Duncan RC: Arch Neurol 50:243–249, 1993.

Simon RP: Arch Neurol 42:606, 1985.

SYRINGOMYELIA   *(see Spinal Cord)*

TABES DORSALIS   *(see Syphilis)*

TAKAYASU'S ASTERITIS   *(see Vasculitis)*

TASTE

Taste receptor cells are modified epithelial cells in the taste buds located in the anteroposterior aspect of the tongue, soft-palate pharynx, epiglottis, and proximal one third of the esophagus. Taste sensation is mediated by the facial, glossopharyngeal, and vagus nerves. Proximal lesions of the facial nerve between the pons and facial canal where the chorda tympani joins the facial nerve result in unilateral loss of taste on the anterior two thirds of the tongue. The greater superficial petrosal branch of the facial nerve carries taste from the soft palate (see Facial Nerve). The lingual, tonsillar, and pharyngeal branches of the glossopharyngeal nerve carry taste from the posterior one third of the tongue and pharynx. The superior laryngeal branch of the vagus carries taste from the esophagus and epiglottis. All afferent taste fibers project to the solitary tract nucleus. Fibers then project to the thalamus, ventral forebrain, lateral hypothalamus, and amygdala. From the thalamus, fibers mediating taste sensation project to the insular cortex.

Salt, sour, sweet, and bitter tastes can be perceived throughout the oral cavity. Taste depends on the adaptive state of the tongue. Even water can evoke a taste if the tongue is adapted to certain substances. When there is a change in either the flow rate or composition of saliva, there may be ageusia (absence of taste), dysgeusia (distortion of taste), or hypogeusia (diminished taste). Therefore when a change in taste sensation is being evaluated, one must rule out conditions affecting production of salivary fluids, for example, Sjögren's syndrome, pan-dysautonomia, and amyloidosis. Olfactory dysfunction must also be considered in disorders of taste.

Taste testing is accomplished with the use of a cotton applicator. The patient should not speak but should point to cards with the words *sweet, salty, bitter,* and *sour* written on them. Causes of an alteration in taste sensation include an upper respiratory tract infection, nasal disorders, head injury with damage to either the lingual nerve or chorda tympani, heavy smoking, hepatitis, following influenza, viral encephalitis, hypothyroidism, diabetes, hypogonadism (Kallman's syndrome), neoplasm, and vitamin A or B_{12} deficiency. Medications that cause a change in taste include antirheumatic, antiproliferative drugs; calcium channel blockers; and drugs with sulfhydryl groups. Cerebellar pontine angle tumors occasionally cause a loss of taste.

Gustatory hallucinations may occur as an aura of psychomotor epilepsy or in alcohol-induced delirium and are usually associated with olfactory hallucinations.

TAY-SACHS DISEASE   *(see Degenerative Diseases of Childhood)*

TELANGECTASIA   *(see Neurocutaneous Syndromes)*

TEMPORAL ARTERITIS   *(see Amaurosis Fugax, Vasculitis)*

TEMPORAL LOBE

The temporal lobe is bordered superiorly by the sylvian fissure and merges with the parietal and occipital lobes. In addition to neocortical areas, it contains the amygdala, hippocampus, and paleocortical areas such as olfactory and entorhinal cortices. Temporal structures contain connections to the thalamus, hypothalamus, striatum, septum, cingulate gyrus, and other neocortical areas. Signs of temporal lobe dysfunction include partial complex seizures, memory difficulty (especially bilateral hippocampal involvement, but nonverbal memory may be impaired with nondominant hemisphere hippocampal damage), aphasia with dominant temporal lesions, agnosias, visual field defects (superior quadrantanopsias), and behavioral or emotional disturbances. The Klüver-Bucy syndrome of placidity, apathy, hypersexuality, hyperorality, and visual and auditory agnosia occurs with bilateral anterior temporal lobe injury involving both neocortex and paleocortex.

TENDON REFLEX   *(see Reflexes)*

TENSILON TEST   *(see Myasthenia Gravis)*

TERATOMA   *(see Tumor)*

TETANUS   *(see Cramps)*

TETANY   *(see Electrolyte Disorders)*

THALAMIC SYNDROMES

The following thalamic syndromes result from infarctions, and each corresponds to a different arterial territory:

1. Inferolateral artery (thalamogeniculate artery) infarcts with posterolateral thalamic lesions involve mainly the ventral posterior nuclear group. Most commonly comes to medical attention with hemisensory loss and pain. Ataxia is present in up to 75% of patients.
2. Tuberothalamic artery supplying the anterior region, including the ventral anterior nucleus and part of the ventral lateral nucleus. Neuropsychologic disturbance is the most common symptoms; dysphasia occurs with left-sided lesions, and hemineglect with right-sided lesions. Mild motor and sensory deficits are common.

3. Posterior choroidal arteries, which supplies the lateral geniculate body. Visual field deficits are the most common feature.
4. Paramedian arteries supplying the paramedian midbrain and thalamus, including the intralaminar group and most of the dorsomedial nucleus. Changes in state of consciousness, coma, confusion with confabulation (bilateral infarcts), and ocular motor abnormalities are frequent with this type of infarction.

The syndrome of Dejerine and Roussy (inferolateral thalamic syndrome) is due to a vascular lesion in the territory of the thalamogeniculate artery. It is characterized by a mild hemiparesis, persistent hemianesthesia for touch, slight hemiataxia and astereognosis, choreoathetotic movements, and pain. *Thalamic pain* occurs contralateral to the lesion and is described as burning, aching, or boring. It is constant, but often there are paroxysmal increases, spontaneous or induced. This pain syndrome *(central poststroke pain)* has also been observed in patients with lesions in the brainstem, internal capsule, basal ganglia, and subcortical parietal lobe. Treatment with tricyclic antidepressants (amitriptyline 10 to 100 mg qhs), or anticonvulsants (carbamazepine or dilantin) are effective. Conventional analgesics are ineffective.

REF: Bogousslavsky J, Regli F, Uske A: *Neurology* 38:837-848, 1988.

Steinke W et al: *Arch Neurol* 49:703-710, 1992.

THIAMINE   *(see Nutritional Deficiency Syndrome)*

THOMSEN'S DISEASE   *(see Myotonia)*

THROMBOSIS   *(see Ischemia)*

THYMOMA   *(see Myasthenia Gravis)*

THYROID   *(see also Graves' Ophthalmopathy, Metabolic Diseases of Childhood, Myopathy, Periodic Paralysis)*

Thyrotoxic crisis is a medical emergency manifested by high fever, tachycardia, hypotension, vomiting, diarrhea, and delirium. It may progress to coma and death if not treated promptly. Crisis may be precipitated by infection or inadequate preparation for thyroid surgery.

Mortality rate is as high as 30%. Management includes the use of thiourea agents, sodium iodide, adrenergic blockers, adrenocorticosteroids, sedatives, and body cooling, as well as maintenance of fluid and electrolyte levels.

HYPERTHYROIDISM

Chronic thyrotoxic myopathy is rare, despite common complaints of nonspecific weakness. Creatine kinase (CK) level is normal or decreased. Electromyography (EMG) reveals short-duration polyphasic motor unit potentials. Neuropathy is rare. Muscle power normalizes as the patient becomes euthyroid.

Thyrotoxic periodic paralysis resembles hypokalemic periodic paralysis. Myasthenia gravis has an increased incidence in patients with hypothyroidism or hyperthyroidism, and vice versa.

Corticospinal tract dysfunction (pathophysiology unknown) rarely appears as an isolated complication of thyroid disease. However, hyperreflexia is common and reflects shortened relaxation time. Acute thyrotoxic encephalomyelopathy becomes evident as an acute bulbar palsy with associated encephalopathy. Brain swelling and focal hemorrhages are seen on pathologic study. Myasthenia gravis often contributes to the bulbar weakness and confounds the evaluation. Symptoms may resolve with achievement of a euthyroid state.

Seizures, usually generalized, may develop or be exacerbated during thyrotoxicosis. Electroencephalographic abnormalities (generalized slowing and increased alpha activity) are seen in 60% of patients with hyperthyroidism.

Psychosis is exacerbated by hyperthyroidism. "Apathetic hyperthyroidism" is common in elderly individuals and comes to medical attention as apathy, depression, and lack of energy.

An accentuation of physiologic tremor by increased sensitivity to sympathetic input is quite common in most patients with hyperthyroidism and involves primarily the upper extremities. Propranolol is useful in treatment.

Chorea resulting from hypersensitivity of dopaminergic receptors may be abolished by a regimen of haloperidol and resolves spontaneously as the patient becomes euthyroid.

Stroke results from cerebral embolism in thyrotoxic atrial fibrillation. Acute anticoagulation therapy may be appropriate.

HYPOTHYROIDISM

Myopathy: Weakness (proximal > distal), cramps, pain and stiffness are common complaints, but objective weakness is less common. The creatine phosphokinase level is often elevated. EMG findings are non-specific.

Myoedema, a percussion-induced local mounding of contracted muscle that relaxes slowly, can be elicited but can also occur in emaciated patients and in some normal individuals. The contraction is electrically silent on EMG.

Muscle hypertrophy, known as *Hoffman's syndrome* in adults and *Kocher-Debré-Sémélaigne syndrome* in children, is rare. Patients complain of stiffness and painful muscle cramps, and the movements are slow and weak. The muscles are large and firm. *Pseudomyotonia*, or delayed muscle relaxation after handshake or percussion, may be present and is differentiated from myotonia by its electrical silence on EMG.

Peripheral neuropathies are mostly median neuropathies at the wrist (carpal tunnel) resulting from mucoid infiltration of the nerve and the surrounding tissue. Eighty percent of patients complain of distal paresthesias. Polyneuropathies are less frequent.

Deep tendon reflexes have slowed relaxation time, but this is also seen in hypothermia, leg edema, diabetes, parkinsonism, drug use, and normal aging.

Ataxia with impaired tandem gait and limb incoordination is common and is attributed to cerebellar dysfunction, although nystagmus and dysarthria are infrequent.

Psychosis is common. In elderly individuals the associated cognitive dysfunction can progress to dementia.

Coma occurs rarely, usually in patients with chronic, severe, undiagnosed disease. Seizures may occur. Emergency management consists of thyroid replacement, corticosteroid therapy, treatment of hypoglycemia, correction of fluid and electrolyte abnormalities and hypothermia, and ventilatory support as needed.

Changes on EEG include slowing of alpha activity and decreased driving response with high-frequency photic stimulation. Markedly reduced background amplitude may be seen in hypothermic states.

The level of CSF protein is elevated in 40% to 90% of patients with hypothyroidism and occasionally >100% mg/dl. Gammaglobulin level may also be increased in both CSF and serum for unknown reasons.

REF: Kaminski HJ, Ruff RL: Endocrine myopathies (hyper and hypo functioning of adrenal-thyroid-pituitary and parathyroid glands and iatrogenic steroid myopathy). In Engel AG, Franzini-Armstrong, C, eds: *Myology*, New York, 1994, McGraw-Hill.

Kaminski HJ, Ruff RL: *Neurol Clin* 7(3):489, 1989.

TIA   *(see Ischemia)*

TIBIAL NERVE   *(see Peripheral Nerve)*

TIC DOULOUREUX   *(see Neuralgia)*

TICS   *(see Tourette's Syndrome)*

TINNITUS   *(see Hearing)*

TOLOSA-HUNT SYNDROME   *(see Ophthalmoplegia)*

TONE   *(see Dystonia, Reflexes, Rigidity, Spasticity)*

TORTICOLLIS   *(see Dystonia)*

TOURETTE'S SYNDROME (DISORDER)   *(see Attention Deficit– Hyperactivity Disorder)*

The DSM-IV defines Gilles de la Tourette's syndrome (TS) as characterized by (1) multiple motor tics, (2) one or more vocal tics present at some time during the illness, although not necessarily concurrently, (3) onset before 18 years of age, (4) duration of more than 1 year without a tic-free interval of more than three consecutive months, and (5) marked distress or significant impairment in social or occupational functioning. The disorder is part of a broader clinical spectrum that includes both transient and chronic tic disorders. Tics occur as frequently as several times per minute, and their characteristics change over time. There is a natural variation in the intensity of symptoms, which wax and wane over months to years. Tics may involve the head, trunk, or extremities. Vocal tics include sounds such as grunts, coughs, clicks, or barks. The utterance of obscenities (coprolalia) is uncommon. Tics may be simple twitches of muscle groups, or complex, such as touching and then smelling the hand, twirling when walking, or retracing steps. They may be voluntarily suppressed for minutes to hours. There is a wide range in severity, and most mild cases do not come to medical attention.

The average of onset is 7 years, but TS may appear as early as 1 year of age. The initial symptom is usually a single tic, most commonly, eye blinking. Although remissions occur (weeks to years), TS is usually lifelong. In some cases symptoms diminish during adolescence or may disappear entirely by early adulthood. Three times as many males as females are affected. There is an association with obsessive-compulsive disorder and attention deficit–hyperactivity disorder (ADHD), each occurring in 25% to 50% of TS patients. TS is currently thought to be inherited in an autosomal dominant pattern with incomplete and sex-specific penetrance and variable expression.

Pathogenesis is unknown. Stimulant drugs used for ADHD may exacerbate or unmask TS. Differential diagnosis includes other disorders with abnormal movements in children, such as Huntington's disease, Sydenham's chorea, Wilson's disease, Lesch-Nyhan syndrome, and myoclonus.

Pharmacotherapy should be reserved for patients with significant impairment of daily activity or potential for self-injury. Clonidine therapy is effective in reducing tics. Side effects include orthostatic hypotension and sedation (early in treatment). Pimozide and haloperidol are equally effective in suppressing tics. Tardive dyskinesia is a concern. When a neuroleptic is given, the minimum effective dose should be used and attempts to withdraw the medication should be undertaken periodically.

REF: Cohen DJ, Riddle MA, Leckman JF: *Pediatr Clin* 15:109, 1992.

Golden GS: *Neurol Clin* 8:705, 1990.

Kurlan R: *Neurology* 39:1625, 1989.

Tourette Syndrome Classification Study Group: *Arch Neurol* 50:1013-1016, 1993.

TOXOPLASMOSIS   *(see AIDS, Abscess)*

TRANSIENT GLOBAL AMNESIA   *(see Memory)*

TRANSIENT ISCHEMIC ATTACK   *(see Ischemia)*

TRANSPLANTATION—NEUROLOGIC ASPECTS
ORGAN HARVEST

The determination of death before organ harvest is based on neurologic criteria. Most current jurisdictions require absence of function of the entire brain (see Brain Death).

CLINICAL SYNDROMES IN ORGAN RECIPIENTS

Organ recipients often have complex syndromes and multiple possible causes and origins of their diverse syndromes. Opportunistic infection must always be considered. Primary neurotoxicity of immunosuppressants may be present but is often accompanied by electrolyte derangements, hemodynamic fluctuations, concurrent corticosteroid administration, and other drug effects. Many CNS symptoms have been reported, but few large series exist. Specific clinical syndromes include the following:

Opportunistic CNS Infection

Infection occurs as a result of immunosuppression; occurs in up to 10% of recipients; mortality rate is high; death occurs 1 month or more after transplantation.

Fungi

Cryptococcus is the most common pathogen and usually becomes evident after 6 months of immune suppression; *Aspergillus* often becomes evident as stroke or encephalopathy; *Candida* usually becomes evident as chronic meningitis; *Mucormycosis* is seen in diabetic recipients.

Bacteria

Listeria is the most common bacterium, usually causing meningitis; *Nocardia* usually causes abscess; *Tuberculosis* is uncommon.

Parasites

Toxoplasmosis becomes evident 1 to 4 months after transplantation.

Viruses

Cytomegalovirus: May cause chorioretinitis. *Varicella:* New infection may cause encephalitis with high rate of morbidity, reactivation produces shingles, either diffusely or in dermatomal distribution. *Human T-cell lymphotropic virus, I:* Causing myelopathy after blood transfusion in heart, bone marrow, and kidney recipients. *JC virus:* Progressive multifocal leukoencephalopathy (see Encephalitis).

Other neurologic syndromes include the following:

Cerebellar dysfunction: Dysarthria and ataxia resulting from neurotoxicity of immunosuppressants.
Demyelination: Central pontine myelinolysis caused by osmotic shifts, frequently during the perioperative period.

Hearing loss: Resulting from cyclosporine-mediated thromboembolic process or from toxic effects of antibiotics.

Language disorders: Reversible; resulting from FK506 neurotoxicity or reversible demyelination.

Malignancy: Primary CNS lymphoma resulting from immunosuppression.

Mental status deterioration: Occurs with cyclosporine use and accompanying diffuse changes on MRI; cognitive slowing, insomnia, delirium, and perceptual disturbances are seen with use of cyclosporine and FK506 in liver recipients; metabolic acidosis can cause coma in kidney recipients.

Migraine: Occurs in bone-marrow recipients as a result of cyclosporine use or hypothesized defect in donor-derived platelets.

Movement disorder: Chorea resulting from cyclosporine use in liver transplantation for Wilson's disease.

Myopathy: Occurs in lung transplantation with use of cyclosporine, azathioprine, or prednisone, along with prolonged response to neuromuscular blockade; myositis is one manifestation of graft-versus-host disease.

Nerve injury: Recurrent laryngeal palsy in heart-lung recipient.

Neurocardiogenic symptoms: Angina and vasovagal syncope are seen in heart recipients, presumably because of reinnervation.

Neuropathy: Reported in a pancreas recipient.

Pain: As a result of varicella zoster or local effects at operative sites; musculoskeletal pain resulting from direct cyclosporine effects in kidney recipients; resulting from oral mucositis in bone marrow recipients.

Seizures: Generalized tonic-clonic seizures occur in bone marrow transplantation with regimen of busulfan, cyclophosphamide, cyclosporine, or methylprednisolone; seen with use of FK506; seen in liver recipients, often with neuropathologic lesions at autopsy.

Sleep disorder: Somnolence syndrome related to radiation therapy in bone marrow recipient.

Stroke and cerebral ischemia: Less common with FK506 use than with cyclosporine therapy in liver recipients; resulting from hypoperfusion in heart recipient.

Taste disturbance: Occurs in bone marrow recipients.

Visual disturbance: Side effects of cyclosporine therapy.

REF: Cilio MR et al: *Arch Dis Child* 68:405-407, 1993.

Eidelman BH et al: *Transplant Proc* 23:3175-3178, 1991.

Estol CJ, Lopez O, Brenner RP, Martinez AJ: *Neurology* 39:1297-1301, 1989.

Lopez OL et al: *Hepatology* 16:162-166, 1992.

TRANSVERSE MYELITIS   *(see Spinal Cord)*

TREMORS

Tremors are regular, rhythmic oscillations produced by alternating contraction of agonist and antagonist muscles. They usually affect the distal extremities (especially fingers and hands), head, tongue, jaw, and only rarely, the trunk. Tremors disappear during sleep. The frequency is usually consistent in all the affected parts, regardless of the size of muscles involved. It is important to observe the amplitude, frequency, and rhythm of the tremor, as well as the effects of physiologic (posture, limb movement, diurnal variation, and so forth) and psychologic factors.

CLASSIFICATION

I. *Action or postural tremor:* Present when the limbs and trunk are held in certain positions or during active movements.
   A. *Physiologic tremor:* Small-amplitude, high-frequency (6 to 12 Hz) tremor seen in normal individuals; exaggerated by stress, endocrine disorders (hyperthyroidism, hypoglycemia, and pheochromocytoma), or drugs (such as lithium, tricyclics, phenothiazines, epinephrine, theophylline, amphetamines, thyroid hormones, isoproterenol, corticosteroids, valproate, levodopa, and butyrophenones) and toxins (such as mercury, lead, arsenic, bismuth, and carbon monoxide). Dietary factors may contribute (caffeine, monosodium glutamate, and ethanol withdrawal). Management depends on the cause; relaxation methods and stress reduction may help if psychologic factors are involved. Beta blockers have been used with some success, particularly in performers with "stage fright."
   B. *Essential tremor:* A postural tremor that often increases with action or intention. It has a frequency of 4 to 7 Hz and usually consists of flexion-extension of the fingers and hands initially, but may progress proximally; the head and neck, jaw, tongue, or voice may be involved. It is exacerbated by emotional and physical stress and diminished with rest, relaxation, and use of ethanol. It may be familial (dominant inheritance), sporadic, or associated with other movement disorders (Parkinson's disease, torsion dystonia, or torticollis). Propranolol is the drug of choice but is contraindicated in patients with

asthma or diabetes and in older patients with heart failure. Start with doses of 10 to 20 mg three or four times a day, increasing dosage if necessary. Primidone therapy is also useful, starting at 50 mg.

C. *Primary writing tremor:* Occurs only during writing. Electrophysiologic studies suggest that it may be a form of dystonia. It may respond to anticholinergic therapy.

D. *Rubral tremor:* A coarse tremor present at rest, increasing with postural maintenance and even more with movement. Suggests ipsilateral cerebellar outflow lesion.

II. Rest tremors.

A. *Parkinsonian tremor:* Coarse frequency of 3 to 7 Hz with variable amplitude, sometimes asymmetric. It occurs at rest and disappears during sleep. It is prominent in the hands, with flexion-extension or adduction-abduction of the fingers. There is also pronation-supination of the hands. Movements of the feet, jaw, and lips may be present. It responds to anticholinergic therapy (see Parkinson's disease).

III. Intention tremor.

A. *Cerebellar tremor:* A tremor of 3 to 5 Hz occurring during the performance of an exact, projected movement and worsening as the action continues. There may be tremors of the head or trunk (titubation). The oscillation begins proximally and occurs perpendicular to the line of movement. Causes include lesions of cerebellar pathways, cerebellar degeneration, Wilson's disease, and drugs or toxins (such as phenytoin, barbiturates, lithium, ethanol, mercury, and fluorouracil).

IV. Other tremors.

A. *Orthostatic tremor,* a tremor of the legs, is present only when standing and disappears with walking. As such, it may be considered a task-specific tremor. It responds to clonazepam therapy, 4 to 6 mg per day.

B. *Hysterical tremor* may be a symptom of conversion disorder. The tremor is often irregular in frequency and may diminish or disappear with distraction.

REF: Findley LJ, Koller WC: *Neurology* 37:1194, 1987.

Hallett, M: *JAMA* 266:1115-1117, 1991.

TRICYCLIC ANTIDEPRESSANTS   *(see Antidepressants, Pain)*

TRIGEMINAL NERVE   *(see Cranial Nerves, Neuralgia, Zoster)*

TROCHLEAR NERVE   *(See Cranial Nerves, Eye Muscles, Ophthalmoplegia)*

TROUSSEAU'S SIGN   *(see Myopathy-Endocrine-Hypoparathyroidism)*

TUBERCULOSIS   *(see Cerebrospinal Fluid, Meningitis)*

TUBEROUS SCLEROSIS   *(see Neurocutaneous Syndromes)*

TUMORS   *(see also Paraneoplastic Syndromes, Radiation Injury, Spinal Cord)*

The presence of tumor within the nervous system is often suspected by the development of subacute or acute focal symptoms. Some tumors, particularly metastases or carcinomatous meningitis, may result in multifocal signs. The combination of location, patient demographics, and neuroimaging often suggests the most likely histopathology (see Table 59 and Figure 43).

BRAIN

Although primary brain tumors occur about five times more often in adults than in children, the central nervous system (CNS) is the second most common site for childhood malignancies. Metastases account for the majority of CNS tumors in adults. Approximately 20% of all patients with systemic cancer have CNS involvement at some time during their illness.

Symptoms and signs of CNS neoplasm may be generalized and nonlocalizing, usually as a result of diffuse edema, hydrocephalus, or increased intracranial pressure. Headaches are variable and may resemble tension or migraine headaches. Most headaches are ipsilateral to the tumor. With increased intracranial pressure a bifrontal or bioccipital headache is common, regardless of tumor location. Seizures occur more often with slow-growing tumors and with tumors in the frontal and parietal lobes. Vomiting occurs most consistently with posterior fossa masses. Localizing symptoms and signs depend on tumor location. Frontal lobe masses may be silent or, if anterior and midline, may produce changes in personality and memory. Third ventricle and pineal region tumors often produce ventricular and aqueductal ob-

TABLE 59
Histological Classification

Neuroepithelial tumors:
  Astrocytic tumors:
    Diffuse astrocytoma
    Astrocytoma
    Anaplastic astrocytoma
    Glioblastoma multiforme
    Juvenile pilocytic astrocy-
      toma
    Subependymal giant cell
      astrocytoma
  Oligodendroglial tumors:
    Oligodendroglioma
    Anaplastic oligodendro-
      glioma
  Ependymal tumors:
    Ependymoma
    Myxopapillary ependy-
      moma
    Anaplastic ependymoma
    Subependymoma
  Choroid plexus tumors:
    Choroid plexus papilloma
    Choroid plexus carcinoma
  Neuronal tumors:
    Ganglioglioma
    Gangliocytoma
  Primitive neuroectodermal
    tumors:
    Medulloblastoma
    Pineoblastoma
    Neuroblastoma
Meningeal tumors:
  Meningioma
  Papillary meningioma
  Anaplastic meningioma

Nerve sheath tumors:
  Schwannoma (neurilem-
    moma)
  Neurofibroma
  Neurofibrosarcoma
Tumors of blood vessel origin:
  Hemangioblastoma
  Hemangiopericytoma
Germ cell tumors:
  Germinoma
  Embryonal carcinoma
  Choriocarcinoma
  Teratoma
Malignant lymphomas:
  Hodgkin's disease
  Non-Hodgkin's lymphoma
Malformative tumors:
  Craniopharyngioma
  Epidermoid cyst
  Dermoid cyst
  Neuroepithelial (colloid) cyst
  Lipoma
Regional tumors:
  Chordoma
  Glomus jugulare tumor
  Chondroma
Metastatic tumors:
  Carcinoma
  Sarcoma
  Lymphoma

From Cohen ME: In Bradley WG, Daroff RB, Fenichel GM, Marsden CD, eds:
Neurology in Clinical Practice, Boston, 1991, Butterworth-Heinemann.

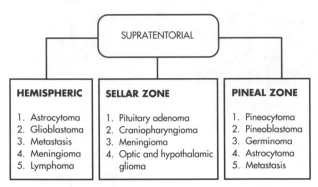

SUPRATENTORIAL

HEMISPHERIC

1. Astrocytoma
2. Glioblastoma
3. Metastasis
4. Meningioma
5. Lymphoma

SELLAR ZONE

1. Pituitary adenoma
2. Craniopharyngioma
3. Meningioma
4. Optic and hypothalamic glioma

PINEAL ZONE

1. Pineocytoma
2. Pineoblastoma
3. Germinoma
4. Astrocytoma
5. Metastasis

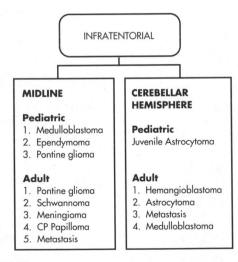

INFRATENTORIAL

MIDLINE

Pediatric
1. Medulloblastoma
2. Ependymoma
3. Pontine glioma

Adult
1. Pontine glioma
2. Schwannoma
3. Meningioma
4. CP Papilloma
5. Metastasis

CEREBELLAR HEMISPHERE

Pediatric
Juvenile Astrocytoma

Adult
1. Hemangioblastoma
2. Astrocytoma
3. Metastasis
4. Medulloblastoma

FIGURE 43
Tumors by location.

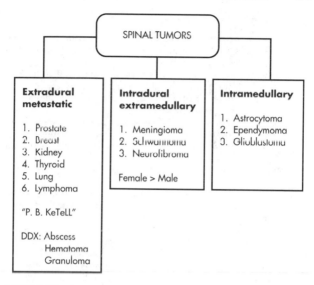

FIGURE 43
Continued.
From AAN: Contemporary neuropathology in Volume six, *Basic neurosciences,* AAN Courses 1993, courtesy of JC Goodman.

struction leading to hydrocephalus. Brainstem tumors produce cranial neuropathies, long-tract signs, and hydrocephalus resulting from compression of the aqueduct.

Once suspected, the diagnosis of a brain tumor is usually confirmed by neuroimaging, either CT scan or MRI. Hemorrhage occurs most often with glioblastoma multiforme and metastatic tumors, especially renal cell, melanoma, and choriocarcinoma. Calcification occurs more commonly with oligodendrogliomas and meningiomas. Skull x-rays remain useful in evaluating bony metastasis; angiography defines vascular anatomy.

Available treatment modalities include debulking surgery, radiation therapy, chemotherapy, and combinations of the three. The late effects of CNS irradiation include radiation necrosis, myelopathy, intellectual deterioration, endocrinopathies, and oncogenesis (see also Chemotherapy, Radiation).

SPINAL CORD

Tumors of the spinal cord and its coverings account for approximately 15% of all CNS tumors. Extradural cord tumors arise from the vertebral bodies and epidural tissues or are metastatic lesions to the epidural space. Intradural tumors are either intramedullary (arising within the substance of the cord) or extramedullary (arising from the leptomeninges or nerve roots). Myelography with CT scanning has been the traditional procedure of choice in the evaluation of spinal cord masses and allows for the simultaneous collection of spinal fluid. Myelography with CT can demonstrate the presence of spinal block, but the upper extent of that may require a second spinal puncture (for example, cervical tap). MRI can differentiate solid from cystic intramedullary tumors and defines whether lesions are intradural or extradural.

Clinical manifestations of spinal masses include local back or radicular pain, myelopathy, sensory complaints, and sphincter dysfunction. On plain radiographic films these masses may produce widening of the interpeduncular distance or of the neural foramina, as well as scalloping of the vertebral bodies. The loss of a pedicle and signs of bone destruction are associated with malignant extradural lesions. Since the majority of spinal tumors are benign and produce symptoms by compression rather than by invasion, surgery is the treatment of choice for most masses.

METASTATIC DISEASE

Metastases to the brain parenchyma are often found at the gray–white matter junction and are typically well demarcated with a zone of surrounding edema. They are usually carcinomas rather than sarcomas or lymphomas. Cancers most commonly associated with metastases, vary according to site, as follows:

Skull and dura: Breast, prostate, multiple myeloma.
Brain: Lung, breast, colorectal, renal, melanoma.
Leptomeninges: Breast, lung, melanoma, colorectal, lymphoma, leukemia.
Epidural (spinal cord): Lung, breast, prostate, lymphoma, sarcoma, renal.

EPIDURAL SPINAL CORD COMPRESSION

Spinal cord compression represents a neurologic emergency. The diagnosis should be suspected in anyone with a known tumor and back pain who seeks medical attention with segmental or myelopathic signs.

Diagnosis can be suspected from the presence of bony destruction if present on plain radiographic films; confirmation can be obtained by MRI, myelography, or occasionally, bone scan. Treatment usually consists of radiotherapy and a regimen of high-dose corticosteroids: load with dexamethasone 100 mg IV, then maintain dexamethasone 24 mg qid (PO or IV) for 3 days; steroids are then tapered over 12 days, decreasing the dose every 2 days (12 mg qid, then 8 mg qid, then 4 mg qid, then 2 mg qid, then 1 mg qid, then 0.5 mg qid). Indications for possible surgery include the following:

1. Occurrence of metastases in a previously irradiated area.
2. Spinal instability.
3. Bony compression of neural structures.
4. Deterioration during radiotherapy, despite administration of high-dose corticosteroids.
5. The need for biopsy when the diagnosis is unclear.

The entire spinal cord should be imaged because 15% to 25% of patients present with two or more lesions.

In approximately 5% of patients with cancer (breast, lung, prostate, lymphoma, melanoma) spinal epidural metastatic disease may progress to spinal cord compression. Acute compression is an emergency and is treated with high-dose corticosteroids and radiation therapy. To establish tissue diagnosis, treat previously irradiated areas, and alleviate bony canal stenosis, surgery is recommended.

REF: Cohen ME. In Bradley WG, Daroff RB, Fenichel GM, Marsden CD, eds: *Neurology in clinical practice*, Boston, 1991, Butterworth-Heinemann.

Fetell MR et al. In Rowland LP, ed: *Merritt's textbook of neurology*, ed 8, Philadelphia, 1989, Lea & Febiger.

Patchell RA, ed: *Neurol Clin* 9(4), 1991.

ULNAR NERVE   *(see also Peripheral Nerve)*

Entrapment at the elbow results from compression of the ulnar nerve as it courses in the elbow joint under the aponeurosis connecting the two heads of the flexor carpi ulnaris. It commonly results from extrinsic compression, from leaning on the elbow (especially in patients with a shallow ulnar groove), or from malpositioning of the arms on operating room tables or the arm rests of wheelchairs. "Tardy ulnar palsy" occurs following an elbow fracture or in association with arthritis, ganglion cysts, lipomas, or neuropathic (Charcot) joints. Symptoms include elbow pain, sensory loss and paresthesias of the fifth and ulnar half of the fourth digits and ulnar aspect of the hand, and wasting of the hypothenar and intrinsic hand muscles. There may be a claw-hand deformity. Marked weakness of the flexor carpi ulnaris suggests that the lesion is above the elbow. There may be tenderness or enlargement of the ulnar nerve (palpable in the epicondylar groove); Tinel's sign may be present at the elbow.

Differential diagnosis includes C8 or T1 radiculopathy, syringomyelia, ALS, lower trunk brachial plexopathy (Pancoast syndrome), and peripheral polyneuropathy. Nerve conduction studies may show conduction block or slowing across the elbow; EMG may show denervation.

Treatment involves removing exacerbating factors by padding the elbow or armchair rests. If this fails, or if motor involvement is found on physical examination or EMG, surgical decompression may be indicated. There is no clear advantage of more complex procedures (such as ulnar nerve transposition) over simple slitting of the aponeurosis of the flexor carpi ulnaris. However, transposition may be indicated in patients with fibrosis from joint disease.

Entrapment at the wrist or hand (Guyon's canal) consists of variable involvement of the deep and superficial branches of the ulnar nerve to the hand, with sparing of the dorsal cutaneous branch that supplies sensation to the dorsal ulnar sensory distribution. The same etiologic factors as for the elbow apply. The EMG and nerve conduction studies should demonstrate involvement of the hand ulnar motor fibers with sparing of sensory function to the dorsal hand.

ULTRASONOGRAPHY

The carotid and vertebral arteries and their branches can be evaluated with ultrasound, that is, sound with frequency higher than 20,000 Hz. Brightness modulation *(B mode)* is based on the transmission of ultrasound through tissues and reflection from tissue interfaces. This imaging technique produces a real-time two-dimensional picture of examined extracranial vessels in longitudinal or transverse view. It allows measurement of vessel diameter and reveals the presence of stenosis or occlusion. High-resolution scans can also determine morphologic features of plaque, such as ulceration, calcification, or hemorrhage. In *Doppler ultrasonography* the ultrasound is reflected off moving targets (erythrocytes). Increased blood-flow velocity in a narrowed segment of arterial lumen (stenosis) is associated with higher frequency shift, which correlates with flow velocities. The best result in vascular ultrasonography can be obtained by combination of these two techniques, *duplex ultrasonography*. It combines advantages of B mode with exact sampling of the site, and systolic, diastolic, and mean velocities are measured in Doppler mode. Compared with angiography, carotid duplex ultrasonography has an excellent accuracy for detection of stenotic process. For arteries with stenosis of more than 50%, sensitivity is approximately 94% to 100%; for occlusions, sensitivity is 80% to 96% and specificity is 95%. However, these results vary considerably, depending on the examiner's experience. Examination of vertebral arteries allows determination of flow direction (for example, subclavian steal syndrome), but morphologic evaluation is not always possible.

Blood-flow velocities in the major intracranial arteries can be examined by *transcranial Doppler* (TCD). It is impossible to visualize intracranial vessels, and atypical anatomic conditions or individual variations may be difficult to distinguish from vascular pathology. In some patients, particular arteries cannot be insonated for technical reasons. Transcranial Doppler has established value in detection of stenosis >65% in the major basal intracranial arteries, in assessing collateral flow, in evaluating and monitoring vasospasm after subarachnoid hemorrhage, in detecting arteriovenous malformations, and in assessing patients with brain death. The accuracy of TCD also depends highly on operator skills and experience.

REF: American Academy of Neurology: *Neurology* 40:680–681, 1992.

Hedera P, Traubner P, Bujdakova J: *Stroke* 23:1069–1072, 1992.

Stewart JH, Grubb M: *Mayo Clin Proc* 67:1186–1196, 1992.

UREMIA

Uremic encephalopathy is most closely correlated with the rate of progression of uremia, as opposed to the absolute blood urea nitrogen and creatinine levels. Clouding of consciousness, ataxia, tremor, and asterixis may be associated with hallucinations, and increased tone and reflexes that may be asymmetric. Tetany may occur that does not respond to calcium. Late signs include multifocal myoclonus, seizures, and coma. The EEG is characterized by low-voltage slowing early; later there may be generalized paroxysmal slowing. Triphasic waves of epileptiform activity are not uncommon. CSF protein level may be elevated, and an aseptic meningitis may occur, accompanied by stiff neck and marked pleocytosis.

Seizures in renal failure are usually generalized but may be focal. They may occur in the setting of uremic encephalopathy, hypertensive crisis, coexistent electrolyte disturbance, or drug toxicity. Seizures of uremic encephalopathy often respond to dialysis. When anticonvulsants are required, dosages must be adjusted. Partial renal clearance usually requires decreased dosages of carbamazepine and phenobarbital. Changes in clearance and protein binding lead to decreased total phenytoin levels with an increased unbound fraction. These changes necessitate free-fraction monitoring for optimal control.

Uremic neuropathy occurs in two thirds of patients beginning dialysis. It is a distal, symmetric sensorimotor polyneuropathy. It is often painful and may be associated with restless legs syndrome. Abnormal nerve conductions may precede clinical symptoms and signs. The neuropathy progresses with great variability over months. It stabilizes or improves with hemodialysis. The greatest improvement seems to occur with renal transplantation. Carbamazepine may alleviate pain.

Patients with chronic renal failure often have symmetric proximal weakness with atrophy and painful stiffness. Serum creatine kinase (CK) and aldolase levels are usually normal but EMG typically shows myopathic changes. This myopathy may be caused by secondary hyperparathyroidism. Rarely, ischemic myopathy occurs with elevated levels of serum CK, severe weakness, and gangrenous skin lesions.

REF: Fraser CL, Arieff AL: *Ann Intern Med* 109:143, 1988.

Ruff RL, Weissmann J: *Neurol Clin* 6:575, 1988.

UROLOGY   *(see Bladder)*

UVEITIS (see Table 60)   *(see also Retina and Uveal Tract)*

VAGUS NERVE   *(see Cranial Nerves)*

VALPROIC ACID   *(see Epilepsy)*

VARICELLA ZOSTER   *(see Zoster)*

TABLE 60
Diseases That May Involve the Uveal Tract and Central Nervous System

Infections

Bacterial
Meningococcus
  Syphilis
  Tuberculosis
  Whipple's disease
  Brucellosis
  Leptospirosis
  Listeriosis
  Borrelia—Lyme disease

Parasitic
  Trypanosomiasis
  Toxoplasmosis
  Ameliosis
  Malaria

Viral
  Cytomegalovirus
    Herpes simplex
    Herpes zoster
    Varicella
    Mumps
    Rubella
    Rubeola
    Subacute sclerosing panencephalitis
    Variola

Fungal
  Aspergillosis
    Candidiasis
    Cryptococcosis
    Histoplasmosis
    Mucormycosis

Adapted from Finelli PF et al: *Ann Neurol* 1:247-252, 1977.
Reference: Nussenblatt RB, Palestine AG: *Uveitis*, St Louis, 1989, Mosby.

Continued.

TABLE 60—cont'd
Diseases That May Involve the Uveal Tract and Central Nervous System

Infections

Granulomatous Disease
  Sarcoidosis
    Wegener's granulomatosis

Collagen Vascular Disease
  Systemic lupus erythematosus
  Temporal arteritis
  Polyarteritis

Neoplasms
  Leukemia
    Metastatic carcinoma
    Reticulum cell sarcoma

Other
  Behçet's syndrome
  Multiple sclerosis
  Sympathetic ophthalmia
  Trauma
  Uveal effusion
  Vogt-Koyanagi-Harada (uveomeningoencephalitic) syndrome
  Bing's syndrome (chorioretinitis, ophthalmoplegia, macroglobulinemia)
  Romberg's syndrome (posterior uveitis, ophthalmoplegia, trigeminal neuralgia, seizures, unilateral facial atrophy)

VASCULITIS

Vasculitis refers to a group of diseases characterized by inflammation of blood vessels. They can be primary or can result from other systemic diseases (rheumatologic disease or malignancies) or some drugs. Classification of the vasculitides is complex; some classifications are based on size of vessel affected or presumed etiology. The neurologic effects of vasculitis are protean, and the following distinct syndromes have been identified:

1. *Isolated angiitis of CNS (granulomatous angiitis)*. Symptoms include encephalopathy, headache, stroke, myelopathy, and seizure. CSF may show increased protein level and lymphocytic pleocytosis. Angiography may show beading and irregularities of large and medium-size vessels. Treatment is with high-dose corticosteroids and cytotoxic agents.

2. *Temporal arteritis (giant cell arteritis)* usually occurs in patients over 60 years of age and comes to medical attention as headache, often localized to temporal or occipital areas. Constitutional symptoms of fever, malaise, and weight loss are common, and the condition may also become evident as sudden loss in vision or jaw claudication. Physical examination often shows tenderness over the temporal artery. Increased erythrocyte sedimentation rate (ESR) and other acute-phase reactants (fibrinogen and C reactive protein) are typical; few patients have a normal ESR. Temporal artery biopsy specimen can be normal because of discontinuous involvement. Pathologic study reveals a vasculitis of branches of arteries originating from aortic arch that are affected in a discontinuous fashion. Treatment is prednisone therapy, 60 to 80 mg every day. Symptoms usually improve in 1 month; dose titration is gradual tapering of corticosteroids based on ESR response and symptoms.

3. *Systemic lupus erythematosus*. Vasculitis occurs in 75% of cases, but it is unclear whether cerebral symptoms are always due to a vasculitis; frequently there are cerebral microinfarcts. Symptoms include neuropsychiatric disturbance (psychosis or depression), stroke, transient ischemic attack, seizures, cranial neuropathy, and myelopathy (rare). Isolated CNS lupus erythematosus may mimic multiple sclerosis. Treatment of CNS lupus erythematosus is with corticosteroid therapy and cytotoxic agents.

4. *Sjögren's syndrome* is a chronic, inflammatory autoimmune disorder primarily affecting lacrimal and salivary glands. Symptoms are dry mouth, dry eyes, polymyositis, myopathy, peripheral and cranial neuropathy, and CNS manifestations (stroke and dementia).

5. *Polyarteritis nodosa* is a multi-organ vasculitis frequently becoming evident as hypertension and kidney, skin, and GI disturbance. Neurologic manifestations are most common in the peripheral nervous system and include mononeuritis, mononeuritis multiplex, or peripheral neuropathy in 50% to 70% of patients. CNS manifestations include seizure, visual dis-

turbance or hemiparesis. Diagnosis is based on the presence of disease in skin biopsy specimen and on results of visceral angiography (renal or mesenteric).

6. *Churg-Strauss syndrome* becomes evident as allergic rhinitis, eosinophilia, and systemic vasculitis. Neurologic involvement may be mononeuritis multiplex.

7. *Wegener's granulomatosis* has involvement of upper and lower respiratory tract, a segmental necrotizing glomerulonephritis, and systemic vasculitis. Neurologic manifestations occur in about 30% of cases via three different mechanisms. A vasculitis syndrome may come to medical attention as peripheral neuropathy, cranial neuropathy, myopathy, or intracranial hemorrhage. Granulomatous invasion through nasal cavity may result in exophthalmos, ptosis, ophthalmoplegia, basilar meningitis, and diabetes insipidus. Cerebral granulomas are rare and become evident as one or more mass lesions. Treatment is with immunosuppressive agents.

8. *Cogan's syndrome:* Rare disease of the young; initial symptoms include interstitial keratitis, vestibular and auditory dysfunction, encephalomyelitis, and polyneuropathy.

9. *Takayasu's arteritis* is a large-vessel vasculitis of the aorta and its major branches. It may result in stroke and amaurosis fugax.

10. *Herpes zoster ophthalmicus hemiplegia* usually becomes evident several weeks after herpes zoster ophthalmicus. There may be vasculitic involvement of the ipsilateral middle cerebral artery with ipsilateral cranial nerve involvement and contralateral hemiparesis.

11. *Behçet's disease:* Recurrent oral and genital ulcers and relapsing vasculitis. Neurologic symptoms occur in 10% of cases and include headache, meningitis, multifocal CNS lesions, and peripheral neuropathy. May mimic multiple sclerosis.

REF: Moore P: *Neurology* 39:167-173, 1989.

Vollmer TL et al: *Arch Neurol* 50:925-930, 1993.

VASOPRESSIN *(see Electrolyte Disorders, Syndrome of Inappropriate Antidiuretic Hormone)*

VEGETATIVE STATE *(see Coma)*

VENOUS ANGIOMA *(see Angiomas)*

VENOUS THROMBOSIS

Cortical vein thrombosis results in headache, seizures, and focal signs. Subarachnoid hemorrhage resulting from rupture of congested veins or extension of hemorrhagic infarction, as well as papilledema, may also occur. Superior sagittal sinus thrombosis is the most common type, and, if the parieto-occipital portion is involved, may produce elevated intracranial pressure, somnolence, and cranial nerve (CN) VI palsy. Contrast-enhanced CT scan shows a "negative delta" sign, which is characterized by opacification of the sinus wall with noninjection of the clot inside the sinus, in only 30% of cases. MRI or magnetic resonance venography may be diagnostic. Venous phase angiography usually shows a filling defect. Other signs of parasagittal stroke or hemorrhage, or both, may be present because of propagation of the thrombus into surrounding cortical veins. Thrombosis may also involve the cavernous sinus (usually as a result of facial or orbital infection; involvement is characterized by facial pain, proptosis, and involvement of CN III, IV, V, and VI), superior petrosal (as a result of otitis media; facial pain is prominent), inferior petrosal (Gradenigo's syndrome with retro-orbital pain and CN VI palsy), lateral (increased intracranial pressure and ear pain), or internal jugular (as a result of catheters or pacemakers, with involvement of CN IX, X, and XI). Vein of Galen thrombosis in neonates after trauma or infection may result in extensor posturing, fever, tachycardia, tachypnea, and death. Survivors have bilateral choreoathetosis.

Causes of venous thrombosis include the following:

1. Trauma: Injury, neck surgery, indwelling IV lines.
2. Infection: Middle ear, sinuses, meningitis.
3. Endocrine: Pregnancy, contraceptives.
4. Volume depletion: Hyperosmolar coma, inflammatory bowel disease, diarrhea, postpartum, postoperative.
5. Hematologic: Polycythemia vera, disseminated intravascular coagulation, sickle cell disease, cryofibrinogenemia, paroxysmal nocturnal hemoglobinuria, thrombocytosis, antithrombin III deficiency, transfusion reaction.
6. Impaired cerebral circulation: Arterial occlusion, congenital heart disease, congestive heart failure, anesthesia in seated position, sagittal sinus webs.
7. Neoplasm: Leukemia, lymphoma, meningeal spread, meningioma.

8. Other: Wegener's granulomatosis, polyarteritis nodosa, Behçet's syndrome, Cogan's syndrome, homocystinuria.

Results of lumbar puncture, if not contraindicated by mass effect, are nonspecific and may reveal increased pressure and increased levels of protein, polymorphonuclear leukocytes (if infection is present), and red blood cells (if hemorrhage has occurred).

Management includes treatment of the underlying cause and supportive care. Anticoagulation therapy is usually employed if there is no major hemorrhage or bleeding disorder. Intracranial hypertension should be controlled (see also Intracranial Pressure).

REF: Ameli A, Bazaar MG: Neurol Clin 10:87, 1992.

VENTRICLES   *(see Computed Tomography, Hydrocephalus, Intracranial Pressure, Magnetic Resonance Imaging)*

VERTEBROBASILAR SYNDROMES   *(see Ischemia)*

VERTIGO   *(see also Calorics, Dizziness, Syncope)*

Vertigo is defined as an erroneous perception of *movement* of self or surrounding or an unpleasant distortion of *orientation* with respect to gravity. Disorders causing vertigo are formulated in terms of distortion or mismatch of vestibular, visual, and somatosensory inputs. Careful questioning can better delineate the patient's perceptions and help differentiate vertigo from other forms of dizziness that result from disturbances of cardiovascular, visual, or motor function.

Examination: Blood pressure measurement (lying and standing), hearing screen and otoscopy, general neurologic examination with special attention to past pointing, ophthalmoscopy, ocular motor examination, and characterization of nystagmus; responses to specific maneuvers (if deemed safe), including tragal compression, rapid head turns, valsalva, rotation in chair, hyperventilation, and postural testing. The latter is performed by abruptly moving the patient from a sitting to a lying position, with the head hanging 45 degrees over the end of the examining table and rotated 45 degrees to one side. This is repeated with the head rotated to the opposite side. The development of vertigo and the time of onset, duration, and direction of the fast phase of nystagmus are noted.

CAUSES

I. Physiologic: Resulting from sensory distortion (for example, change in refraction) or intersensory mismatch (such as motion sickness or height vertigo).

II. Pathologic: Based on localization within vestibular pathways.

A. Labyrinths: Otitis media, endolymphatic hydrops, otosclerosis, cupulolithiasis, viral infection, perilymph fistula, trauma, toxicity (for example, from antibiotics).

B. Vestibular nerve and ganglia: Carcinomatous meningitis, herpes zoster.

C. Cerebellopontine angle: Acoustic neuroma, glomus, or other tumor; demyelination, vascular compression.

D. Brainstem and cerebellum: Infarct, hemorrhage, tumor, viral infection, migraine, Arnold-Chiari malformation.

E. Hemispheric connections: Temporal or parietal dysfunction (for example, seizure), psychogenic (especially severe vertigo without nausea or nystagmus).

F. Systemic and Metabolic: Anemia, intoxication (such as ethanol, anticonvulsants, diuretics, and other medications), vasculitis (for example, Cogan's syndrome of deafness, interstitial keratitis, and systemic vasculitis), metabolic derangement (for example, thyroid disease).

III. Other causes of vertigo. Psychogenic vertigo has features of rotational or linear movement rather than isolated lightheadedness. It often begins gradually, is associated with anxiety, and terminates abruptly. Forced hyperventilation may provoke vertigo. When a patient complains of severe rotational vertigo without nausea or nystagmus, a psychogenic cause is suggested. Cases in patients with chronic, constant dizziness are usually nonorganic.

SPECIFIC FORMS (SEE TABLE 61)

Acute peripheral vestibulopathy (other terms include viral labyrinthitis, vestibular neuronitis, and peripheral vestibulopathy) is associated with spontaneous vertigo, nystagmus (fast phase away from the lesion), and nausea or vomiting, or both, lasting hours to days. The environment seems to move in the direction of the fast phase (away from the lesion). There is a subjective sense of self-motion in the direction of the fast phase. The patient may fall to the side of the lesion during Romberg testing. Past pointing is to the side of the lesion. Symptoms and signs may be brought on by hurried movement ("positioning") but not necessarily by maintaining a particular position ("positional").

TABLE 61
Localization of Vestibular Dysfunction

	Peripheral	Central
History	Sudden onset; episodic; duration ≤days; intense vertigo; marked exacerbation with head movement; auditory symptoms (often unilateral); neurologic symptoms absent	Insidious onset; continuous; duration up to months; mild dysequilibrium; little or no exacerbation with head movement; no associated auditory symptoms; associated neurologic or vascular symptoms
Examination	Neurologic signs absent; *spontaneous nystagmus:* rotatory component, not vertical; *positional nystagmus:* latency before onset (≤45 sec), habituates, conjugate, uniplanar, attenuates with visual fixation	Associated neurologic or vascular signs; *spontaneous nystagmus:* horizontal or vertical, less often rotatory; *positional nystagmus:* immediate onset, no habituation, may change direction with different head positions, no change with visual fixation

Hearing is usually normal. A variable residual deficit of one peripheral vestibular system (labyrinth, nerve, or both) may persist. With a unilateral fixed deficit, central compensatory mechanisms intervene and vertigo and nystagmus decrease and may resolve. Acute peripheral vestibulopathy may recur (see below). Viral causes are held to be most common. Bacterial suppurative ear infection should be excluded.

Perilymph fistula is usually due to spontaneous rupture of the inner ear membranes with resultant vertigo that may be aggravated by changes in position. It is associated with a fluctuating hearing loss. The fistula may occur during strenuous activity or Valsalva maneuver. The patient may hear a "pop" in the ear at the moment of rupture. The attacks are discrete and short-lived. The therapy is bed rest. If this fails, surgery may be required.

Central vestibular vertigo resulting from lesions of the vestibular nuclei or vestibulocerebellar pathways have vertigo and nystagmus, often accompanied by diplopia, dysarthria, weakness, sensory loss, involvement of cranial nerves V and VII, and pathologic reflexes. Acoustic neuromas are usually associated with hearing loss, tinnitus, and occasionally, involvement of other cranial nerves, including VII and V.

Drug-induced vertigo is due to effects on the peripheral end-organ or nerve and may be due to aminoglycosides, furosemide, ethacrynic acid, anticonvulsants (phenytoin, phenobarbital, carbamazepine, and primidone), some anti-inflammatory agents, salicylates, and quinine. Drugs may produce only dysequilibrium when the damage is bilateral but can produce vertigo when the damage is asymmetric. Some agents also produce hearing loss.

Meniere's disease that results from endolymph hydrops is characterized by severe episodic vertigo, vomiting, fluctuating or progressive hearing loss, distortions of sound, tinnitus, and pressure or fullness in the ears. Recovery is usually within hours to days. The interval between attacks often ranges from weeks to months. Low-salt diet and diuretics are considered most helpful. Surgical therapy (endolymphatic drainage or vestibular nerve section) may give lasting relief but should be considered only as a last resort.

Benign paroxysmal positional vertigo is a symptom that usually indicates benign peripheral (end-organ) disease. Vertigo and nystagmus, often with systemic symptoms such as nausea and vomiting, occur when certain positions of the head are assumed, such as lying down on the back or side. Symptoms are usually transient (<60 seconds). Latency is usually several seconds but may be as long as 30 to 45 seconds. Signs and symptoms include fatigue after onset and do not recur until there is a change in position. Nystagmus is most commonly torsional toward (upper pole) the undermost ear during positional testing. With repetitive maneuvers, signs and symptoms lessen (habituate). Therapy consists of repetitive positioning exercises to stimulate central compensation or a liberatory maneuver. Elderly patients compensate more slowly. Vestibular suppressant medications generally do not help.

Laboratory studies: Brain imaging (CT, MRI) with attention to posterior fossa and temporal bone; MR angiography with attention to vertebrobasilar circulation; caloric and rotational testing quantify vestibular function. Audiogram and auditory evoked potentials detect associated cochlear or brainstem dysfunction.

Management: Generally, management during acute vertigo includes bed rest, avoiding sudden head movements, clear fluids or light diet if tolerated, and reassurance. Vestibular suppressant medications such as antihistamines and benzodiazepines (see Table 62) and antiemetics may be useful in acute peripheral vestibulopathy, in acute brainstem lesions near the vestibular nuclei, and for prevention of motion sickness. These agents are of no benefit in chronic vestibulopathies. After the acute phase (approximately 1 to 3 days), a graded program of exercises hastens the adaptive recalibration of the vestibular system to provide better ocular motor and postural control and reduce vertigo.

REF: Baloh RW: *J Am Geriatr Soc* 40:713–721, 1992.

   Brandt T, Steddin S, Daroff RB: *Neurology* 44:796-800, 1994.

   Sharpe JA, Barber HO, eds,: *The vestibulo-ocular reflex and vertigo*, New York, 1993, Raven.

VESTIBULAR DYSFUNCTION   *(see Vertigo)*

VESTIBULOCOCHLEAR NERVE   *(see Cranial Nerves, Hearing, Vertigo)*

VESTIBULO-OCULAR REFLEX   *(see also Calorics, Vertigo)*

The vestibulo-ocular reflex (VOR) generates eye movements that compensate for head movements. Head movements, voluntary or caused by locomotion, are sensed by the semicircular canals and otolith organs (utricle and saccule). Signals from the vestibular end-organs are combined with visual information in brainstem vestibular and ocular motor centers to create the appropriate control signals sent to the extraocular muscles. Adequate vestibular function results in eye rotations nearly equal and opposite to head movements and maintenance of a stable image on the retina, allowing high visual acuity. Overall vestibular function involves cerebral cortical centers and a spinal cord relay and processing of sensory input and motor outflow. Thus vestibular disorders (peripheral or central) can result in eye movement abnormalities or more subtle disorders of postural control and spatial orientation.

TABLE 62
Medications Useful in Treating Symptoms of Acute Vertigo

Drug	Dosage	Route
Dimenhydrinate (Drama-mine)	50-100 mg q4-6 hr	PO, IM, IV, PR
Diphenhydramine (Bena-dryl)	25-50 mg tid to qid	PO, IM, IV
Meclizine (Antivert)	12.5-25 mg bid to qid	PO
Promethazine (Phenergan)	25 mg bid to qid	PO, IM, IV, PR
Hydroxyzine (Atarax, Vis-taril)	25-100 mg tid to qid	PO, IM

IM, Intramuscular; *IV*, intravenous; *PO*, by mouth; *PR*, by way of rectum.

VOR *testing:* After integrity of the neck is assured, bedside testing of the VOR is best accomplished in the following ways: (1) Rapid, passive head rotations (unpredictable, high-acceleration) are applied while the patient fixes his or her gaze on a stationary target. The examiner watches for a corrective saccadic eye movement which occurs after the head rotation only if the VOR has not adequately maintained gaze. (2) A more continuous high-frequency, low-amplitude head oscillation is applied while the examiner views the optic disc with an ophthalmoscope. If the VOR is intact, the disc image should appear stable to the observer.

Head rotation in comatose patients with a normal VOR results in compensatory controversive eye movements (see Calorics).

Quantitative evaluation of the VOR involves measuring eye movement responses to controlled head perturbations and calculating the VOR *gain,* defined as eye velocity divided by head velocity.

REF: Leigh RJ, Brandt T: *Neurology* 43:1288–1295, 1993.

VISUAL FIELDS

The visual field (VF) can be conceptualized as an "island of vision in the sea of blindness." The peak of the island represents the point of highest acuity, the fovea, whereas the optic disc (blind spot) is a bottomless pit in the midst of the island. Visual field testing is performed with stimuli of various size, color, and intensity. There are various manual and computerized types of perimetry, but confrontation is the mainstay of clinical testing.

The characteristic features of visual field deficits have high localizing value (Figure 44). Retinal nerve fiber-bundle lesions cause defects originating from the blind spot and respecting the horizontal meridian. Arcuate deficits occur with segmental lesions of the optic nerve. Cecocentral deficits suggest an optic nerve lesion. Chiasmal lesions produce bitemporal defects. All retrochiasmatic lesions cause contralateral homonymous hemianopsia or quadrantanopsia, which increases in congruence (similarity between the eyes) as the lesions approach the occipital lobe.

REF: Bajandas FJ, Kline LB: *Neuro-ophthalmology review manual*, ed 3, Thorofare, NJ, 1988, Slack.

VITAMIN DEFICIENCIES   *(see Nutritional Deficiency Syndromes)*

VON RECKLINGHAUSEN'S DISEASE   *(see Neurocutaneous Syndromes)*

WALLENBERG'S SYNDROME   *(see Ischemia)*

WEAKNESS   *(see Ischemia, Lambert-Eaton myasthenic syndrome, Motor Neuron Disease, Myasthenia Gravis, Myopathy, Neuropathy, Periodic Paralysis, Spinal Cord)*

WEBER'S SYNDROME   *(see Ischemia)*

WEBER'S TEST   *(see Hearing)*

WEGENER'S GRANULOMATOSIS   *(see Vasculitis)*

WERDNIG-HOFFMANN SYNDROME   *(see Hypotonic Infant Motor Neuron Disease)*

WERNICKE'S APHASIA   *(see Aphasia)*

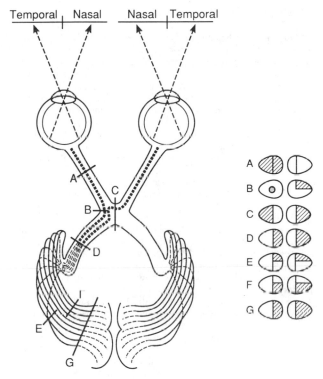

FIGURE 44
Diagram showing the effects on the fields of vision produced by lesions at various points along the optic pathway.

WERNICKE-KORSAKOFF SYNDROME   *(see Alcohol, Memory Nutritional Deficiency Syndrome)*

WEST SYNDROME   *(see Epilepsy)*

WILSON'S DISEASE

Also known as hepatolenticular degeneration, Wilson's disease is an autosomal recessive (chromosome 13) disorder of copper metabolism. The basic defect is unknown. Age at presentation is usually between 10 and 40 years. Behavioral or personality change, dysarthria, ataxia, and abnormal movements (chorea, athetosis, tremor, or rigidity) are common neurologic presentations; the classic "wing-beating" tremor is no longer common. Hepatic dysfunction is identifiable in nearly all patients, and cirrhosis may be apparent early in the course. Other clinical features include hemolytic anemia, joint symptoms, renal stones, cardiomyopathy, pancreatic disease, and hypoparathyroidism. Kayser-Fleischer (KF) rings are present in more than 90% of patients and are virtually pathognomic. They are brownish discolorations at the corneal limbus consisting of copper deposits in Descemet's membrane and may be visible only under slit-lamp examination. "Sunflower" cataracts may occur.

The diagnosis is made by observation of the KF rings, low serum level of ceruloplasmin, elevated 24-hour urinary copper excretion, and increased level of copper in liver biopsy specimen. Serum copper measurement is often normal. Although the diagnosis may be relatively easy, Wilson's disease must be suspected in children and younger adults who come to medical attention with unknown hepatic or CNS syndromes.

Treatment consists of chelation with D-penicillamine; initial dosages about 0.5 g per day in children and 1 g per day in divided doses for adults, and a low-copper diet to minimize acute worsening caused by mobilization of copper stores. A regimen of pyridoxine, 25 mg per day, is given to counter the antimetabolite effect of penicillamine. Acute or delayed hypersensitivity reactions to penicillamine develop in up to 20% of patients receiving treatment but may be overcome in some cases with a reduced dose and concomitant administration of corticosteroids. Trientene, a chelator, and zinc salts, which block GI copper absorption, may be of use in patients who cannot tolerate penicillamine. Patients with advanced disease may require liver transplantation. Levodopa may be of some benefit in reversing neurologic symptoms not improved by penicillamine.

REF: Danks DM. In Scriver CR et al, eds: *The metabolic basis of inherited disease*, ed 6, New York, 1989, McGraw-Hill.

Starosta-Rubinstein S et al: *Arch Neurol* 44:365, 1987.

WITHDRAWAL SYNDROME *(see Alcohol)*

WORD DEAFNESS *(see Agnosia)*

WRITER'S CRAMP *(see Dystonia)*

XANTHOCHROMIA *(see Cerebrospinal Fluid)*

ZOSTER

Varicella-zoster virus is the infective organism in varicella (chicken pox) and herpes zoster (shingles). Varicella is usually a benign disease of childhood. Rare complications include meningoencephalitis, acute cerebellar ataxia, transverse myelitis, and Reye's syndrome. Although full recovery from the first two complications is common, rare permanent deficits include paresis, seizures, and cognitive changes.

Herpes zoster (literally, *girdle*) represents reactivation of latent virus demonstrated on pathologic study in the trigeminal and dorsal root ganglia. Herpes zoster is most frequent in those with weakened cell-mediated immunity, particularly elderly and immunocompromised individuals. At particular risk are patients with lymphoma who have had radiation therapy and splenectomy and patients with AIDS in whom disseminated disease usually develops. Typically zoster becomes evident as pain in a single or several adjacent dermatomes; pain may precede the vesicular eruption by up to 3 weeks. Rarely the pain occurs in the absence of any rash (zoster sine herpete), leading to considerations of carcinomatous, lymphomatous, or diabetic radiculopathies. Associated findings include altered sensation in the involved dermatome; fewer than 5% of patients have segmental weakness. The CSF may show an elevated protein level and a mild lymphocytic pleocytosis. Diagnosis is established by the presence of typical rash, Tzanck smear, direct immunofluorescence study, viral culture, or comparison of acute and convalescent titers. On pathologic study the acute phase of herpes zoster consists of a hemorrhagic inflammation of the affected dorsal root ganglion and nerve root, which sometimes involves the spinal cord and leptomeninges.

Zoster most commonly involves the dorsal root ganglia at vertebrae T5 to T10. When zoster affects the cranium (20% of cases), 90% of cases are in the trigeminal distribution and 60% of these involve the first division, *herpes zoster ophthalmicus*. Complications include corneal involvement (with anesthesia and scarring), internal or external ophthalmoplegia, iridocyclitis, and optic neuritis (rare). The prognosis for improvement of oculomotor disturbance is excellent, whereas return of lost vision is minimal. The *Ramsay Hunt syndrome* describes zoster of the geniculate ganglion, which becomes evident as painful vesicles on the tympanic membrane and external auditory canal, a peripheral cranial nerve (CN) VII palsy, and variable CN VIII dysfunction.

Complications of zoster also include myelitis, encephalitis, cranial nerve palsies, and granulomatous angiitis. The latter is the most common of these syndromes and becomes evident as hemiparesis contralateral to the ophthalmic involvement weeks to months later. It may represent a vasculopathy due to viral reactivation in trigeminal branches innervating cerebral blood vessels.

Postherpetic neuralgia is a syndrome of persistent dysesthesias and hyperpathia persisting beyond healing of the zoster vesicles (usually beyond 1 month). The pain has the following components: (1) a constant, deep burning pain, (2) paroxysms of shooting pain, and (3) sharp pains after light stimulation (allodynia). On pathologic study the condition is associated with a localized small- and large-fiber sensory neuropathy and may result from reorganization of inputs to the second-order neurons. Postherpetic neuralgia is rare in patients under 50 years of age but occurs in as many as 50% of patients over 60 years of age and in 75% of those over 70 years of age. It resolves within 1 month in 90% of patients and in half of the remainder, by 2 months. Only about 2% of patients have persistent pain, which may last for months or years.

Acute zoster is treated symptomatically in patients with normal immunity. Oral acyclovir therapy accelerates cutaneous healing but has no effect on acute neuritis or postherpetic neuralgia. In the immunocompromised patient, parenteral acyclovir is more effective than vidarabine in preventing dissemination and accelerating cutaneous healing. Corticosteroid therapy may reduce acute pain and the risk of postherpetic neuralgia, but evidence of effectiveness is inconclusive. Treatment of postherpetic neuralgia consists of application of capsaicin 0.75% ointment five times per day for at least 4 weeks and amitriptyline therapy, up to 10 to 150 mg per day. Resistant cases may respond to trancutaneous electrical nerve stimulation, carbamazepine, neuroleptics, or surgical blockade.

REF: Carmichael JK: *Am Fam Physician* 44(1):203-210, 1991.

Terrence CF, Fromm GH. In Olesen J, Tfelt-Hansen P, Welch KMA, eds: *The headaches*, New York, 1993, Raven.

EPONYM INDEX

A

Addison's disease (Coma, Dizziness, Muscle Disorders, Myopathy, Olfaction)

Adie's syndrome (Autonomic Dysfunction, Pupil, Reflexes)

Alport's syndrome (Retina and Uveal Tract)

Alström syndrome (Retina and Uveal Tract)

Alzheimer's disease (Alzheimer's Disease, Chromosomal Disorders, Dementia, Memory, Myoclonus, Olfaction, Parkinson's Disease)

Amalric-Dialinos syndrome (Retina and Uveal Tract)

Anton's syndrome (Parietal Lobe, Occipital Lobe)

Apert's syndrome (Craniosynostosis)

Argyll-Robertson pupil (Pupil, Syphilis)

Arnold-Chiari malformation (Craniocervical Junction, Developmental Malformations, Hearing, Nystagmus, Vertigo)

Avellis syndrome (Ischemia)

B

Babinski's sign (Degenerative Diseases of Childhood, Parkinsonism, Reflexes, Spasticity, Spinal Cord)

Babinski-Nageotte syndrome (Ischemia)

Balint's syndrome (Parietal Lobe, Occipital Lobe)

Balo's sclerosis (Demyelinating Diseases)

Bassen-Kornzweig syndrome (Nutritional Deficiency Syndromes, Retina and Uveal Tract, Spinocerebellar Degeneration)

Batten-Mayou (Retina and Uveal Tract)

Batten's disease (Myoclonus)